LIFE ON THE LINE

LIFE ON THE LINE

Selections on Words and Healing

EDITED BY

SUE BRANNAN WALKER

&

ROSALY DEMAIOS ROFFMAN

Negative Capability Press

Mobile, Alabama 1992

NEGATIVE CAPABILITY PRESS
62 Ridgelawn Drive East
Mobile, Alabama 36608

Copyright © 1992 by Negative Capability
All rights reserved
Printed in the United States of America

Cover Artist: Nall Hollis
Cover & Graphic Designs by: Guillermo de Borja Narvacan IV "Gumby"
Typography & Page Design: Betsy Luther

FIRST EDITION
ISBN 0-942544-16-1 HBK ISBN 0-942544-15-3 PBK
Library of Congress Card Number: 91-091330

CONTENTS

FOREWORD BY Karl Shapiro

ACKNOWLEDGMENTS

INTRODUCTION BY Sue Walker

ODE TO HEALING by John Updike

CHAPTER 1 - ABUSE

CHAPTER II - DEATH & DYING

CHAPTER III - ILLNESS

CHAPTER IV - RELATIONSHIPS

CHAPTER V - MEMORY

CHAPTER VI - RITUAL AND REMEDIES

CHAPTER VII - WHITE FLAGS FROM SILENT CAMP

CHAPTER VIII - WITH HOPE FOR LIFE

POET

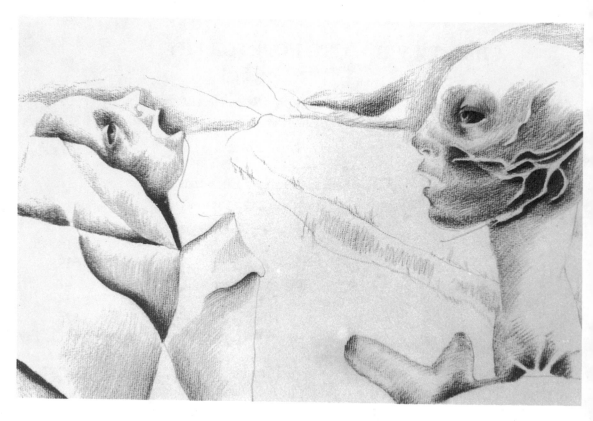

Drawing: Pencil on paper by Pfeiffer-Towner

FOREWORD

There have been more claims about poetry, true, half-true and false, than about any other art. One of the true claims is that poetry has restorative or healing properties. This has been recognized since antiquity, when Aristotle introduced the idea of purgation. The poet could arouse in his audience the emotions of pity and terror, in order to purge them. Man is taught by suffering, according to this prescription. The overtones of such a doctrine are not only "medical" but religious. Poetry is not only a form of therapy; it is a vehicle of prayer.

This anthology of poems and prose is a rich contemporary documentation of the theme of poetic redemption. If the pain of reading these pages sometimes overshadows the pleasures of art, so be it. The title of the collection is the best explanation. The *line* is the demarcation between life and death, the ultimate anxiety of everyone. For poets and writers the expression of this anxiety might be called the writing-cure. In writing there is a process of dislodgment of the pain by making it available. To use a term which has become somewhat vulgarized in our time, it is the art of sharing. The reader is forced to participate. Accident, abuse, murder, abortion, paralysis, cancer are not the sweets of poesy, but they lie at the frontiers of consciousness and are a large part of the materia poetica of the serious artist.

The prevalence of the tragic and the pathological in great works of literature has misled many theorists into the belief that art is symptomatic of psychic disorder, whereas it is the opposite. Art is a reaching for wholeness by way of the assimilation of the pathic into the joyousness of the unified being. Great poetry mourns for fragmentation and prays for recovery and reunification with the healthy soul. If this borders on sentimentality it is one of the risks of the belief in wholeness, with art, music and poetry as handmaidens to the purgation of evil and the restitution of the unified being.

KARL SHAPIRO

ACKNOWLEDGMENTS

We gratefully acknowledge the permission granted by the following authors and authors' representatives to reprint poems and excerpts from their publications.

Dannie Abse: "Tuberculosis" from *White Coat, Purple Coat: Collected Poems 1948-1988*. Copyright © 1991 by Dannie Abse. Reprinted by permission of Persea Books, Inc.

B.B. Adams: "Marriage" from *Hapax Legomena* (Edwin Mellen Press). Copyright © 1990 by B.B. Adams. Reprinted by permission of the author.

Maggie Anderson: "The Thing You Must Remember" from *Cold Comfort* (University of Pittsburgh Press). Copyright © by Maggie Anderson. Reprinted by permission of the author.

Richard Beyer: "To Majorie-Remembering" first appeared in *Kentucky Poetry Review*. Copyright © by Richard G. Beyer. Reprinted by permission of the author.

Phillip Bollier: "All Hallow's Eve" first appeared in *Negative Capability*. Copyright © by E.P. Bollier. Reprinted by permission of the author.

Gerald Cable: "Mortality Tables" first appeared in *Southern Poetry Review*. Copyright © by Gerald Cable. Reprinted by permission of Martha Farris.

Leo Connellan: "Origins" from *New and Collected Poems*. Copyright © 1989 by Leo Connellan. Reprinted by permission of Paragon House.

Colleen Connors: "You Will Learn Lessons" from *The Rules of Being Human*. Reprinted by permission of the author.

Peter Cooley: "Winter Light" from *The Company Of Strangers* (University of Missouri Press). "The Last Gift" from *The Room Where Summer Ends* (Carnegie Mellon, 1979). "For Allissa," "The Elect" from *Night Seasons* (Carnegie Mellon, 1983). "The Loom" and "The Last Self Portrait" from *The Van Gogh Notebooks* (Carnegie-Mellon, 1987). Reprinted by permission of the author.

Jack Coulehan: "The Sorrow Of The World", "Skinwalkers", "Deep Images", "Anesthesia", "The Man With Stars Inside Him" and "Medicine Stone" from *The Knitted Glove* (Nightshade Press). Copyright © 1991 by Jack Coulehan. Reprinted by permission of the author.

Barbara Crooker: "On Losing My Anterior Cruciate Ligament" first appeared in *The Pharos*. Copyright © 1990 by Alpha Omega Alpha Honor Medical Society. Reprinted by permission from *The Pharos*.

Rita Dove: "Roast Possum" and "One Volume Missing" from *Thomas and Beulah* (Carnegie-Mellon University Press, 1986). "Reading Hölderlin On The Patio With The Aid Of A Dictionary", "Grape Sherbert" and "Anti-Father" from *Museum* (Carnegie-Mellon, 1983). Copyright © by Rita Dove. Reprinted by permission of the author.

Carl Djerassi: "I Have Nothing Left To Say" first appeared in *Negative Capability*. Copyright © by Carl Djerassi. Reprinted by permission of the author.

Nan Fry: "From Persephone's Letter's To Demeter" and "Riddle" from *Relearning The Dark* (Washington Writers' Publishing House, 1991). Copyright © by Nan Fry. Reprinted by permission of the author.

David Ignatow: "For My Daughter", "For My Mother Ill", "With The Door Open".

Judson Jerome: "Liking What You Do" from *Jonah and Job* (John Daniel & Co. 1991). Copyright © by Judson Jerome. Reprinted by permission of the author.

Norbert Krapf: "Coming To Terms With April Snow" first appeared in *Images* and was included in *A Dream Of Plum Blossoms*. Copyright © by Norbert Krapf, 1985. Reprinted by permission of the author.

Carolyn Kremers: "The New Students" is from *Place Of The Pretend People*. Copyright © by Carolyn Kremers. Reprinted by permission of the author.

Glenna Luschei: "Visiting Hours" is from *Unexpected Grace*. Copyright © by Glenna Luschei. Reprinted by permission of the author.

Peter Meinke: "Untitled" from *The Nighttrain and the Golden Bird* (University of Pittsburgh Press). Copyright © 1977 by Peter Meinke. "The Guru" from *Nightwatch on the Chesapeake* (University of Pittsburgh Press). Copyright © 1987 by Peter Meinke.

Anne Meisenzahl: "The Lone Woman" from *What's A Nice Girl Like You Doing In a Relationship Like This* (Crossing Press). Reprinted by permission of the author.

Richard Moore: "Words & Healing: What's In It For The Poet?" includes "The Dolls" by W.B. Yeats from *The Collected Poems Of W.B. Yeats* (London: Macmillan and Co., 1950), pp 141-142 and his note on it, page 531. Quoted by permission of A.P. Watt Ltd. on behalf of Anne Yeats.

Alice C. Nagle: "The Whistle" first appeared in the *Walrus* (Mills College, Oakland, California, 1989). Reprinted by permission of the author.

Mary Oliver: "University Hospital, Boston" from *American Primitive* (Atlantic-Little, Brown, 1983). Copyright © by Mary Oliver. Reprinted by permission of the author.

Alison Reed: "At The Bedside Of A Dying Grandfather Who Once Played The Violin" first appeared in *The Fiddlehead*, Spring 1986. Reprinted by permission of the author.

Elspeth C. Ritchie: "Spring Lettuce" first appeared in *The Radcliffe Quarterly*. "Paratrooper, Ft. Bragg, N.C." from *Military Medicine*. "AIDS" first appeared in *JAMA*, 1989; 262: 3134. "Tearing Through The Moon" first appeared in *JAMA, 1990; 263: 2040*. Copyright © 1989-90 American Medical Association. "Hospital Sketchbook" first appeared in *The Washington Woman*. Reprinted by permission of the author.

Danielle D'Aunay & Charles B. Rodning: "Patient-Physician Interaction: Healing Power Of A Covenant Relationship" first appeared in *Human Medicine* Vol. 4 No. 2 Nov. 1988 (Toronto, Ontario, Canada). Reprinted by permission of the publishers.

Karl Shapiro: "The Leg" and "The Figurehead" from *Collected Poems 1940-1978* (Random House, 1978). Copyright © by Karl Shapiro. Reprinted by permission of the author.

Bernie Siegel: "Shopping List For Change" *Peace, Love & Healing* (Harper and Row, 1989). Copyright © by Bernard S. Seigel. Reprinted by permission of the author.

Liubov Sirota: "Your glance will trip on my shadow" was published in *New York Quarterly*.

William Stafford: "For A Lost Child" and "Right To Die" first appeared in *Field*. "A Memorial: Son Brett" first appeared in the *American Scholar*. Reprinted by permission of the author.

Lamont B. Steptoe: "Parts" from *Mad Minutes* (Whirlwind Press, Camden, New Jersey, July 1990). Reprinted by permission of the author.

Gerald Stern: "Bob Summer's Body" from *Lovesick* (H&R, 1990, 86)."The Sacred Spine" is from *Paradise Poems* (Random House). *Reprinted by permission of the author.*

Vivian Smallwood: "The Participant", "The Denial" and "The Wake" and *And Finding No Mouse There* (Negative Capability Press, 1983). Copyright © Vivian Smallwood. Reprinted by permission of the author.

John Updike: "Ode To Healing" from *Facing Nature* by John Updike. Copyright © 1985 by John Updike. Reprinted by permission of Alfred A. Knopf, Inc.

Peter Viereck: "Hospital Window" first appeared in *New Letters* January, 1991. Reprinted by permission of the author.

Sue Walker: "What No Lips Can Tell" first appeared in *Red Dirt*. "Patty Cakes and Poetry" first appeared in *The Alalitcom*. "Gliderman" and "Live Old Soldier, Live" from *Traveling My Shadow* (Negative Capability). Copyright © 1982 by Sue Walker. Reprinted by permission of the author.

Gerald Weissman: "The Age Of Miracles Hadn't Passed" from *The Doctor With Two Heads* (Alfred A. Knopf, Inc. 1990). Copyright © 1990 by Gerald Weissman. Reprinted by permission of the author.

A careful effort has been made to trace the ownership of poems used in this anthology in order to obtain permission to reprint copyrighted materials and to give proper credit to the copyright owners.

If any error or omission has occurred, it is completely inadvertent, and we would like to make the correction in future editions provided that written notification is made to the publisher: **NEGATIVE CAPABILITY PRESS.**

John Updike

ODE TO HEALING

A scab
is a beautiful thing—a coin
the body has minted, with an invisible motto:
In God We Trust.
Our body loves us,
and, even while the spirit drifts dreaming,
works at mending the damage that we do.
That heedless Ahab the conscious mind
drives our thin-skinned hull onto the shoals;
a million brilliant microscopic engineers below
shore up the wound with platelets,
lay down the hardening threads of fibrin,
send in the lymphocytes, and supervise
those cheery swabs, the macrophages, in their clean-up.
Break a bone, and fibroblasts
knit tight the blastema in days.
Catch a cold, and the fervid armies
swarm to blanket our discomfort in sleep.
For all these centuries of fairy tales poor men
butchered each other in the name of cure,
not knowing an iota of what the mute brute body knew.

Logically, benevolence surrounds us.
In fire or ice, we would not be born.
Soft tissue bespeaks a soft world.
Yet, can it have been malevolence
that taught the skinned knuckle to heal
or set the white scar on my daughter's glossy temple?
Besieged, we are supplied,
from caustic saliva down,
with armaments against the hordes,
"the sling and arrows," "the thousand natural shocks."

John Updike

Not quite benevolence.
Not quite its opposite.
A perfectionism, it would almost seem,
stuck with matter's recalcitrance,
as, in the realm of our behavior, with
the paradox of freedom.
Well, can we add a cubit to our height
or heal ourselves by taking conscious thought?
The spirit sits as a bird singing
high in a grove of hollow trees whose red sap rises
saturated with advice.
To the child as he scuffles up an existence
out of pebbles and twigs
and finds that even paper cuts, and games can hurt,
the small assemblage of a scab
is like the slow days' blurring of a deep disgrace,
the sinking of a scolding into time.
Time heals: not so;
time is the context of forgetting and of remedy
as aseptic phlegms
lave the scorched membranes,
the capillaries and insulted nerves.
Close your eyes, knowing
that healing is a work of darkness,
that darkness is a gown of healing,
that the vessel of our tremulous venture is lifted
by tides we do not control.
Faith is health's requisite:
we have this fact in lieu
of better proof of le bon Dieu.

INTRODUCTION

Is there a connection between healing and words? This question first arose for me when dealing with the death of my father and mother. I kept searching for something to read that would address my grief as I pondered the difference in coping with my father's slow dying from a stroke and my mother's sudden death in an automobile accident. Was one death easier to accept than the other? This quest toward understanding confronted pain. The concomitant need to heal resulted in this anthology. The writers presented here were asked: What is the relationship that exists between healing and words?

The answers we received enrich us with profound moments of anguish, despair, suffering, and with a movement that accepts or transcends the pain. Healing seems to be a process that differs from person to person though the experience of it is universal. It incorporates anger at times. It needs, if not requires, a lot of love. It reaches out, through words, to meet anguish in others.

This book relates the experience of 228 writers as they address the relation between healing and words. Their situations differ, but the attempt to transcend sorrow is poignant and real. The truths in these stories, essays, and poems make us weep, scream, laugh sometimes, and understand. It is, in essence, a compendium of lives on the line. Working on this anthology was an experience that I will never forget. It has taught me patience with myself and with others as they suffer and endure. It has taught me the grace of love and provided an education in pain and a knowledge that there is a movement beyond it that makes the struggle worthwhile.

This project enabled me to work with Rosaly Roffman who was introduced by Dr. Jack Coulehan. Their reach toward healing appears in these pages along with other authors who made this book happen. May the poems, stories, and essays of these lives on the line speak to you and heal you.

Sue Walker, Publisher

LIFE ON THE LINE

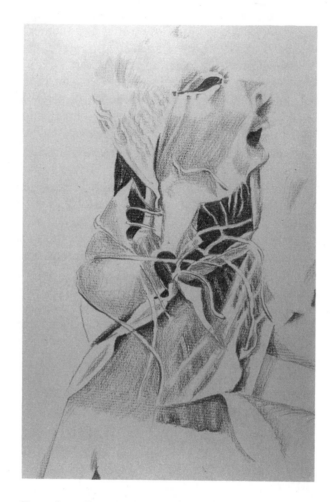

Drawing: Pencil on paper by Pfeiffer-Towner

CHAPTER I

Abuse

How do we keep living, when living is dangerous, when things happen that make our hearts retreat? I write as a way of looking for an answer. I leave these notes about the search.

Jeannine Atkins - "These Notes"

Anya Achtenberg

GENESIS

She sat on the stoop and looked out at all that had been made.
The heavens glimmered through the black smoke,
the vegetation withered as it struggled through the concrete
and fat pink earthworms wriggled blind,
cut in two by boys with army knives.

Her father worked all night at the factory
and slept in the day when she was awake,
so she had to be very quiet
and wait for the schoolbus outside on the stoop.
She tried not to be in the house alone when her father woke up
because sometimes he thought she was her mother.

She knew what he wanted
and didn't want to make him mad
but each time it happened
she could see a sad crazy bird fly past the window
and hurl itself into the river.

That day she stared down from the stoop
at an earthworm severed from itself,
one part inching toward the stubbly grass
and the other careening down the sidewalk
without its other half,
its cut end exposed for the first time to the world.
Then she remembered
she had left her science book on the table
near where the coats hung in a row.

When she entered, all light fled.
When he grabbed her, she fled further into the darkness,
and his voice was not soft and the fruit was not sweet
and she had not been able to name it for a long time.

She came back into the light
with her book and her bruised mouth
and rushed into the big yellow bus before it pulled away.
Then the sky opened up,
the storm's strength lodged the bleeding halves of earthworms

3

between the blades of stubbly grass,
and she decided to tell.
She saw each face
of each child in the bus like someone she used to be,
and the darkness broke in the sky
as the yellow bus pulled up to the school.

Then she clearly heard,
as she stood on her thin legs in front of her teacher,
her own voice work its way into the air.

Jeannine Atkins

THESE NOTES

In second grade I sat in the back row, second from the right, by the coat rack. I remember how my eyes widened when Mrs. Dunwoody raised her yardstick. The sound as it split the air was louder than the sound it made as it smacked Jimmy Scanlon's hands and desk. She wanted Jimmy to pay attention.

When it was winter, I breathed in the smells of wet jackets, leggings, and plastic boots. Quizzes and arithmetic papers were passed to the back. Sometimes I was allowed to collect them and given the key to grade them. I marked the perfect papers with a star-shaped stamp I pressed on a pad of red ink. Mrs. Dunwoody used her yardstick to make lines on the blackboard so that she could show us how to form script letters. She drew margins as we did with our rulers. The boys who were caught talking without first having raised their hands, or who laughed if the yardstick slipped on the board, sat in the front row for easy access. She picked up the stick from the chalk tray. The boys leaned back in their chairs as the stick cracked down. Sometimes they smiled. Maybe they thought she was a joke. Maybe they smiled out of embarrassment or pain. At the time I didn't think I needed to know. The choices I'd made as an even younger girl about who I was, about what I would let myself do, would keep me safe in back. I could think of nothing that would be worth hearing the air snap inches from my eyes. I was even more afraid of the possible next step: being sent to the principal. Even walking by his closed door on the way to the lunchroom made me nervous. In the playground, the teachers talked to each other, sometimes looped their arms over girls' shoulders, and asked us, "What did you do with your tooth?" or "What's the name of your horse?" as we ran, neighing, up to them, pulling on imaginary reins. The principal walked alone with his arms crossed over his chest. He wore a black suit. His power lay in his secrecy; the things that happened in his office were myths. What we did not know, we learned from him, might really hurt us.

***

As I begin to write down these memories of my body, I find that I want to mock the girl I used to be. I dislike her conventional goodness. The disobedient boys are more appealing. Mrs. Dunwoody is a sad cliché, and Mr. Santoian was clearly a lonely man. I make myself put these judgments aside. I have chastised the girl in the back row before for her over-caution, and I've missed the complexity of the scene because I was busy disliking her. It's true that my timidity has weakened me, but I like that girl now, stamping stars on her own papers and wrists, pretending to be the teacher, pretending to be free. I can let her be.

But remembering still makes me afraid. I loved Mrs. Dunwoody, and I don't want to see how she flushed as she spun around to the chalk-tray for the stick, how much she needed the attention of the whole class on her, how frustrated she let a little boy make her feel. I don't want to see her violence. I breathe deeply to keep my body from tightening against the pain in that classroom. I want the story I used to tell: that it was in her classroom that I learned to write. There we added and did take-aways, worked in phonics books with a picture of a lamb on the cover, and got a new coloring book at the beginning of every month. We practiced script, filling whole pages with letters; I loved making s's, though they got sloppy by the end of the row. Papers were sent back if you didn't dot the i's; she insisted that it wasn't a letter if you forgot the dot, so I made rows of scalloped lines, then went back and poked dots all over the paper. She noticed if you missed even one. I don't remember writing, actually forming these letters into words, as a class activity, but Mrs. Dunwoody allowed Heather Ramsay and me to sit together at indoor recess and write books on folded arithmetic paper. Like the books we read, these had more pictures than words. We brought these to her desk and she let us use the stapler to bind them.

I also loved Mrs. Dunwoody for her hair. Everything else in that room seemed ordinary enough, but her blue-rinsed hair reminded me of fantastic elements. Her dresses were long and discreetly patterned, her arms had loose flesh that wobbled when she raised them, and her shoes were dark and practical. But she must have loved blue, and loved her hair, to dye it, and that self-confidence made me feel secure and hopeful about adulthood. I could imagine her leaning back on the beautician's chair, letting her large head settle into the beautician's hands. And, as the rest of us might stare at the ceiling and say, "Cut it just below the ears," she said, "Blue, please. I want it blue."

***

When I was eighteen, I was raped. For years, I stayed the cautious girl in the back row. Even my fear was secret, like the writing I showed only to Heather, opening my desk at the beginning of recess, and, just before the bell, putting it back in.

I finished college and became a school teacher, I never used a yardstick, but I've felt my face warm with anger when kids weren't paying attention or didn't want to follow the beautiful order I'd planned the night before. The violence I've committed most often has been the violence of negligence. There were hearts I couldn't open to, tragedies I didn't attend to in days crowded with about a hundred high school students. I know what it's like to feel like you're failing people, and simultaneously, to be full of rage at them.

And I've been like Jimmy Scanlon, too, wanting to wreck someone else's plans, to talk out of turn, to have things my way, and even to force somebody to pick up a stick—to feel the power of making another person furious. I've often pretended that I didn't know what that was like: I was invested in looking perpetually innocent. And when I admitted that I know Jimmy too, I know what it's like to be hit, then I could respect the meek girl in the back. She suffered but she survived. I did not think I could. Sometimes I did not think I did. I have had to look at her pain directly to be able to see the courage alongside it.

***

Now I'm writing a book based on what happened when I was raped, and what happened afterwards. In the fifteen years since I was raped, it's been a struggle to remember that it's not wise to let my pain sit still in me. It hurt to sit so quietly in the back row, pretending I was safe, believing that safety came from hiding. Now I've found not safety but release from pain by exposing myself in the open air. Pain won't change unless I let it move, and writing is motion. Writing touches and pushes out the pain. How do we keep living, when living is dangerous, when things happen that make our hearts retreat? I write as a way of looking for an answer. I leave these notes about the search.

Phyllis Beauvais

BODY BONDING

She screams, lunging
with dog teeth for my bared neck I duck
under her chin   I cling
close as a koala   mold to her body
tight as a leech

rolling side over side   smashing
our heads against cushions
we are sheltered by nurses counsellors
therapists   we are safe in the flailing
she howls and I hold

Mommy she is watching her mother
throw her sister against the crib
Daddy she is tied to a post in the cellar
her father is beating her
over the head with a bat he is
killing her kitten

her terror is a torrent
I am her bandied boat her raft in the hurricane
her mother her mouse her mealy rat
scruffed in the jaws of a terrible cat

I hold her grown body   hold
as she should have been
held
waiting
until she comes home

Barbara Williams

CARVING

This is the anger poem that won't come
the one that keeps burying itself deeper
deeper

as if I'm burying the hatchet
literally   in my self
again and again   the pieces
getting smaller and smaller
their number increasing

I'm a heap of shards   bone
and flesh   splintered and sliced
I'm a mound of dead matter
picked clean by the scavengers

so clean you can carve it
into a work of art

this is a love poem
for you, Daddy

Judith Hirshmiller

HAUNTED

You will not leave me
dreams of decisions
that i did not want to make
houses that i had to leave
children scattered
that i had to garner
who keep changing sizes & houses
you are clinging to me
against my will
you who in the beginning
i clung to
fearful that you would not
want me
then when i cracked
& the hate seeped in
i tried to shake you off & you
suddenly realized that it was i
who was strong i the survivor
how i churned with loathing
for you as your face turned to me
& your hands opened
but memories of love kept me guilty
guilt & love & hate & loathing
to wake each day with the dread
of those eyes that grasp
& tho you are gone
you will not let me go
you keep trying to mend the web
you ripped for all those years long ago
of my dreams & i gather courage
to leave
only to wake in another time & place
knowing that you will be there
& that i will leave again

David Starkey

ACCIDENTS

When I was eight, I broke
a vase Mom bought on her honeymoon.
Blood squealed
in her puffy cheeks. Trembling
she gripped my arms, "God,
what a mistake
your father and I made."

I kept stray cats in my bedroom
until they howled for food
and Mom would throw them out.
She hated crippled life.
Still, in late spring I fed
the fledgling jays
fallen from our backyard elm.

I was seventeen.
She was fifteen probably, though
she claimed to be the older one.
She'd been hanging out
in Smokers' Corner after school.
"Just a runaway with an attitude,"
she said when I asked her name.

I thought the door was locked.
Her nipples were red peppers
between my tongue and teeth.
Mom was wrapped in her house robe;
"Get out! Get out for good!"
But I couldn't stop,
I was a root pushing for air,

and I was still growing.

Bernadette Darnell

PAY ATTENTION

My mother was very small.
But she had such big feet.
Sometimes she'd take off her shoe
and smack me with it
if I didn't pay attention.
The world is full of fools
she'd say. Smack.
Don't you be one.

When I was growing up we lived in a house
with flowering trees and neighbors who spoke
in the lilting vowels of the Azores.
In the morning the men walked down the hill
to tan hides in the red brick factories.
They carried their lunches in metal buckets.
They left their black cars shining in the sun.

Once or twice a factory blew up.
The women threw on their embroidered scarves
and ran down the hill to the front gate.
Nobody from our street ever died.
In the evening the fathers walked home,
washed their faces and necks at the sink,
ate supper and sat under the trees.
When the streetlights came on we would sleep.

I went away from that street; the world
was rough and dirty and full of fools.
A woman was murdered under the highway.
It's a place where the boys take you.
They tell you she comes back,
looking for her shoe. Smack,
they hit the roof of the car
and scare the shit out of you.

It makes you feel small.
I should have listened to my mother.

Susan Luzzaro

NECESSARY ACTS

I crawl in the dark to the phone—
the clock reads 3:15.
I pick up the phone & hear
the rapid breathing, the slimy
click, click, click,
of a man beating off.
I hangup. Relieved—
so many worse things can happen—
have happened. My mother
can never forget to lock
the backdoor again.
I check my own locks,
my father installed for me, at the time
he was worried about me,
was telling me how I could
use my keyring for a brassknuckle.
Maybe the locks, maybe the key-ring
can save me now—my father cannot.
Once I made my son sell off his 22,
it was I who believed, like a teenager,
that we were invulnerable.
My mother was the best shot
in Decorah. If you wanted
a varmint killed, or stew meat,
you just called Katherine.
Her brothers would call her
to shoot the squirrels away
from the birdfeeder—till one day
she told me she hit a cardinal,
accidentally, as it was lighting,
she cried she said to see the scarlet feathers,
the scarlet ribbons of blood,
spread out across the snow.
When she moved to the city
she told my father to pack away the gun—
as if it were for country use only.
Sometimes I imagine her trying
to get to it, to unpack it
in those last dark & frantic minutes.

This morning I ran alone in the tall bamboo at the river bottom. Small birds rattled the dry reeds, a torn maroon blouse lay misshapen in the mud—I refused fear— though my son had warned me about the campsite in the bushes, the brown-bag bottles, the cigarette butts—I looked instead for the white winged egret to lift out of the shallow, soiled water—listened for the communal cry of the killdeer. My pace was all leap & joy—each footfall a reclamation—as if to say this world is mine as well.

> But the phone rings again,
> the night seems a century long,
> & I have a gun in my nightstand so powerful
> it frightens me.

Pat Schneider

LUCIA THERESA

Nicaragua, 1985

Lucia Theresa is raped
by eight soldiers
first with their cocks
then with the barrels of rifles.

Her young sons watch from the corner.

The soldiers explain:
they are punishing Lucia Theresa
for the escape of her little daughter.
The child ran naked into the street
and hid in the home of a neighbor.

I write about mothers and daughters
and say the name: Lucia Theresa.

Her name is a name for women:
faces of women refugees on the evening news,
bodies of women sleeping on the floor
of the train station in New York City,
women raped, disappeared, dismembered,
women telling their little girls to never walk alone
on any street in any town at night,
women denied jobs at the top of corporations
women intimidated into wearing high heel shoes
at Massachusetts Mutual Insurance Company,
women nameless in the housing projects
all across this land where Ronald Reagan
told the bitter lie: there is no hunger here.

So I name her name because I do not know
what else to do:

Lucia Theresa.

Carolyn Page

JUDGE

Raw wind sweeps me up the stone steps
to the court house.
Strangers gawk as the complaint is read.
My legal aid attorney whispers to the
judge, shows him my flowered diary
to His Honor's attention.
A recess of good reading is followed by:
"Bailiff, clear the courtroom."
My lawyer says it's going well.
"It appears he likes the way
you've, uh, documented it."

"Meet with me in chambers?"
The judge smiles benignly and motions.
I wonder what he wears beneath those robes,
which description of cruelty he's savored most.

"It seems he threatened you
if you didn't give him ..."
"Yes!"
"And how long on your knees?"
"An hour or two."
"If you don't mind my asking,
how did he manage to ..."
"But I do mind, Your Honor."

An hour later I have my decree.
Next day my diary is returned to me.

Two weeks later, ten at night
His Honor calls, suggests we meet
for drinks at his house.

Ellen Herbert

"ALL OUR SINS AND GRIEF TO BEAR"

When I remember my childhood, it's as though I stand outside our kitchen's bay window, looking in at my family sitting around the table, eating Saturday breakfast. No matter how I try to press these memories down, they remain solid in my mind, the details of life then more real than things that happen to the grown-up me: the smell of frying sausage in dewy morning air, the soft scuffling of Mattie's bedroom shoes on the kitchen's hardwood floors as she traveled from stove to table serving us our hard scrambled eggs and mounds of grits, a well of melted butter in their center. Father in his white, starched shirt, would stand, take his watch, attached to his pants by a shiny fob, out of his pocket, flick the watch's lid with his thumb, and look at the time. There were clocks all over the house, but whenever we suspected any of them were off, we asked Father to check his watch. He controlled our world, and when he held his watch, he held time in the palm of his hand.

Sarah, my older sister, sat closest to him. Mama never came to breakfast. Mattie, our colored maid, hovered about the table, serving and retrieving dishes. She never stood still in Father's presence, nor did she sing or hum when he was home. I loved her and her hymns, for they were the music and religion of my childhood. She didn't know all the words to her songs, but what she knew she taught to me.

There I was around the table, farthest from Father, the fringe of the Beacham family, Little Pearl, youngest, on the rung just above Mattie. Nowadays I try not to think about our life in Kingston, N.C., but when I do, I pretend that life happened to someone else. Even back then, when we were together as a family, I wished I wasn't one of them. I wanted to trade places with another little girl, any other little girl. I wanted to be anyone, but who I was.

This is all kind of funny because children we knew envied Sarah and me. Growing up during World War II, times were hard for everyone, but the war'd been good for Father's business. He'd gotten government contracts to supply the Marine Corps with tobacco from his auction house, so we actually prospered then and afterward. Girls would rush up to Sarah and me at school to open our coats and admire what we were wearing. People thought Father spoiled us, and in a way, he did. They also thought we were snooty because we rarely asked other children over to our house.

I overheard Mrs. Hargett, our neighbor, say once at a Christmas party that the only folks in town good enough for the Beacham girls were each other. What she didn't know. The problem with Kingston people is they think they've got you figured out from the time you start to walk. They want to say the whole of you in one sentence. "Oh, she was always a pretty one;" or "He's been sneaky since he was three and stole an RC Cola out of the cooler at McThenia's Shell Station." Towns like Kingston don't allow for a person to change. You are who you are from birth to death, and they will shoehorn you into their summing up sentence of you, no matter what you do.

But Sarah and I were spoiled. For our shopping pleasure, Father had set up charge accounts for us all over town. If we wanted to buy something really big, like a winter coat, we had to get his permission first, but for a sweater or blouse, we could have what we wanted. He felt bad for us because Mama drank, so letting us throw money around shopping was his way of making it up to us.

Although sometimes over breakfast, he'd protest our spending yet another Saturday shopping. "You two have enough stuff to outfit the armed forces and all the orphans of London," he'd say. "Why don't you stay home today?"

And we did have a lot, but we wanted to be in town for more than just gathering things to wear. We liked to be out and about; we liked not being stuck at home with Mama on the day Mattie left early. As usual, Sarah had a way around any objection Father might come up with.

"Mama could use a new bathrobe," she'd say, pretending to wipe her mouth in order to hide her sly grin behind a napkin.

Since Mama rarely went out of the house, she lived in bathrobes. At the idea of seeing her in a new one, Father sent us out with his special blessing. "Get her something real pretty, girls," he said, unfolding some bills from his money clip and handing them to Sarah. His fingertips had a permanent brown stain from the tobacco he handled at his warehouse, and his money always looked old and faded as though it'd gone through a wringer washing machine. "Buy your mama something that will snap her out of her funk," he went on.

To him, Mama was always in a funk, but to us, she was just into gin, which he'd switched her to from bourbon. He told Mattie gin didn't go through your system fast as bourbon, and you couldn't smell it easily on someone's breath.

"She'll drink it if she doesn't have anything else," Mattie told us one day as we helped her smash bottles in the overgrown corner of our backyard.

We lived on almost an acre of land. Our house on Midday Lane, one of best addresses in Kingston, was last in a row of large houses that sat on the hump of a hill with a rolling lawn in front and a big U-shaped drive. Because Midday Lane was a dead end, we had neighbors, the Hargetts, only on one side. Father sent men from his warehouse to mow and trim our front lawn with its carpet of lush grass, azalea bush hedge, and pink mimosa trees. Mattie kept the petunia and zinnia flower beds of the back yards. In the corner of the backyard, on the side away from the Hargetts, Father let nature have her way. The men didn't mow there nor did Mattie tend it, so it'd become overgrown. Sarah and I thought of it as our own North Carolina jungle of pine seedlings and honeysuckle vines.

"Why don't you clear away that area?" Otis Hargett asked Father once, nodding to the wild place as the two men stood on either side of the hedge.

"That's the girls' favorite hide-out," he told Otis. "They made me promise not to touch it."

It was true that it was one of our places, but we could never get Father to promise anything of the sort.

"You let those girls rule the roost over there," Otis went on to say, which was exactly the impression Father wanted him to have.

I knew that was odd: the way Father wanted to be thought of as henpecked, a sucker for his daughters' wants and wishes, but he knew, and we knew, the truth. WHAT WILL PEOPLE THINK ruled Father's mind. Even when I was little, I understood that. WHAT WILL PEOPLE THINK came foremost in my mind, too. Sarah, hating to be cut off from the rest of the world, chafed under the secrets of our household, but I didn't. Better isolation then for people to know.

Father made sure Mattie took Mama's bottles in an old burlap bag to the overgrown part of the yard. There she broke them against a big rock. The rock was Sarah's and my favorite place. Sometimes in the evening we'd come and sit side-by-side on it. Slivers of broken glass that made their way out through the weave of the burlap sack lay in the weeds around the rock and sparkled like jewels in the twilight. We pretended we ruled this magic kingdom from our rock throne. We'd sit, hugging our knees, listening to the crickets, frogs, and trucks shifting gears down on Highway 17. Lightning bugs came out, glowing off and on like caution lights, as daylight drained away.

Father would call from the back porch for us to come in, but he never walked out there. The rock was our safe place. One summer we even painted our initials on it.

Father made Mattie break the bottles so they wouldn't clunk around when the trash men picked them up. He didn't want one falling out and rolling down Midday Lane when they emptied our cans into their truck. As if the Hargetts didn't suspect what Mama did with her time. Once when they were having a wedding reception for their niece on their lawn, Mama stumbled out back. Just across from the striped tent their caterers had set up, she squatted in Mattie's pink and purple petunia bed and relieved herself.

After she did that, I wouldn't walk out our front door for weeks. I'd sneak out the back as if to avoid someone waiting to accuse me of being the daughter of the woman who peed in front of the Hargett's wedding guests.

Our house was a beautiful old victorian, one anybody in town would have been proud to live in. Father kept up the exterior to a fare-thee-well, having it painted a brilliant white every summer with robin's egg blue trim. A leaf didn't fall in the front yard that one of the colored men from the warehouse wasn't catching it before it hit the ground. Its splendor meant little to me, though. I would've settled for a more modest house and sober mother.

Father felt the way I did. He did all he could to keep folks from knowing what life was like within our freshly painted walls. We were alike, he and I, but not Sarah. She could even laugh at times about Mama's shenanigans. "What she does is what she does," Sarah said. "And I can't help what Mama does." Sarah was the one who went out back to Mama the day of Hargett's reception. She pulled up Mama's underwear and led her back in the house. From our second floor bedroom, I stood watching them, peeking out a crack in the drawn curtains. Had my sister managed to walk on the parlor's ceiling, I couldn't have been more amazed at what she'd done.

19

I did enjoy helping Mattie, though, with the breaking of the bottles. In our jungle, no one could see what we were doing. With the bag filled to capacity, I took it high over head and flung it against the rock. At the moment of impact, I felt like Hercules in all his glory. I liked to be first to crack a new load, because the first whack against the rock, when the bottles were still intact, make a noise loud as thunder. As the bottles became more pulverized, the sound lessened. Sarah and I argued over who got to be first, so Mattie made us take turns. We could hardly wait for Mama to drink a sack load full.

I knew something was wrong with Sarah the summer she stopped caring about breaking the bottles. "Oh, you go 'head," she said to me early on in May of her last summer.

"She's eighteen and gettin' too old for such thing," Mattie told me at the rock. "She's worrying over what to wear when she goes out with Mr. Wesley tonight."

But that wasn't true, and Mattie knew it. We both felt something happening in the house, what with the sickly sweet odor of vomit lingering in the air. Mama threw up often. Whenever we heard her retching in early morning, Father said later over breakfast that she'd eaten something that hadn't agreed with her. But the summer Sarah drowned, the vomit odor never left our house. Whenever I opened the front door, the odor greeted me, causing my stomach to knot. And the odor wasn't from Mama being sick all the time, either; Sarah was sick now, too.

One morning when I heard Sarah in the bathroom, I went in to her and said, "We've got to get you a doctor."

"No doctor," she told me before I led her back to her bedroom. I went back to the bathroom and got a wet washrag. Folding the cloth over her forehead, I watched the rise and fall of her breathing.

Mattie came in. "You all right, Sarah?" she asked and knelt beside her.

"We've got to get her to a doctor," I said again.

"No doctor," Mattie told me.

Mattie knew something I didn't. I stared at Sarah. For all her illness, she'd been looking so beautiful, more womanly, with her figure filling out like a pin-up's. I kept staring at her while Mattie stroked her hair and hummed "Amazing Grace."

In that moment, I knew. My fears about things we never talked about were confirmed in that moment in time, as I stood beside her white canopied bed in the room Father had insisted she have. That confirmation divided my life. I came to look upon everything that happened to me until then as "before" and the rest of my life as "after." *I once was lost, but now am found / Was blind but now I see,* Mattie sand, as if it was a good thing, but I didn't want to see. I wanted not to know.

Until she turned thirteen, Sarah and I shared a room. I was afraid of the dark, so plenty of nights I crawled into her twin bed next to mine, where we slept like two entwined vines.

But when she turned thirteen, Father said she needed her own room. "You're a young lady now," he told her. "You don't want to share a room with your little sister."

Putting it that way, Sarah wasn't sure if she did want to stay with me. When she saw the ruffly canopied bed he bought for her, she moved her things into the new room. The first night she slept away from me, I waited an hour or so after everyone had gone to bed. Then I put on socks so I could walk the hall and not be heard. I moved like a shadow over the hardwood floor toward her room. My plan was to beg her to let me come in and stay the night. I would tell her I'd heard something scary outside my window. I'd describe the sound, maybe even make it for her. My sound would resemble a bat's wings flapping in flight or an owl screeching, but I would say that it could be a thief scratching on my screen, trying to get in.

As I reached for her door knob, I heard noise in her room. This was not my imagination. I heard Father's voice and Sarah's; their words I could not make out, but I could tell he was hurting her.

That night has haunted me all my life. Why didn't I knock and ask if she was all right? Why didn't I burst through the door and tell him to stop? I know the answer to that: I didn't tell my father to stop anything. At eleven years old, I was afraid of him.

I backed down the hall and stayed awake all night and nights to come.

Father made Mattie take me downtown to see Doctor Banks. He sent a note along with her to be given to the doctor. On the bus ride there, I took the note out of Mattie's purse and read: *Pearl's started looking like an old hoot owl, Paul. Can you give her something to help her sleep?*

Father was right in what he said. I hardly recognized my reflection. Looking back at me from the mirror was a long, pale face with a dark crescent moon beneath each eye.

Doctor Banks shone a light in my eyes, ears, and nose, examined my throat until I gagged, and listened to my heart with his stone-cold stethoscope. I was afraid when he sat down behind his desk to write out a prescription. I knew whatever was wrong with me was my own fault.

"Do you like chocolate?" he asked, surprising me with the harmlessness of his question.

I nodded my head.

He proceeded to tell Mattie how to make egg milkshakes, which he explained, "would put some weight on me." The other thing he recommended was exercise, swimming specifically.

Father signed Sarah and me up at the "Y" for lessons. After I learned freestyle well enough to swim back and forth across the narrow end of the pool, I did sleep better, but not well enough to drown out his footsteps down the hall to her room nor his soft knock at her door.

Time passed. I never asked Sarah about Father's visits, she said nothing to me about them, and I didn't tell Mattie. We all walked a wide path around those nights. Looking back on it, I realize I couldn't do anything about what he was doing to her, but back then, when I was nearly twelve, I thought we were all more connected. I thought that if I did things just right Mama wouldn't drink and Father wouldn't hurt Sarah.

I tried to keep things perfect in my room. My shoes had to be lined up in the closet with the toes pointing north. Above them, all the hangers had to go in one direction with the blouses and dresses on them buttoned and zipped. The moment I woke in the morning, I jumped up and made my bed. The quicker, the neater I made it with tight hospital corners, the closer I would be to perfect and, thus, keeping things right around the house.

"Don't make your bed this morning," Mattie might tell me, "I need to change your sheets."

But I made it anyway. What I wore, what I said, what I ate had to be perfect. No wrinkles, saying unkind words, or bruised spots on my banana would keep me from perfection. Nights when I heard Father's footsteps in the hall or mornings when Mama threw up, I told myself I had to do better. Then I added another requirement, like keeping all the books in my bookshelf alphabetized, to my list. If something got out of control, if they did those things I was working to prevent, I tried harder.

My right eyelid started twitching. Father didn't send me back to Doctor Banks, but everytime he saw it twitch, he told me to stop it. And I tried to, but I couldn't.

"You're doing it on purpose," he said to me one morning when my eyelid fluttered out of control. The twitching was the strangest sensation; it was as if something entered my body and moved the lid without my permission.

"Stop it," he yelled, and he never yelled. Filling up with fear, I watched to see what he would do next, but my eyelid was not afraid. It kept right on going as if to sass him. He brought his cup down hard against the table and broke it, the milky brown coffee spurting up to sully his shirt.

He jumped up. "There, see what you made me do," he said. He'd been in a terrible mood ever since the day before when Mama'd gotten a ride with Mrs. Hargett to our Arbor Day celebration at school. She hadn't been drinking, but since she seldom went out anymore, she didn't know how to dress. She'd worn her bathrobe as a coat. Mattie, who was supposed to make sure Mama didn't leave the house, had been grocery shopping at the time. Father really yelled at Mattie, too.

Yelling got him upset. He said often he didn't believe in it. I'd heard him tell Mr. Hargett, and it was usually true, that ours was a household in which a harsh word was seldom spoken. I liked that: a harsh word was seldom spoken. *And seldom is heard a discouraging word/And the skies are not cloudy all day.*

But the morning when my eyelid went dancing, he yelled—louder than I'd ever heard anyone yell—for me to stop. His voice went up to our high, high ceiling and spread out to the tiny roses on the kitchen wallpaper. I ran into the little room off the pantry where Mattie slept when she stayed overnight. I lay on her narrow cot, pressing my face into the soft bed linens that were full of her smell. I loved the way she smelled. I'd had my face deep in her bosom off and on all my life. Whenever she wasn't there and I needed to be close to her, I came into her room and lay on her bed.

Sometimes when she had the day off, I got scared she wouldn't come back. She wasn't a slave, she wasn't a daughter. If she wanted to, she could go home and not come back to me. When I was little, I woke early on Mondays, the morning after her day off. I ran downstairs, found her in front of the stove or behind the ironing board, and threw my arms around her, joyous that she'd returned.

I couldn't remember when she didn't work for us. Sarah told me that when I was born, bottle milk made me sick, so Mattie came here and nursed me. Late afternoons when Mattie got ready to leave for the day, sometimes I became scared she might not return. To keep me from crying, she would hold me for awhile and tell me her version of how she started working for us. Everytime she told it, she used the same words, so her story, our story really, became like scripture to me.

"When I came to you, my little boy, my little Willie, had gone to Jesus. Woke up one morning and he'd gone to Jesus so quiet in the night. Hadn't even cried out to his mama on his way. Jesus must've took him before the sun came up, in that early cold time of mist when it's not night, and it's not day. I cried and cried over little Willie. Only baby I ever had that came out of my body." Then she would hug me to her. I filled up with her delicious smell, waited for her to go on or prompted her by saying, "Then Mr. Clifton came to Big Willie…"

Mattie would smile. "Then Mr. Clifton came to Big Willie and said, 'Sorry 'bout you losing your baby.' Big Willie nodded. Then Mr. Clifton said, 'You reckon your wife'd come take care of my baby?' Big Willie nodded. Then I came here and saw you and knew I'd gotten me another baby. Jesus sent me another one. A pale one this time." With that, we would laugh.

The day of my eye twitching, I heard Father say to Mattie, "Keep Pearl home from school today and straighten her out." Mattie made me my favorite breakfast, pancakes, and we sat in the bay window, letting the sunshine settle on us, pressing through our skin, warming us to the bone. I was so happy to be with her and for us to have the house to ourselves. Under her gaze, my worries spilled out of me. We sat there all morning while I talked and talked. I told her how I'd tried to be perfect, about my shoes and hangers and keeping the books in alphabetical order.

To everything I told her, she nodded and said, "Uh-huh." That's all she said. "Uh-huh." Her words came out like a song, like a hymn she was humming. "Uh-huh." Her sounds washed over me as if they were cleaning me off. I kept going. I told her about all the things I'd been walking a wide path around, about Mama and Father and Sarah.

Finally after I'd said everything three or four times and sat looking at my reflection in the greasy syrup shine of my plate. She said, "It's a wonder with all that on you, my Pearl, your whole body isn't twitching."

Then she asked me if I knew the Lord. Well, I did, sort of. All I knew about Him I knew from her. We didn't go to church. Mama'd been an Episcopalian, but Father said Sunday's were his day of rest, and Mama was usually recuperating from Saturday night, so we didn't go to church.

"I'm not sure if I do or not, Mattie," I told her.

"You believe?" she asked.

I nodded. We got on our knees, and she prayed. She had me ask Jesus to come into my life. I closed my eyes and brought my hands together with my palms touching as she was doing.

Mattie's hands were beautiful. The tops of them were ashy black, gnarled as a tree trunk. She had a story for every scar and lump. When I was little, I would hold her hands and trace the lines and rub the rough places while she told me stories about picking tobacco or working in the kitchen of the Kingston Hotel. Her hands held a brilliant surprise, too, for when she turned them up and opened the palms, they were pink as the inside of a seashell.

I felt her lean closer to me and her fingertips come to rest lightly on my eyelids. All the while she sang soft and low. *Just as I am without one plea, but that thy blood was shed for me.* Then she said, "Satan be gone. I claim this child for the Lord." At that, she pressed the hard pads of her fingertips against my eyelids.

Right then, with my eyes still shut, I saw a bright glow and felt something like an electric charge from her touch. Shortly after that, we got up. I helped her clean the kitchen while we sang happy songs: "Bringing in the Sheaves," "The Church's One Foundation," and "I Come to the Garden Alone."

I walked around the rest of the day feeling lighter. when Father came home that night, I ran up to him and told him, "My eyelid's not going to twitch anymore."

"Good girl," he said.

And it didn't. Mattie's fingertips and Jesus healed me, but they didn't heal me from worrying about what was going on around me. I've been a champion worrier all my life. Mattie would tell me, "If you worry, why pray? And if you pray, why worry?" But I did both, still do, with the two acts balancing me, somehow.

Sarah didn't worry over what all was going on. I remember once, though, she tried to stop Father. She found the key that fit her bedroom door. Actually, I was the one who found it, but I didn't know what it was or meant at the time.

Sarah and I were in the attic one rainy afternoon in summer when the air was thick enough to choke on. Steam was rising from the gabled rooftop outside the dormer windows. Great beads of sweat dripped from our foreheads, burning into our eyes. We ripped up old shirts of Father's and tied them around our heads. How neatly Sarah tied hers. The cuffs stood out stiff on either side of her forehead, their cufflink slits looking like snake eyes. In even that ridiculous garb, she looked the part of a beautiful twenties flapper. I danced the Charleston, or what I thought was the Charleston. She laughed at me, and when she did, her eyes shut and her dimples deepened.

We liked the attic, heat and all. It was another place where no one else ever came. That day I found the keys, I was looking for some music sheets to use as fans. I was back in a corner where old furniture was stacked, opening and shutting drawers, dust flying in the air so I could taste it. When I slammed one drawer shut, I heard something, a clanging. I took the drawer out, reached in, and pulled out a ring of large, heavy keys.

"Looky what I found" I said, holding them up.

"Let me have them," she yelled, the laughter gone from her voice.

I flung them at her, and she scrambled for them. "Damn you," she said. "Why'd you do that?" She reached beneath the old sofa that was losing its stuffing and pulled the keys out. Coming to her feet, she held them up to the light of the dusty window. Then she ran downstairs with them.

I followed her to see what she would do. She stood at her bedroom door. Our house had thick wooden doors with eyeball-size keyholes. The keys from the attic were long and heavy with fancy curlicues on the end. One by one she tried each key until she found the one that fit her door. She took it off the ring and to the bathroom, where she washed it in the sink, dried it, and put it in her pocket as though she'd found a great treasure.

"It's only an old key, Sarah," I said.

"No, it's not," she told me.

A few nights after that, I heard Father knock at her door, but she didn't let him in. He knocked harder, calling her name over and over. "Sarah, Sarah, please Honey, open the door." His voice echoed through the dark and stillness of the house. Her door didn't open. I stood at my own door to listen, but I heard only my Father. If she said anything to him, I didn't hear it. He kept up his calling and knocking. He got louder.

That night Mama'd actually come down and eaten dinner with us. She did that sometimes. So she wasn't passed out; I knew she was hearing what I was hearing. Finally, he stopped.

The next morning he was sitting at the kitchen table when I came to breakfast. Sarah hadn't come down yet. Several times he stood and pulled his watch from his pocket. After opening it and checking the time, he'd snap it shut with a sigh.

We heard her footsteps on the other side of the kitchen's swinging door. "I'm not too hungry," she said and walked in. She grabbed a piece of toast from a plate on the table and turned to walk out, barely breaking her stride.

From the ironing board, Mattie started to say something about how she needed to eat, when Father jumped up from the table. He caught hold of Sarah's wrist. She leaned in his direction and hunched over a little.

When he looked at her, his green eyes had a sad cast to them. "Don't do me this way, Sarah," he said, loosening his grip on her.

She pulled away and bolted through the house. He followed her while I followed him. She went out, leaving the front door wide open. He came to stand in the doorway and watched her run to the bus stop. The stooped way he stood with his square jaw down, the beaten look on his face made me feel sorry for him. Why wouldn't she let him in? I went to him, put my arm around him, and hugged him. He pushed me away as though he were swatting a gnat.

"Go on to school, Sister," he said.

One night, not too long after that, I heard Sarah turn the key in the lock and let him in.

The day she drowned, I went into her room and lay on her bed. I pressed my head into her pillow and smelled her sweet Shalimar perfume. When I put my hand under the pillow to cradle it, I felt something. It was that old key.

To this day I still have that key. I keep it in my dresser drawer wrapped in the note, soft and faded from time, that she left for me. She wrote the note before she and Wes went to the beach that day. She knew she wasn't going to be coming home.

Several months before she drowned, I sensed something awful was going to happen. Our house felt as though a hurricane was coming with that sick odor lingering and the heavy stillness of everything. Father was gone a lot, and Mama almost never came out of her room. By then I was sixteen and had met a boy, Ernie Ballou. I went out often with him. We'd meet at the other end of Midday Lane. He thought I didn't let him pick me up at the house because I was ashamed of him, when, in truth, I was ashamed of our house and everyone in it.

More than anything, I regret those last months with my sister. She started fighting with Mattie and me over little things, and when she fought, she fought like a tiger. She'd scream at me over nothing.

"You wore my new shoes, you little jerk," she said to me one day, holding a black pump by its heel.

"No, I didn't. I swear."

Yes, you did," she screamed. "See how it's worn right here."

"Sarah," I told her, "how could I wear them when I don't wear nylons yet. Couldn't you see me prancing around in high heels with my anklets on?" I felt like crying. "Please believe me."

At that, she melted, put her arms around me, and told me she was sorry.

Looking back now, I saw that in the weeks leading up to her drowning, a calm came over the house. In that time she must have decided what she was going to do. Stupidly, I told myself her trouble had been resolved. I wish now I'd told her how I loved her, how I couldn't have gotten through life on Midday Lane without her, but I didn't.

August 16, 1946 she walked out into the Atlantic Ocean as far as she could go and let it take her. That day was the only time I ever saw Father cry. Mama asked for a bottle to be brought to her bedroom where she drank in the dark. Mattie and I stared at each other over the funeral crowd bearing platters of food for our family.

I liked the church service for Sarah. She would have liked it, too. Well, maybe not the preaching, but certainly all the flowers. I liked the preaching. I knew where we as a family had gone wrong. We never went to church together. We were a family who didn't know the Lord. Satan had a strangle hold on us.

Mattie was the only person who talked to Sarah and me about Jesus. She sang hymns, told *Bible* stories, and was a missionary to us as surely as if our house had been in deepest Africa. After my conversion in the kitchen the day when my eyelid was mad calm, I tried to get Father to take us to church, but he refused. I was too shy to go by myself. Sarah liked Mattie's stories about Daniel in the lion's den, Ruth and Naomi, and, especially, Samson and Delilah, but she didn't see the need for church like I did. She thought she was strong enough to live life alone on her own strength. For myself, I knew better.

The day after she drowned, I couldn't face another mourner. By dying, Sarah succeeded in bringing people into our house. She would have loved it, but I didn't. For one thing, I began to see the interior of our house through new eyes, the way other people were seeing it. As much as Father'd kept the outside up, the yard, etc. in good order, he'd done nothing with the inside. The wallpaper was peeling in every room, and except for Sarah's canopy bed, we'd not had a new stick of furniture since I'd been born. I felt ashamed, too, that with my sister gone, WHAT WILL PEOPLE THINK still came foremost in my mind. Father was caught up in keeping guard over Mama and her behavior. He'd enlisted my help to do so, but I'd gotten tired of following her every move.

So I went in the bathroom, ran a tub of cool water, and got in. Father came to the door.

"Come on out, Pearl," he said. "I need you. Come go to the funeral home with me and help pick out a casket."

I moved down in the water so that the back of my head and ears were beneath its surface. I liked the way water muffled Father's voice and all the other sounds in the house: high screechy female voices downstairs, the scraping of chairs, the clanging of pots. I entangled my fingers in my pubic hairs, which reminded me of seaweed, and waited. I heard through the water the stamp of footsteps as he walked away from the door.

Later Mattie knocked, then let herself in. She rolled up a towel, situated it beside the tub, and knelt on it. I grinned up at her.

"You ever been baptized?" she asked down at me.

I shook my head under water.

"It's not too late," she said. "Long as you're living, it's not too late."

I sat up in the tub. My skin was wrinkled and pale from soaking so long. Mattie turned on more water. Our tub was large and set up from the floor on thick claw feet.

"Come sit up here," she said, pointing to a spot closer to the front of the tub. I moved where she told me. I felt her hand come into the small of my back for support. Slowly she brought the pink palm of her other hand over my face and closed off my nose.

"I baptize you in the name of the Father, the Son, and the Holy Ghost," she said.

I shut my eyes and let myself go, as she guided me back. The water folded over me. Even during my swim lessons, I'd never liked the feeling of water covering my whole face, but this time I didn't mind. I wasn't afraid. I prayed the water had taken Sarah as gently.

When Mattie brought me up, she said, "Congratulations. You're a soldier of the Lord now." Then she sang. *Mine eyes have seen the glory of the coming of the Lord.*

I sang the words I knew along with her while I got out of the tub and dried off. A breeze blew in through the window. It seemed as though it was the first breeze we'd had that entire summer. I stood in front of the window and let the cool air dry me. Tingling all over, I felt cleaner than I ever had.

I shed something of my old self in the water: the fear I had of Father, the idea that he controlled time, that I had no say in my life. All these were washed out of me. In her own way Sarah had freed herself, and so could I. With Mattie's help, a few days after the funeral, I ran away with Ernie Ballou and started my life over.

I would like to believe I made a clean break with everything that'd happened in Kingston; I would like to say I never look back, but I do. During my day, decades of time and hundreds of miles separate me from Midday Lane, but night builds a bridge to that life, and I am there again. In my sleeping household, I lie in bed with my eyes closed, and in the silence hear footsteps in the hall.

Maryrica Lottman

HIS PALS SPINNER AND PADDLE-FOOT

" '*Clutch Cargo!*' " little Tom yelled, imitating a TV announcer, " 'with his pals Spinner and Paddle-foot! In another exciting adventure!— *The Lost Gold Mine!*' "

Peggy the social worker was sitting on the chair beside him. "You mean cartoons?" She smiled with her mouth only.

Tom nodded, re-explaining it all to himself:

"Paddle-foot is the dog. Spinner the boy is ten, twice as old as me. One time Spinner dipped his fingertips in red paint and dotted freckles over his nose because that was the way he wanted to be. He made himself! He has a big head full of brains. Spinner doesn't have parents, Clutch Cargo is all. He goes everywhere with Clutch—Asia, Africa, Alaska.

"Paddle-foot is Spinner's weiner dog. He has long ears to hear everything, and afterwards they flop over to cover the secrets he's been told. His body is a sausage. He can worm his way into places Skinner is too fat to go. But sometimes Paddle-foot gets stuck. One time he came out of a hole with seaweed dangling from his ears, one time with burrs covering his fur, and one time with a bucket on his head. One time near 'The End' he thought he was the king of Morocco. One time he played the ukelele and sang in a high dog voice, and Clutch and Spinner plugged their ears. Paddle-foot can be all the things that Clutch and Spinner can't be, stupid and silly, and crafty too. But Clutch and Spinner will risk their lives to save him from a crocodile, from counterfeiters, or from a dog catcher. Paddle-foot is worth swinging from a vine to rescue. He can swim, and if you toss him he can fly. His ears drag on the ground, and sometimes his belly.

"Clutch Cargo is a genius. He can fix the boat engine, trap robbers, outsmart a spy, cook stew in the jungle, talk with Indians, and lasso the end of the dock to keep the motor boat from running away with Spinner in it."

Peggy the social worker clicked her tongue. She told Tom to stop talking to himself. "Talk to me," she said. She looked at herself in the mirror. Through the glass Tom could hear the whirr of the video camera. He knew that it was a one-way mirror, and that Peggy's supervisor, who knew everything, was watching them from behind it.

"Tom, sit down on the floor with me," Peggy said.

She dumped herself down on the floor and pulled him by the hand. She was fat, and it was hard for her to breathe. Her stomach sat heavily on her knees, and she exhaled like a bull, blowing gusts through her nose.

"I've talked with your friends," Peggy said. "You said they got 'sick with germs' from 'playing in bed' with your neighbor. What's his name? Mr. Carlson?"

She knew everything, so why was she asking him, Tom wondered.

Peggy reached out.

Tom smelled the wet pit that grew under her arm. She gave him two rag dolls, a pink one and a blue one. The dolls were almost real between their legs, under their clothes. He could stick his finger in the pink one, and a wiener stuck out of the blue doll.

"How about you, Tom? Did you play in bed with Mr. Carlson?"

Tom looked into the mirror for the supervisor who knew everything, but he saw only himself.

Peggy asked him again about his neighbor.

Tom sucked his thumb and thought. Mr. Carlson drove kids to the zoo, had rabbits and candy. Once Mr. Carlson stuck a rolled dollar bill in his nose and blew blue smoke through it. He said he had been everywhere in the world, and he could prove it. He had money from everywhere in the world. Kids called him Clutch Cargo. He looked just like Clutch, everyone said so. Big and with blonde hair and a wide forehead and a square jaw. Tom's father too had said, "Clutch Cargo!" and snorted.

Peggy didn't want to hear about Clutch Cargo on TV cartoons.

Tom nodded. They were re-runs from a long, long time ago. He thought about how on *Clutch Cargo* real mouths move the mumbley cartoon lips. He shivered a little. It was a real mouth.

Peggy asked him about the other kids. Did he know what Mr. Carlson had actually done to them?

He knew, he thought so. But he couldn't say. It was like a thought in the toes of his shoes. If he took them off, he couldn't tie them back and for the rest of his life he would have to go barefoot, even over glass. It was like his belly-button. If he uncurled it, all his air would bleed out. Clutch Cargo and his pals Spinner and Paddle-foot! He couldn't remember. But Peggy knew, so why was she asking him? Why did she want him to remember? She kept asking him and making him, leaning towards him.

Tom closed his eyes. He put his hands over them in case he wanted to cry. Peggy kept touching his hands and saying his name. He wrinkled his eyes tight together, till he could feel ruts traveling across his forehead.

"Tom?"

He made Peggy and her pestering disappear.

When he opened his eyes, two clowns were standing with their hands on their hips in the middle of the room. They had whooshed out of the air. One was pink, the other was blue. They were both three times taller than Tom, and they had four fingers like a stuffed Donald Duck or a Mickey Mouse. The pink clown, who had a rolling pin, resembled Tom's mother, and the blue one wore his dad's bow tie. The pink clown wiped her red eyes with her hair. It was hanging half in front of her face. The blue clowns's pajama pants buttoned like sailor's trousers.

The first thing the pink clown did was to bug her eyes at Tom. She broke out crying again. She tried the knob on the supervisor's beige plastic floor, pulled on it hard. The blue clown jumped on top of her, humping and groaning, and pulling on the knob with her. He called her Honey. He put his feet up on the door around the knob and pulled hard with his whole self. It wouldn't budge. He got down. He dusted off her bottom. Then they both stood in front of the supervisor's mirror, primping. The grease paint on their faces had already started rubbing off on their collars. The pink one pushed out her lips and rolled her rolling pin against them.

The blue clown said in Carlson's voice, "You tell us!"

Tom felt his face go red, like swollen crying eyes. He didn't know what had happened to him. He couldn't explain it. He wiped his eyes.

The blue clown nudged him and snickered, man to man. He stuck two gloved fingers between his pants buttons. "Down there. Did you wee-wee on yourself in kindergarten? Is that all that happened?"

Tom nodded.

The clowns turned to squint at the mirror. They shrugged their shoulders, scratched their heads, and turned to scowl at their son. "You lied to us!"

"Talk up, Tom," the pink clown said, "or we'll throw you down the manhole."

"What manhole?" he asked.

The blue clown moved the chair away. "There!"

Tom saw it, the sewer manhole in the middle of the floor. It hadn't been there before. He had the sneaky feeling that someone for sure was watching all three of them.

"The secret of what Mr. Carlson did to him," the pink clown said, "is in his belly button!"

Tom had checked his belly button just that morning, and it had looked okay, curled up like a snail asleep.

The blue clown grabbed him by the ankles. He turned him upside-down and walked him on his hands wheelbarrow-fashion over to the sewer hole. He held him headfirst over it. "Spill the beans!"

Tom's pink tongue hung in the sewer air and its bumps grew slimey. The air was wet with garbage smells. It stuffed his nose, and he pinched his nostrils shut. His shirttails were pulled out of his pants. The blood rushed into his head and ran into the roots of his hair upside-down. It ran into his closed eyes too and invigorated them. Now he could see farther. He could concentrate for longer than ever before. All the big pieces of the past year slid to the bottom of the sewer and the little pieces stayed on top. He turned his head, and the piece shifted again, like inside a kaleidoscope. He shook his head to rattle it. He turned it to the right and left. He craned his neck, touched his chin to his chest, and looked up. Up above him the blue clown's feet loomed bigger than his head, and the pink clown, bent over backwards with her head stuck between her legs, stared at Tom.

Tom's neck stretched like a Slinky. Pieces of suspended dust were tumbling slowly into the distance, and the light was playing on them. Someone held a flashlight at the other end of the sewer.

The blue clown held him by one heel.

"There's a man talking behind Clutch," Tom said in his own words, not the TV announcer's. "Sit close to the TV. You can see that behind his thin cartoon lips the wet insides of real lips are smacking. A real tongue with bumps is resting, like an alligator's back waiting under the water. Even Spinner has real inside-lips. You can't trust what real-live people will do. But Paddle-foot doesn't talk, and he doesn't have a tongue.

"Behind the screen there's someone bobbing paper cut-out figures pasted on popsicle-sticks. The tropical landscape stays still behind Clutch Cargo, Spinner, and Paddle-foot. They bob up and down, across the screen, through the swamp, like solid people. It's just a layer over real life. They're puppets run by people. They're not cartoons.

"Even though Clutch explores the jungles in Florida and meets beardy professors that get kidnapped and have daughters, all the same he's my neighbor, Mr. Carlson. When he shows me his tongue, he thinks that's a good enough clue about what happened. But I can't guess. He puts his mouth against the screen and says letters. The screen fogs up. He says, 'Read it, Tommy boy.' "

Peggy said, "Read it."

"I can't read. Just ABC's. I press my nose to the TV screen. I don't want to cuddle with Clutch in bed anymore, but Peggy tells me to look and see. What happened. Worse than peepee. A mouth somehow wanting to eat me."

Peggy touched him.

Tom started to spell the letters out loud so that she could hear him and make the words. She held his hand. She could make some sense out of it. But the ABC's faded into the cut-out trees and snow-capped mountains, into oases, palms, peaking waves, grass huts, and the scenes from everywhere Clutch has ever voyaged. Clutch bobbed out of the jungle and vanished off the edge of the screen. He was a ghost walking through a wall.

Tom was shaking. Behind him, the arc of the light from the eye of the camera was like his peepee. He could hear the machine whirr and his brain think. The light hit the wall and showed Clutch in black and white and all swollen, reddish. *Come here*, Clutch said. Tom had to. *Open your mouth.* Tom's hair burned at the roots, and it felt as if it were growing. What Clutch was doing should never happen to a little boy. But it could happen to a little girl. Clutch's touching him made the long, pretty hair braid itself into pigtails with bows. Clutch kissed him. The little boy winced and disappeared. Tom had made himself into a little girl again, just as he had when Carlson had unzipped himself on the sprawling bed.

The little girl named Tom touched the wall where Clutch was playing with Spinner and Paddle-foot. The shadows from the camera light danced on her hand. She ran her fingers across the wet plaster. It was soft, wet, and cold like her own goose-pimpled flesh. She poked her fingertips into Spinner's freckles. Any minute now the camera would turn off. Now was her one and only chance. Now while it was big and clear she could see and say it, show and tell, that it was real and not TV. It had happened to her, to Tom. Now while the head of Clutch Cargo was swollen twice the size of her. *Come closer.* He made her. Peggy wanted her to feel it all and tell about it, so that eventually it wouldn't be so scary anymore. It would be just an evil thing that had happened and was no more. But now it was nasty. It made him bug out his eyes. The insides of his nose, bloody and full of fizz, itched him. *Open your mouth.* Clutch unzipped himself. *Wider.*

The little girl Tom touched the TV screen. She put her face on Clutch's face horrid, cold, hot and wet. Carlson smelled of tobacco. He had a wide blank forehead and a square jaw and eyes that told nothing. He had hair as yellow as pee. He swelled up. He was too big to be just a grown-up man. She pressed her mouth to the episode on the screen. *Put your hands behind your back. Close your eyes.* She did what Clutch whispered in her ear. His breath tickled her neck. *Open your mouth.* Her eyes were closed tight, pretending to be asleep. Clutch pulled down his boxer's.

But she put her hands behind her head and parted her long hair. Her eyes in the back of her head saw the camera and the supervisor who knew everything. The light whirred. The beam heated up the back of the little girl Tom's head. It splashed a picture there where he himself couldn't see.

"Tom?" Peggy said.

She pulled his hands away from his eyes. He couldn't remember, for fear that he himself would disappear.

***

Lisa M. Peck

FANTASY

66 Why?" is the question that I keep asking myself. Why are they doing this to me? I just don't understand. I wish that someone would come and rescue me from this terrible experience and take me out of here to a better place in time. I really don't like the things that they are doing to me. I am feeling really scared and my whole body is shivering inside.

I am in my mom's bedroom on her bed in the middle between Eddie and my mom. Mom is trying to talk to me calmly so that I will relax and just let Eddie do what he wanted to do with me, while my mom is, in a way, giving him encouragement, like saying that it is o.k. for Eddie to do what he wants to do with me.

It felt to me that she actually gave permission for this guy, who is not my father, to do terrible things to me. To me it felt that she was on his side. She didn't even bother to tell him to stop after she saw what I was going through. She was just right there not saying one word to this guy. All I remember her saying was, "Just don't hurt her," while in my mind I felt alone in a very dark shell trying to get out by sticking my head out, but every time that I did stick out my head I was getting hurt even more."

But eventually down the road I was rescued by some caring people, and I have come out differently than what I expected. I now like myself for who I am.

Elizabeth Michaels

APRIL 12, 1986
Saturday
8 P.M.

I have not written an entry since March. I still don't know how to write this entry ... have debated whether to do so and don't know if I'll keep it if I do.

Joseph is accused of raping a man and is in jail. I look at those words and say goddamn ... and it's a crazy mixture of pain, pity, anger, and confusion...and yes, even, love. He is my brother...and I have always wanted to understand him. I have tried so hard to...and now realize that what little understanding I have will be all there is...and I cry.

Details? There is no need ... a police report states what was supposed to have happened. Joseph neither hid or destroyed any evidence. The only debate is whether the other guy was unwilling—or if brutal sex was their idea of enjoyment. Was enough money not paid? If the first is true, it means Joseph literally waited to be arrested. The other means a self-revenge even more brutal than the act.

No matter how many times I tell myself I can't, I still try to understand.

Genius. "Your brother is a genius. I don't understand why he makes the grades he does," Joseph's professor asks. I had been appointed to pick up his exam since I had a class in the same building. His physics' professor searched my face for some type of response to a blunt statement about the red "F" glaring off the paper I was holding. As Joseph's sister, he thought I would know the answer. The prof never realized how many times I had said, "I don't know." Joseph could do anything he wanted and neither family, friends, nor professors ever understood why he chose nothing ... preferred nothing. Instead, he devoted countless hours to magazines which he never wanted to throw away and dreamed of a life filled with success.

Isolation. I remember Joseph proudly introducing the one friend he had at our father's funeral. The guy stayed maybe twenty minutes—having arrived only thirty minutes before the mortuary closed. He had other things to do.

Moods. Joseph either loved or hated you from moment to moment...and you never knew when it would change. One instant he could be stringing a set of Christmas lights that had been on his first Christmas tree as a child and the next shattering china plates on the floor while my mother cried and begged him to stop ... and my elderly father stood frightened in a corner.

Blindness. Both Joseph and my parents refused to ever see that he had a mental problem. Eventually, my other brother and I had to leave home to maintain our own sanity. To suggest treatment was to start an emotionally, and frequently physically, violent argument. The only "sin" of his my parents would vaguely acknowledge was his homosexuality, and they always clung to the belief he would get over it. Otherwise, there were "no problems"—except for a "bad temper" due to his "feeling poorly," the irritating habits of others or simply someone else "trying to start an argument." In short, my parents needed help as badly as Joseph.

Hugs. I probably haven't hugged Joseph a dozen times in the last twenty years. He believed hugs to be stupid and overly sentimental. The times he allowed someone to touch him…to really touch and be near physically and emotionally, is almost non-existent.

As soon as I heard Joseph was in jail, I was on the next available flight. In spite of everything that had happened, he never doubted I would be there … and maybe I wasn't quite prepared for the fact that he was right. Within twenty-four hours, I was sitting across from him, talking into the prison booth's telephone and looking at him through a thick pane of glass. He did not look like the other prisoners, my neat brother with stylish wire-rim glasses, but that didn't surprise me. It was the conversation that ignored everything going on. Joseph acted as if this were a normal visit, and refused to discuss the present situation. Did I have a good flight? Find his apartment? Like driving his car? Have a problem finding the jail? Plan on seeing any of the sights in the city?

Then he told me I must go to a wonderful bookstore that he knew I would love. It was the same one where he had gotten the poetry books for my birthday. They had everything. "You'll love it. Go. Don't come all the way out here and not go. It's not hard to find."

Two days and five, fifteen minute visiting periods later, I went to say goodbye. I had closed out Joseph's apartment and various banking accounts, the sum of which was around a thousand dollars. His car was packed, and I was about to start a sixteen hundred mile drive home. He asked if I had completed his list of things to do and I said yes, having finished the final items that morning. Joseph became angry I had not done them sooner. I asked him if he wanted me to get him a private lawyer.

"No, don't be an idiot."

I found myself in the middle of old patterns … old angers. But I said, "I love you." There was a silence. Then, he added: "The only thing I want you to do is get yourself through school and get your Ph.D. … and write." He said, "Did you go to the bookstore?"

"Yes."

"Didn't you like it?"

"Yes."

"I knew you would. That's your world."

The guard announced over the loudspeaker that visiting time was over. Again I said, "I love you." I put my hand to the glass and for a moment Joseph looked at it. Then he put his hand to mine, hung the phone up, mouthed goodbye, and walked away.

M.S. Leavitt

I'M NOT JOSEPH

Joseph wore a technicolor coat and God was on his side when they threw him in jail. I wore a pin-striped suit and a silk tie and God and I hadn't spoken in a long, long time.

That's not true. I had spoken to Him, but He didn't return my calls. Maybe I wasn't home. Maybe it doesn't matter 'cause I ain't Joseph.

Nobody told me about the pain of blue skies seen through chainlink fences as the mist sparkles on razor wire deftly designed to slice flesh to the bone. Nobody told me that the dawn hurts.

Nobody told me that there were too many heartbeats to the minute, too many hours and too many days. The sound of the watch ticking on my arm bangs slowly in the back of my head like some caller in a minaret sounding off the hours with deadly precision. Nobody told me it hurts when your heart is out of step.

Nobody told me how pride stings when they search you. "Strip down. Bend over. Smile." Nobody said it would hurt to say your name. I ain't Joseph.

She cried when I left. So'd my mother and family and friends and former lovers, each tear scratching my hollow veneer. I can handle it.

One more tear. One more silent whimper. I can handle it.

The sound of metal bars sliding to the left claws the soul like fingernails on a blackboard, only the sound seems to call out SINNER as it lumbers to a stop. Silence. I can handle it. Silence.

Nobody told me the sound of the stars in the night was loud enough to burst the eardrums as if the one voice of every man who had gone before me was now singing in concert, a fugue flickering to moonlit madness. Too loud, too damn loud.

Nobody told me of the pain in the first visit, or all the ones after that. You see it in their eyes. The separation. The hurt. And in that silent hug you can hear their eyes denying words of forgiveness that trickle from their lips.

"How are you?"

"Fine."

How can you say you watched another man get raped and you couldn't say anything? How do you describe a cluster party and what it looks like to view the slow motion beating of someone as frail as you feel? They drop like a blanket that folds slowly over itself and the blood doesn't make a sound.

"I'm fine."

You talk about nothing because nobody wants you to worry. You talk about nothing because they cannot understand. You talk about nothing and the words hurt. Nobody told me that words can rip bits of your heart away. Rip. Tear. Bleed. Hurt.

Nobody told me that dreams haunt you like a cruel lover sneaking into your bed and that the walls and eyes and ears of this place swallow you bit by bit until nothing remains but a shadow of who you once were. Nobody told me those shadows hurt.

So everything is fine. Don't worry about me. Did you like the bookstore? How's my car? Do I have a future? Don't worry about me, I can handle it. Did you get my letter? Will you write to me? I'm doing fine.

Nobody told me about the pain.

Blanche Woodbury

MY BROTHER

My brother lives in a box of cigars.
Each day every day
he lifts the lid to peek at the world
and hopes the world won't notice.
Bristles grow on his face and throat.
He smells, fears soap.
He never throws his loose hairs away
but carefully keeps them, dirty and dark,
in the teeth of a green plastic comb.

Long ago he spent years committing incest.
I survived but we never mention it.
He's thirty-five now and still lives with our mother.
My favorite joke when I visit is to talk
of the time I stabbed his thigh with a fork
and sent him screeching around the table
for ruining my first perfect crayoned picture.
We pretend to laugh. And the scar
does not go away. Migraine headaches
take me back to the fork, to the fort
he built under cool pines
where he wouldn't let me visit
unless   I would   and I did

Now he does his best to repel.
He rots his teeth, sucks his cigars,
growls and belches and gets fat.
Each night every night
he grows a little smaller inside.
One morning my mother, weeping,
may find he's flickered out at last,
a tiny gray heap in an ashtray.
I'll visit, leave the jokes behind,
bring instead a perfect crayoned picture
to wrap around his coffin.

Kim Bridgford

WHAT YOU MIGHT SAY
IF A FRIENDSHIP ENDS UNHAPPILY

It's not hate that I feel for you,
Although you might expect it
Just as you always expected extremes.
It was unpredictability
You couldn't swallow—
In short, human behavior—
And so you saw everything
As betrayal. And, oh, the scenes—
Tragedies all—
That I couldn't help interpreting
As a deficiency in myself.

Friendship is not
A constant shattering of teacups,
Dragon fire, the whole holy mess.
I still can't quite believe
What you were willing to do
To keep yourself gold.
Meanwhile, a bruise started growing
In the center of my psyche—
Purple and sloppy and infinitely rare—
Until finally, my friend,
I had to get the hell out.

CHAPTER II

DEATH
&
dying

*For I share in the life of all who live
And the death of all who die.*

Vivian Smallwood
"The Participant"

Peter Cooley

THE ELECT

Many the shadowless under the rose leaves
untrembling midmorning.
Many at early evening
the wings, ochre, henna, cinnabar,
which continue, unseen, singing
when night, never stirring, takes the air.

In this garden out of time
the stillborn until their moment linger.
Their souls climb the white down
of little tubers, footless; they suck
mouthless the orris root. Hoarfrost
their spoor foreshadows them, burned off by noon.

And from this place we called the child to us
that you might carry it
to give it up. And spare her breath
this life, the agony of body, the next, the next, the next.
Tonight on the long, clear wing of her voice
the soul of our daughter walks out
between the thorns, uplifted, no one

warbling her absence, everlasting.

Elisavietta Ritchie

NATALIE

Long before science could sex a fetus,
I figured you female, gave you your name.
Three months into a sort of life,
salamander stage, you gave little hint
of the brilliant beauty you might
become at six, sixteen or thirty.

The doctor warned: *It's not growing right.*
So I wasn't surprised, that New Year's Eve,
when I bled like a calf under the farmer's knife.
All for the best, to be sure, for us both,
lost embryo, who would not stick
to my persnickety womb.

After the doctor's curved blade had scraped
your imperfect fragments away, and I awoke,
asked what they'd done with you.
Don't worry, my dear. But what curious taste …
I wanted you back to inspect, perhaps
preserve in a jar of formaldehyde

like my biology teacher's fetal pig.
Too late, the shocked doctor replied.
Perhaps a more appropriate course:
a pint-sized plot in the garden beneath
a salmon azalea or lavender hyacinth
to fertilize at your own time-release pace.

Not plunked in a graveyard with strangers,
or dumped in a pit with the hospital waste.
Too tiny for priestly blessing.
Big enough for my tears.
Each year now seems to bring
a new loss to mourn,

but I'd mostly forgotten
that old one in a distant town.
My leftover child, who gave
no promises, no expectations,
why today do you float in my brain
like a salamander reborn in flame …

44

Edward William Stever

SONOGRAM AT FOUR MONTHS

My unborn child
pauses,
sucking her thumb,
peers out at me
as if to say,
"I know something
you don't ..."

Skeletal as death
she hovers in an ocean
of beginnings,
a breather without gills,
drowning into life.

Blind as she is,
she sees
distances
and depths
that swallow
even the stars.

Meg Baxter

SECOND CHILD

Footsteps on my belly
lighter than the kick of butterfly.

You—safely curled in
that balloon I bore before me—
seldom thrust out an arm
to pierce my night's sleep.

Those were your best days ...
before the trauma of your travel
through my tight tunnel

until the light revealed
your alien chromosome.

Doll-still,
you close your Asian eyes.

COMING TO TERMS

That year when my baby was dying, writing was the only religious thing I could do. But words were flimsy, so common. I wanted other materials. Alabaster. Soapstone. Marble. Something fresh and pure and clean and untouched. Like the baby. Pink, waiting for shaping. Full of beauty, just by existing. Photographs couldn't capture her; even a drawing was flat, one-dimensional, square. The baby needed roundness, weight, to be made whole. She needed to float up whole from something already perfect, like stone.

This impulse to find art in her was an expression, a way of keeping something that was going to go away, a way to make beauty from tragedy. To get to the heart, the art, only symbols could provide perspective, distance to see her in focus: clearer, more perfect, orderly, simple, than she was herself. White and pink rose petals where there was skin, tulip mouth.

The baby was brand new. New as a bud, as fragile. All expectancy, waiting to bloom. Enclosed, self-contained. Some buds never opened; they remained in that state of waiting. I've seen roses die like that. Slowly falling over to one side, a head fallen asleep on a chest, petals still folded like hands in prayer. I have thought they were pretty; it was a pretty death, and I liked keeping these remnants in vases around the house for the shape and mood of them.

***

Rosie lived seven and a half months and was, every day, silent. A baby who didn't cry. Without voice. My job as her mother was to interpret this silence, make sense, accommodate her unspoken needs, imagine her unspoken wishes. The silent baby was surrounded by talk. Endless discussions about the quality of life, in meetings with experts, doctors, priests, psychics, philosophers. That was all right; silence was worse. Her silence, and other people's cautious quiet, the insignificant talk that surrounded it; any conversation that wasn't about her was insignificant.

Time went, and no one talks about her anymore. I move on. I swallow down deep, to make her stay away, so I can pay attention to the task at hand, my job, my other child, making love, caring about others and their pains, sorrows and grief. I am choked by the lump of words.

I write stories. Behind everything, she throws a shadow. In the story of the restaurant date, the couple isn't arguing about money, they are missing their baby who died. In the vacation tale, expectations go unfulfilled because they can't forget Rosie; now far away, they still must speak of her or go crazy. But they have already talked so much. Unanswered questions will always be so; any guilt has no choice but to be assimilated. Words can accomplish this much: re-examination, clarification. The living ease each other, it's not your fault, it's no one's fault. Felicitous catch phrases temporarily make sense: Her life has (our lives have) purpose and meaning. But what, what? Can I name it? The purpose this sorrow serves, this feeling of loss, this emptiness, longing. This potent desire to make meaning, words all I have.

***

So much time went by waiting for Rosie to die. You can't live that way. You have to pretend that death is far away, not imminent, or why invest in anything? But in the case of Rosie, it was impossible to pretend. What could I hope for, sad and exhausted at the thought of her going on the way she was, alive, not alive, in ruinous limbo? If some doctor could have said, one year, five years, a normal lifespan (if it were just the same mystery we all endure), I could have pretended for Rosie the way I pretend for myself. I could safely assume she would be alive in the morning when I went in to get her. I could stop thinking about death all the time. The thought of her living a long time was the other monster, and during those days and months I mostly held on tight to a vision of a future, soon, without the weight of caring for this very sick baby. The idea could bring relief. I could imagine myself after. Except I felt guilty. What mother hoped for her baby's death? Crazy. And the few times I'd looked in on her and found her breathing invisibly, thinking she had died finally, my feeling had not been relief. It was fearsome sadness. A pit, a fall, horror as anyone would feel, looking in on a death. She forced me to look through and feel it, feel it, because I knew this was preparation, all the false alarms, for when Rosie really would be dead in there.

Wanting neither, her death nor her life, having no good choices, I was forced to live in the present with Rosie, without expectation. I learned to enjoy holding her, smelling her, looking at her. Each moment whole, complete in itself because there was no future. I found there could be peace in such a state when it was genuinely achieved. Not easy because we are so conditioned to plan ahead, look forward, project, imagine, fantasize. There could be none of that with this baby. So I learned to sit still and just be with her. In love with her.

***

I comfort myself with words. She is sacred and holy and permanently innocent. Perfect. She doesn't suffer.

William Stafford

FOR A LOST CHILD

What happens is, the kind of snow that sweeps
Wyoming comes down while I'm asleep. Dawn
finds your sleeping bag but you gone.
Nowhere now, you call through every storm,
a voice that wanders without a home.

Across bridges that used to find a shore
you pass, and along shadows of trees that fell
before you were born. You are a memory
too strong to leave this world that slips away
even as its precious times goes on.

I glimpse you often, faithful to every country
we ever found, a bright shadow the sun
forgot one day. On a map of Spain
I find your note left from a trip that year
our family traveled: "Daddy, we could meet here."

William Stafford

A MEMORIAL: SON BRET

In the way you went you were important.
I do not know what you found.
In the pattern of my life you stand
where you stood always, in the center,
a hero, a puzzle, a man.

What you might have told me
I will never know—the lips went still,
the body cold. I am afraid,
in the circling stars, in the dark,
and even at noon in the light.

When I run what am I running from?
You turned once to tell me something,
but then you glimpsed a shadow on my face
and maybe thought, why tell what hurts?
You carried it, my boy, so brave, so far.

Now we have all the days, and the sun
goes by the same;
there is a faint,
wandering trail I find sometimes, off
through grass and sage. I stop
and listen, only summer again—remember?—
set off like other strangers

The bees, the wind.

William Stafford

RIGHT TO DIE

God takes care of it for
everyone, once. And armies
figure it out, wholesale,
for others, in the air, on the ground,
at sea.

Living, though, is a habit
hard to shake, and they don't
move the heavy stuff at you
till later when you are about ready,
usually, any time.

Still, maybe I'd help,
knowing what I do about need and
the grim alternatives; maybe
I'd be very kind when the hurt eyes
turn, suddenly loud, toward me.

Mark Scott

WHEN I DIE

When I die, shall I tell you what to say?
I think about it all the time.
Do this first: look at all the notes I made.
And the sheets of calendars I saved.
You won't find certain things,
so don't worry about covering me.
Say that I knew a baseball from a cycling cap.
Say that I knew what was going on
on my side of the table.
Say I lied where my feelings were concerned—
without compunction say it.
When it comes to friends, hesitate,
but say that I had too many,
and none but my father depended on me.
Him I didn't let down, not even now:
even today's accomplishment he envies.
Say that for a model I used my mother:
those whose hearts I broke were always
welcome around me in the kitchen.
In the notes you'll find very little
to go on, since I never took down
the depths. I doubted their existence
beyond my sixteenth year. That I never
set out to hurt anyone is a lie
that bears repeating nonetheless.
But to tell the truth that I was not
different—this will get you (and who
shall you be?) borne away on the wings
of disbelief. Add that I loved myself.
Add that near the end. Tack it on
just before you close, not because I did,
but because it will kill my father.
He is, I know, afraid of dying,
but he wants to be immortal.
Our secret lay in not dying daily,
but in wishing to, and telling no one.
Add that to the end.
Then bury me beside my brothers.

Susan Jacobson

DORK

The kardex said: *admitted for*
right index amputation / S/P
gunshot wound / suicide attempt /
bilateral craniotomies / restraints /
contracted / pressure sores (decubiti /
on right lateral aspects of buttocks,
knee, anklebone / non-verbal / Rancho IV
level (unmeasurable mental functions) what is known
as a dork on the neuro floors.

I took his vitals while
it was still dark and later
fed him his breakfast.
He ate the sweet things,
refused the eggs—
he was very hungry—
but we didn't get to AM care
until late morning, telling
the secretary we'd be in there a while.

He stank, of course—they always sweat.
The scarring on his temples
was hardly noticeable—
someone had done a good job closing—
black hair, gray eyes, thin,
tiny hipped barely buttocked,
with the uncurving characteristic hands,
no expression except perhaps sadness.

He wasn't so much contracted
as fiercely fetal,
could be unbent with
enough pressure, patience,
if you talked softly
for long enough.
His eyes shifted from
straight ahead to right,
looked right at you
when you talked to him.
I have no idea if he saw us

or, if seeing, knew us
as human, like himself,
but he looked at us
when he spoke.

We bathed him slowly, thoroughly.
Sherry redressed the sores—
he wasn't very strong,
I could hold him still for her—
changed the bed, passing him
back and forth between us,
decided to go whole hog
and shave him, snitched
a rinsette from another room
and shampooed his stiff
smelly hair with enema soap,
massaged his back—
he relaxed all over—
talking away the fear.
(It was fear.)
He held his bandaged
wounded right hand
tight to his chin, but
we managed to stuff a pad
into the crook of his elbow
where the skin was breaking down,
raided the linen room
for soft bath blankets,
cranked up the bed
so his persistent stare
would see the skyline,
tied his hands down,
and we finished.

We stood together
at the foot of the bed
two women separated
by twenty years,
united by nurturing,
and saw / heard him
take a deep breath
and sigh.
I have heard dogs
heave great sighs of satisfaction,

their heads on my lap, eyes closed,
in a daze as I stroked their ears,
and horses, when I brushed them,
have fallen asleep standing up,
drunk with pleasure, with touch.

Was it cruel to be
so gentle with you
when we must send you back?
How long does it take
a man to chew off
his right index finger?
What despair, self-hatred,
rage remains after
you have blown away
your frontal lobes?
Were you protesting
your rehab treatment,
that storage place
for the terminally alive,
being handled, talked over
like a sack of potatoes?
Did you lie on one side
until perfect circles of pain
burned through your thin flesh?
Is the word protest appropriate?
How about the word soul?

That contented sigh.
Your eyes closing in sleep.
Your face rosy as a child's.
That sigh.

Mary Alice Ayers

THE INFINITE DARK

He only saw the window, tenderly alight within, and the infinite dark leaning like water against its outer surface, and even the window was not a window, but only something extraordinarily vivid and senseless which for the moment occupied the universe....

(Apologies to James Agee)

What does this mean? A father, a child of a father, had been thinking about his father who was dying and then he was thinking about infinity, about dark, about water, about life. Water had long been a symbol for life, for life everlasting. But death and the outer darkness—what does this mean? A teacher explaining the writing of a man is much like a preacher explaining the will of God. Neither can be analyzed; there isn't one answer that can be labelled "meaning." And how explain literature, which attempts to explain life, to children who haven't yet experienced it, who haven't lived? And this story was about life although apparently about death. Explain that.

Among the fourteen-year-old children who were learning about the story was one who was learning about a death and the death was her own. The doctors predicted that she would die before Easter, and they had told the parents and the school this. Part of Karen's neck had been taken out in September. She had found the lump there herself, but the doctors had discovered that the lump was merely what had surfaced from a long tube that coiled downward into the chest. They took out the lump and left the tube because too much else was involved.

So an unexpected death became part of a curriculum that had been planned to include a major work on the subject long before the girl's condition became known. Books had been purchased, and it would have been too obvious to ask for a new text now, well into the term.

The girl's condition itself was understood by all, the end to it also known. Yet nothing could be said. When she began this year, her first teaching, they had told the teacher, Ann Blake, to ignore the illness, not to treat the dying girl any differently. If Karen brought up the subject on her own, it could be discussed with sympathy yet detachment.

But she didn't. However, the subject came up in the required literature; first in a short story they read before the long story about the "infinite dark." In this first tale, a man had tuberculosis; this disease had to be explained to them—that it was the cancer of the nineteenth century. It had been greatly feared, and many people had died of it, including many famous writers. A boy asked what in other circumstances could have passed for a perfectly acceptable question—is he going to die? The only response that came to his teacher was the cliché, that we are all going to die, that in life we can be sure only of our death, and more of the same.

But the answer might as well have been the answer to another question for all the attention they paid to it. Many of them looked at Karen. She noticed them looking at her. She smiled at her teacher. Karen was an attractive girl, more so when she smiled. She was built boxy, square jaw and square body, but the loss of weight caused by her illness and the hospital stay had rounded off the corners. There was an appealing softness to her now that she had lacked the end of August. She still had, though, the same beautiful skin, clear, and clear grey eyes. The boys had not discovered her prior to the discovery of malignancy, and now they were not likely to; no fourteen or fifteen-year-old would want to fondle a breast that covered a cancer.

Karen smiled, accepting of both her condition and the attention it caused. She could smile because she had faith. Her parents believed in prayer, and in the healing power of Christ. Karen had undergone a healing, and she was certain she would live. Ann Blake herself believed in healing, that it could be self-caused; this was possible if an individual had an immense desire to live because he had to accomplish something. She wanted to give Karen that desire.

This was a goal entirely her own; it had nothing to do with pedagogical theory, with what she had learned in her education courses. In these, a great deal had been made of the central question in education—whether the child was a machine to be trained or a soul to be awakened. There also had been much discussion about all the problems today's teacher would encounter—sex in the schools, drugs in the classroom, racial conflicts in the community. But nothing about a dying student; nothing about how a teacher should react to this crisis, more serious than any of the other difficulties. It was a special challenge, but this teacher enjoyed challenges. Ann Blake had gone into teaching later than most, age thirty, because she had wanted children and was childless. She had been married twice and was again husbandless. She was, therefore, more than willing to make of these children her whole life. With these emotional needs, she could see Karen as almost heaven-sent, if Karen could be saved.

That morning the girl had been able to produce only two sentences of creative writing when the requirement had been at least a page. She had said she hadn't felt well, had trouble breathing, asked whether the beginning had possibilities, whether it might be a story. Her teacher told her, using the principle of positive reinforcement so important in the theory of behavior modification, that she was a natural writer; perhaps she might someday be great if she worked hard.

"Is he going to die?" The question was still with them; Karen was still smiling. Miss Blake, reminded of Karen's breathing problems, gave names and specifics of some good writers who had died of what was then called consumption: Keats ("mortality weighs heavily on me"), Browning, Chekhov, Mansfield. Another writer had survived a bout with lung disease, H.G. Wells. In his twenties he had one tubercular lung and a damaged kidney when he decided he was tired of being sick and would never be sick again. He never was.

As she was speaking, every particle of the teacher was willing her student to do a Wells and not a Keats, to fight to live and to win. They went back to the story; then they read the long one about the infinite dark. Karen successfully answered a reading comprehension question—the infinite dark was eternity where the man who wrote the story imagined his father was.... The term wore on.

Karen told her teacher that she enjoyed writing; it wasn't a strenuous activity, and it could be done anywhere—at home, at the doctor's, in her sick bed, or in Radiology at the hospital, waiting. In class, Karen spoke up more, and shared her writing freely. Hyperactive as the students could be during readings, they were motionless for Karen's papers. For them, however, their attention reflected merely curiosity, whereas for the teacher, her stillness was caused by wonder—at a creative talent producing regularly despite the decay of tissue and the demand of pain.

Possibly the class wondered too about the reason for the sudden achievement, but more certainly they wondered about the date of the writer's death. No one sat next to her; the teacher was advised by one student that her mother had told her that cancer was caused by a virus, and therefore was contagious; much like the common cold, it could be caught. That Karen was in a quarantine situation was evident because of the empty chairs surrounding her; unfortunately, there were more seats than students in this particular class. There was a need, therefore, to do more group work, to force cooperation and participation. The idea worked; Karen came up with good ideas and gained new respect from the others in her group, and they reacted with less horror to her presence. Perhaps everything, even the most sickening, could be borne if given time to become familiar.

They started studying poetry, and Karen wrote poems easily. Poetry writing made her feel as good as story writing, she told her teacher. She did her poetry research paper on Millay's "Childhood is the kingdom where nobody dies." The paper was read from behind the lectern, which was centrally positioned at the front of the room for the occasion. Karen's topic shocked those students who hadn't been aware of her choice. Fear of the unknown, death, was again a living presence. The paper was well-written, but Karen had failed to see the message of the poem. What did it mean? It was saying that in life sometimes people are dead to each other, "Who neither listen nor speak...." A man and a woman had had a quarrel, and they were not talking. The pain of life can be worse than the pain of death. It was fortunate that this could be said. Family argument was next brought up as a topic for discussion, and the class ended on that note of intimacy; a universality shared was the family.

Discussions like that eased the strain, lessened the constant concern over Karen's condition. It wasn't forgotten, but by November it was less talked about, less reacted to. Then, a week before Thanksgiving, Karen went into the hospital where they removed one lung. Ann called to ask about what she was reading, and whether she was writing. She did not ask for a prognosis, as others did. The parents in turn did not refer to the illness as terminal. They truly believed she had been healed, and that the process was just taking longer than had been expected. Their daughter was not seriously sick; she had just had surgery to correct a painful condition.

Karen returned in mid-December looking not at all well. She was very thin. The doctors knew how much she wanted to live a normal life, so they let her try. Some of them apparently could see the miraculous possibilities of self-will.

Karen had a new batch of writing efforts for her teacher. Most were fragments of stories; too much imagination had been given to the openings so that what was created was an unreality. Karen had been so romanticized by them that she hadn't been able to go on with the action; she had described fireworks, waterfalls, tornadoes, canoe trips, desert camels, overgrown jungles. Yet everything moved and had a sort of riotous life to it even so—color was everywhere. Karen herself was now lacking in color; she was very white. Also weak; she didn't accept criticism. "I don't want to be boring," she protested.

"But you must be real; these scenes are not. They can't be real to you or to any reader."

"I felt good when I was writing them."

But Karen agreed to take a little bit of action at a time; where there had been a waterfall, she would describe a stream and a picnic beside it. Family happiness.

They were still in poetry and were reading Shakespeare. Surprisingly, the sonnets were not too advanced for them, and with some explication, they went over quite well. One of these brought up for the first time for these ninth graders, raised for them for the first time, the question of the immortality of art. Artists created perhaps because they craved eternal life. A great book might live forever, even though the writer of it himself could not. "So long as men can breathe, or eyes can see / So long lives this and this gives life to thee." The work, the child, had outlived the parent, by almost four hundred years in this particular case.

Christmas arrived and with it a three-week vacation. Ann Blake enjoyed the rest but not the separation from her students. She missed them, despite the fact that she recognized she was not an especially good teacher. She credited herself with stimulating a few, blamed herself for several failures, and noted that most had been content to remain in the middle stretch. She had thought she had awakened one creative talent, Karen, but now, removed from the situation, she wondered if the efforts put forth by the dying girl didn't appear greater than they were simply because she wasn't expected to do anything, to be anything; she was not expected even to be living, never mind writing. Her own problems—sense of self-insufficiency and absence of enduring ties—weighed more heavily as the days wore on. It was a relief to hear the exciting news that Karen's parents had given her a horse for Christmas. Everyone thought the gift was an absurdity, carrying faith too far; the girl was too weak to ride at all, never mind to ride well. Ann Blake was thrilled by it; the parents had great belief in the miracle of Karen's living to ride her horse in the spring shows. When she visited, Karen had to show off, and she jumped the mare, which, in addition to being a superb animal, was also a trained hunter.

Scarcely had Karen's classmates and their parents recovered from that interesting piece of news when they had to contend with the shocking report of the death of Holly Martin, a pretty fourteen-year-old who hadn't been as pointed in her avoidance of Karen as had the others. Two states south at a lakeside resort, a motorcycle had caught her in the middle of a road and tossed her over a hedge and onto a field. The accident was hit-and-run, and they never found the rider. Most of her classmates attended the funeral, including Karen. Holly's body had been badly broken in the fall and her face shattered because she had landed full on it; therefore, the coffin was closed. Karen found the closed coffin very upsetting; she wanted to see Holly for the last time and didn't care if she was in bits and pieces. Her teacher explained to her that she wouldn't be seeing the girl she remembered but only remnants, a reconstructed entity, not a personality but a mannequin. That didn't satisfy.

Weeks later, Karen's depression had changed to an extreme excitation—she could talk of nothing else—whenever she had an opportunity to bring up the name of the dead girl she did so. The injustice of it was what rankled, and whenever she talked about Holly her jaw blocked off a perfect square. Her teacher warned Karen's parents about what was happening; what if her condition was aggravated by this needless worry? Time for another cliché, and Miss Blake told Karen, "She has gone to a better place; she is at peace; she is with God."

January got off to a wet, dreary start; they suffered through two weekends of solid rain from Friday night through Monday morning. After the second one, Karen came to Miss Blake with a finished story. It was the longest piece she'd done, and it was about Holly—"About how she died and about what she thought when she was dying, between the bike and ground."

Her teacher started the story before lunch and did not eat anything, could not, after reading it. Karen could not have been aware of the well-known and much-praised poem about the stewardess falling 40,000 feet to her death from a plane over Kansas, yet the story was exactly like it—the girl as she fell thinking about all that had happened to her. It was a story within a story—the accident described—a young boy hadn't been looking, wasn't drunk or high on drugs, just hadn't been looking—and then the hurtling through the air over the road and over a hedge and a brook and then finally dropping. But the thoughts of the girl dying from an accident were the thoughts of the girl dying from a malignancy, and why shouldn't they be? The creator and the created might well reflect on life in the same way since the death they faced was the same, only the means whereby they would experience it different. An unreal moment in the story was Holly's considering the irony of her unexpected death when the expected death of a classmate exactly her age had still not occurred.

At the bottom of the last page, Karen had printed in block letters, "SO LONG LIVES THIS AND THIS GIVES LIFE TO THEE." And in a classic hand beneath it, "With gratitude to W. Shakespeare."

Her teacher suggested that she submit the story to young-reader publications. In May, it won a magazine-sponsored high school writing contest. Two other stories had not been accepted but had elicited words of encouragement. If not a career, Karen at least had a distraction going. Whether the writing had helped her, or the new horse, or her parents' faith, or her healing, whatever, by the summer, she looked new and alive, radiant, tenderly alight within, well beyond the grasp of the infinite dark, and Ann Blake felt like a mother, partly responsible for new birth and for hope of immortality. Nobody had to die, she decided—she might undertake a research project, write a paper, on chronically ill writers who had been helped by a surge of creativity.

Karen lived through that school year and lived into the summer and lived on into the next year. But what happened? She forgot her teacher. She did not even speak to her in the halls—unless she was spoken to first, and then she responded not unkindly, but from a distance. What was strange, finally, was not that the cancer had been arrested, healing or no, not that the creativity had been continued, teacher-inspired or no, but what was strange was that the girl had forgotten someone who had worked with her, cared for her, had even prayed for her—the student had forgotten the important role her teacher had played in her life. The teacher found it hard to say to herself that perhaps her part had not been such an important one. Divorced husbands were lost to her, and children by them were lost to her, and now a student she had wanted to be her child was lost to her. Was there no permanent feeling to be found anywhere—even right in the face of death? Here was the infinite dark then. Here was explanation galore, of literature, life, death, whatever. What the dark was. "Who neither listen nor speak." It must be the living of the moment that counted, not what came after. Maybe there was no after, only the dark now, and no connection. No matter. The moment had to occupy the universe.

Cullene Bryant

MISSA SOLEMNIS

The altar boy holds the long taper high in the air, his extended arm quivering, standing on tiptoe in order to reach the top of the white Paschal candle. The priest meets the coffin at the door, says a brief prayer and proceeds with the mourners down the aisle. He approached the altar table and bows to the crucifix while the men place their burden near the lighted candle. Then the priest turns and faces the people.

Kyrie: *Lord have mercy upon us.*

Joshua stares at her face. He has never seen such stillness, such heaviness, such impassive leaden weight as he sees in those closed eyes, that set mouth, those rouged cheeks. He imagines he can see her breathing. He waits for the rise and fall of her chest, the gentle lifting that would signify breath, life.

He and his wife were the first to venture from Trinidad to Canada. His plan was to bring all five of them, all five brothers and sisters and finally his parents, even though they complained they were too old to make such a change. He hadn't realized how lonely it would be. Edmonton, hardly a large cosmopolitan centre, had a fair sized Muslim community but not a large black district. He settled in Sherwood Park, a predominately white, anglo saxon, bedroom community where he most certainly did not belong. But the rent was cheap. His wife cleaned houses, something he abhorred. She picked up after other people's spoiled children, washed out their bath tub ring, scrubbed greasy pots left soaking in a cold sink because the woman of the household was out working at an office job so that she could buy another TV for the family room or a second car.

He and his wife sacrificed for the ones back home. In this rich country they lived simply without the amenities they saw others enjoying. But when he felt exhausted, cheated, bitter, Angela cheered him.

She was the one he brought over first. Nothing broke her spirit. For her Canada was a great adventure. She adjusted almost too quickly to this alien country. In her graduating year she became a high school cheerleader and runner up as Queen of the prom and in nurses' training won a scholarship. But to his relief she also held to the old traditions. On Sundays after church the house was filled with the aroma of roti, and her hot curry was the best he had tasted since leaving home.

But now as he bends over the coffin he shakes his head at the senseless loss. Why? His wife nudges him to go back to the pew and sit down. The line of her classmates had already formed behind him. They had all come, all the girls and the two young men who graduated with her from the school of nursing. Joshua is touched.

Dies Irae: *Day of wrath and doom impending.*

Joshua sat uncomfortably in the plush chair of the Jubilee Auditorium. He still hated suits and ties. But in this cold country even in summer one would freeze dressed in a cotton shirt so light that it flapped in the breeze and allowed currents of air to rush up under the arm pits. He readied his camera, pulled it out of its case and set it on his lap. The pianist struck the first chord of Handel's "Largo" and the audience rose to its feet. There she was, marching down the aisle with the other girls in their starched white uniforms and new white noiseless shoes and cradling an armful of red roses. She stared straight ahead to the stage where the chairs sat in rows awaiting the graduating class. He knew she must be wondering where he was sitting but she dared not look from side to side as she moved down the aisle. She kept in step and remained smiling as she looked for her seat. He regretted that in a few more days she would be doing the same thing again, holding flowers and walking down another aisle to another tune and dressed in a white wedding dress. But he could not be there.

When they arrived on stage there was a rustle of white uniforms as the girls found their correct chairs and squeezed beside each other. They waited until everyone was in place and then they sat in one graceful movement. He wondered if she was looking for him now. Their dark faces wouldn't be so hard to find. She had told him to sit up close so he could take pictures. They would be sent for everyone to see. Her day of glory.

Credo: *He was crucified dead and buried and descended into Hell.*

The police came right into his office and told him she had already been rushed to emergency. He didn't wait to call his wife or anyone. They asked him questions: the young officer, the medical examiner, even the doctor staring down at his shoes in the Quiet Room.

"Where was she going?"

"To the airport. She was flying to San Francisco."

"Would the family consider donating her cornea? I know it's a hard time for you but ..."

"I don't know ... Yes ... if it helps somebody else."

"Did you want to make some telephone calls? Would you like a priest? Did you say she had relatives in San Francisco?"

They offered to let him see her before they turned the respirator down but he refused. Then they brought her clothing to him in a brown paper bag. A nurse, crying, slipped the crucifix she had been wearing into his hand. The young policeman drove him home. "Yes. They had the driver of the other car. Bud Fraser. A young kid. Drunk. Yes. He was badly hurt. No. He wasn't dead. Yes. They should raise the driving age. Of course. Bud Fraser would go to court. Yes. A senseless waste. If I can be of any further assistance ..."

When he got home he tore up the graduation pictures.

Consecration: *When we eat this bread and drink this cup we proclaim your death.*

He breathes the heavy odor of burning candles and flowers mixed with the musty smell of the church and he feels confused and dizzy as if he had inhaled ether. He concentrates on what her last moments might have been like hoping that by re-creating the scene in his imagination he will undo the horror of her death. At least he will fabricate a quick and painless end.

The taxi driver probably got out of the car to help her with the suitcases as she dragged them across the sidewalk. One of them contained her wedding dress. Joshua remembered the day she and his wife had gone shopping. "Seed pearls ... sweetheart neckline antique satin ... dropped waist." Words he never used, couldn't visualize. But still he knew it was the perfect dress for a San Francisco wedding.

Would she have sat in the front seat to be friendly? The back would have been safer. After she told him, "international airport," she probably would have stopped talking. Instead, she might have rehearsed the name she was soon to enjoy to the click of the metre: Mrs. Greene, Mrs. Sam Greene, Mr. and Mrs. S. Greene. The bride and groom were to fly home to Trinidad immediately after the wedding. She complained to Joshua that he hadn't used an instamatic camera so that her mother could see the photos of both special days. A close-up of Angela wearing her nurse's cap, smiling but not too broadly, smiling and gazing into the future, smiling and thinking of the inner-city hospital where she would work. Not for her some smart, sophisticated clinic where all the patients had nose jobs. A formal portrait of Angela and Sam cutting the wedding cake and kissing at the same time, his hand on top of hers guiding the knife. The camera flashes. She blinks. Opening her eyes she is blinded not by the quick sparkle she expected but by an explosion of hard yellow beams that jostle, plunge and thrust at the taxi's window and then with one final lunge break through the glass.

Pastoral Prayer and General Intercession
Events June 20/90

6:00 Anne Bradley, a two year old girl, died of smoke inhalation when her parent's farm house burned to the ground.
8:00 A helicopter, part of a search and rescue team crashed in northern Ontario. There were no survivors.
8:30 Bud Fraser undergoes spinal cord surgery.
9:30 A bomb threat closes down the International Airport for over an hour.
10:15 Sam Greene flies in from San Francisco.
11:45 The doctor tells Mr. Fraser that Bud is paralyzed from the waist down.
13:40 Angela Armstrong is buried from St. Anthony's Roman Catholic Church.
15:00 Olga Barovsky, Russian gymnast, defects while touring the States.
15:30 Sam Greene flies back to San Francisco.
17:00 A busload of Japanese tourists overturns outside of Mexico City.

Agnus Dei: *Lamb of God who takes away the sins of the world have mercy upon us.*

The kneeling bench is hard against his bony knees. At first his foot cramps and then his whole leg falls asleep. Joshua tries to discreetly perch his backside onto the edge of the pew and then to ease gently into this seat, but he miscalculates and falls noisily back into place.

This sudden clumsy lack of control reminds him of the boy. Joshua wanted to kill him. It didn't take long to find out which hospital admitted Bud Fraser. He wanted to stand over him in the bed and threaten him, quietly so no one would hear, just the kid. Torture wouldn't be good enough. Obeah. Joshua was sure his grandmother would remember. He wished he had brought some of the dirt from Angela's grave to sprinkle on the kid's head. Obeah. The curse.

The nurses come and go like phantoms on rubber soled shoes, only their uniforms rustling when they walk. For a moment he pretends that one of them is Angela. She would have nursed a boy like this, soothed his brow, held his hand, probably given him a rosary or lit a candle for him at mass. One of the nurses scurrying down the hall sees him leaning against the wall.

"Excuse me, Sir. Can I help you?"

"No thanks," he says and pretends to start moving away.

In the end he doesn't go into the boy's room. He only stands at the doorway, his hands in his pocket, clenching and unclenching his fists. He watches. The angry well rehearsed words stick in his throat. His hands relax. He leans against the wall. He has not cried in all this time but now…. The kid is sitting up in a wheelchair, staring out the window. He can't be more than sixteen, his arms skinny, resting on the handles, his hands white, frail, fingers long, lifeless. He wears the hospital gown and a baseball cap.

Benediction: *Go in the peace of Christ.*

The priest breaks the bread and then lifts the host and chalice. The congregation rises and forms a quiet orderly line moving slowly towards him. Joshua's wife is the first to receive. He lets her go before him in deference. The spray of roses tremble as he passes the coffin. He wants to reach out, pick one of them and place it over her crossed hands so that her resting place will smell of at least one flower. If only he had not brought her to this cold country of no spring and short summers, this city fed by a muddy river whose waters, after the endless winter, taste of run off. Here she would never have walked with a basket of fruit on her head or swayed her hips to the calypso rhythms of a steel drum. He squints his eyes like the quick shutter of the camera, trying to imprint her face forever on some empty blank space in his brain.

He moves away and stands in front of the priest. Cupping his palms together to receive the host, he extends his hands. He hears the priest, "The body of our Lord Jesus Christ, broken for you."

When the mass is ended the priest raises his arms in a final blessing and descends the steps of the sanctuary. The altar boy genuflects before the crucifix and extinguishes the Paschal candle.

Cathy Blackburn

PATTERNS

I.

To keep the house, each sister knitted,
wound skeins of color against the Thirties.
She learned economy from the stitches,
then found it easy to spend just enough.

When she tried to teach certain patterns,
I lacked her touch, so I studied the years
on the backs of her hands and memorized
those fingers working the yarn into sense.

Returning even now to the measured street,
everything is larger, smaller than memory.
My daughter points to the place, carefully
insists this house was her grandmother's.

I am part of my mother's unfinished business.
She repeats herself in my vision.
I try to rest in her chair, think her thoughts.
The rocker clicks like needles, works the dark.

II.

The days when motion is the only rest,
I look for the rhythm of certainty.
But dreams tip selectively, protect
the heart from repeating too much at once.

Through the words, I am returning to myself.
Language is becoming mother, without tongue,
perhaps, but not voiceless, after all,
a way of listening for a way back.

Marilyn Elain Carmen

MOTHER'S DAY BLUES

Momma
I carry your picture with me
wherever I go
right there in my wallet
next to my Preferred Master Charge
and American Express

Momma
I'd prefer to be able to call you
on the phone
instead of talking to your picture
when I need you
or to be able to stop by after work
to have a cup of tea with you

Marion Arenas

HOSPITAL VISITS, 1955

Aren't you glad it isn't you? Mother said,
gray faced in the white bed.

And I was glad it wasn't me,
glad I was young and pretty,
not sick, not fifty, not dying.

Give me a cigarette, oh give me a cigarette.

We can't, we told her, my brother John and I,
because of the oxygen, we said,
and because of the tubes in your nose.

When she closed her eyes we hurried off,
to let her rest, we said.
We hurried off to one of those
California restaurants where we could lounge
all afternoon, where we wouldn't hear
her pleading, and with the warmth
of martinis spreading in our bellies,
we smoked Luckys and ate avocado sandwiches
and talked about everything
but Mother's cancer.

Kiss me, Mother said, and I did,
wanting to wipe my mouth.

Take me home with you. Give me a cigarette.

We can't, we said, *you've had an operation.*
When you're better we'll take you home
and you can smoke again.

My brother and I talked about our marriages,
glad to be free for a time from them,
from our duties, our work, our other people,
surprised at our pleasure in each other,
surprised at our same blue eyes,
our same hands, our same taste in gin,
our same Lucky Strikes.

From the elevator we heard Mother
call our names down the hall:

John! Marion! Where are you?
Give me a cigarette! John! Marion!

But she had pulled out all the tubes
from her arms and nose,
so the nurses made us leave.

We called the restaurant Our Club,
smiled through our smoke-and-gin haze
and talked of other times together:
our serious tree climbing as Tarzan and Jane,
school dances where we were too tall
and too shy so we danced with each other.

Where have you been?

Hung over, guilty, afraid she knew,
Heavy traffic, we said, *very heavy traffic.*

I'm so glad you're friends. I'm so glad.

She closed her eyes.
She didn't speak again.

Days later she was close to comatose.
The nurse taught us to shout
to make her stir. Then she barely breathed
and didn't stir and we stopped going,
sure she wouldn't know, couldn't hear,
didn't see, was really gone.

She died three days later.

I went East, John went North,
grieving, busy, we hardly wrote each other,
seldom called, and were never alone again.

Laura Pollard

FOR MY MOTHER, WHOSE FRIEND IS DYING

All around me in the trees were talented people
munching vegetables and discussing literature,
while I stood happily in my too-big pants, drinking beer,
messing around with stuff on the grill,
talking about the Duchess of Windsor's jewels.
You taught me this, a confidence in what I have to give.

When it was me in that white bed, blood cold as stones
falling through a tube into my arm, you sat like a sentry
with the nurse by my side. I think of your crouching
through that first night, knowing you might not get a chance
to finish the book you'd begun in me. You held my heavy hand
and spoke in my deaf ear of home.

Perhaps you think you pulled me back like taffy,
but Mother she is dying.
I know there is no reason.
Don't turn the fierceness of your love
against yourself this time,
don't blame yourself because you can't
reach into your brown purse,
grope among the Kleenex and paper scraps
and cigarettes, and pull out life.
This pride of yours is terrible,
don't do this, Mother.
You must let her death be no reproach to you.
Just sit by her bed.
What you have to give, I swear,
is loaves and fishes.

Sue Walker

WHAT NO LIPS CAN TELL

Lips carved in yellow jasper,
are what remains of Queen Tiye's face—
a fragment, given by Harkness
to the Metropolitan Museum.

Some say that heads of the dead sing
the way sea waves are misunderstood.
Thirty-eight years—and what remains
is a mouth full and smooth, a piece
of Egyptian stone, Dynasty 18—
the idiom of art.

My mother's shattered face
last lay on a white silk pillow;
the cut above her eye oozed.
Leaning over the coffin, I kissed her cheek;
it was cold and hard,
thin lips painted wrong—
the work of an awkward mortician.

This month the groundhog saw its shadow;
in March it snowed.
Bundled in the coat my mother gave me,
I walked before the sun got up,
strolled along the shore,

argued with the freezing wind,
the ocean, and tried to understand
what no lips can tell.

Margaret Robison

LETTER POEM

Mother, the tree across from me is such
a fire against the sky.
And underneath, leaves—the summer shattered overnight to fall.
A month now you've been dead.
What difference does all we never said make now?
A flock of birds flies past the white
church steeple, back again.
The sky behind them is a watercolor in deep grey.
Everything has grown more vivid in this light
and papers rattle restlessly against a fence
like letters left unmailed—

Dear Mother, what I meant to say was this …
Dear Mother, don't you know …

Geri Rosenzweig

SNOW ON THE PATH

Something is taking my mother
from the world; she calls it light.

Last year it slipped a white
hook to her mind to capture

a word on the tip of her tongue.
Lately it wakes her before dawn,

cradles her thin body along
a path of wildflowers in serene

fields covered years ago
with asphalt. If there's snow

on the path, she wears the green
coat she loved at nineteen

but the air is mild, she's happy,
her father's alive, her mother

smiles beneath the trees' frosty
branches. When it seems as if a river

of light fills her bones
and she could float like a speck

in the wind, she forces herself
to leave her wide bed

and go down to the emptiness
of the kitchen where she brews

tea, listens for the screak
of her iron gate, the chink

of milk bottles delivered
to her red-tiled doorstep.

Lamont B. Steptoe

THERE IS A HOUSE

There is a house
with all the rooms filled with Momma
with all the days filled with Momma
but there is a river
that separates me from this house
it is a wide river
a river so wide that
it must be called a sea
yes, a sea
a sea so wide
that it must be called time
yes, time
a time so wide
that it must be called death
yes, death

Pamela Portwood

GRANDMOTHER'S GIFTS

Shoes, purses, slips, nightgowns, hose, scarfs,
my father's mother has left the things
which cannot serve after death,
and my mother would spare me this sorting.
Now when she opens her own drawers,
my mother keeps throwing things out.

Handkerchiefs drawn with Arizona maps, hearts,
cactus, these come in a box, Christmas
presents and memories from my grandmother
forwarded early and late by my mother.
I stroke the music box, raise its lid,
unpack the mail-order gifts, finger
the crossword books with her return address.
I never knew she worked them as I do.

I hug the negligee I will never wear
to my chest, cry for the silliness of her gifts,
wonder if I can resolve these puzzles:
her unexpected death, my grief,
the love which did not rest on who
I was or what I did.
How little we knew each other
and how little it mattered.

In memory of Mae Portwood, 1902-1986

Marine Robert Warden

ROCKY MEADOW

A delphic sun smokey and pine scented
grass of the meadow ripe yellow wheat
open space where life seems most certain
but death gnaws away inside each fallen log
and I think of one day 40 years ago
when my grandmother died and I cried
while sitting on the toilet in our bathroom
my father heard me and came in quietly too
"I loved her" I said but he said nothing
his hand gentle on my shoulder no word
just his small hand more eloquent than a word

Kathleen Patrick

A PROPER DISTANCE

Outside an auto showroom,
cold sun pours across plate glass.
I glance at my reflection
against a sloppy street and squint
when I think I see your face in the crowd, Grandma,
your hair up, the way it was when I was five
and you held me on your lap
all soft arms and powder.
I saw you, as in the dream portrait
one night weeks after the funeral,
standing in the picture window,
your body illuminated by lightning.

I walk home, calling you down from the dirty sky,
from the heaven I cannot touch,
the place where my uncles said you were happy.
They cried only when they thought we weren't looking.
Putting the years back in place,
I pass a rusted Chevy smothered with snow.
Loneliness crowds my throat.

Grandmother, please fill a hot tub for me,
kneel down, the way you used to,
your apron against the porcelain,
and scrub my dirty toes again.
Make me clean enough for church,
clean enough to learn your prayers,
to be Catholic enough for you.
Do anything. I want to believe.

The world has turned to crystal.
All the saints have climbed trees
and frozen there.
It has dropped below zero and everyone
I know would give anything to melt;
it's been years since we've all relaxed.
Grandma, I can't believe
you look down through gray clouds
and see us floundering.
But I must believe in something.

Lately, at night, you come back,
a gift from the dead,

a second chance for us. You seem
unimpressed with life this time;
you speak slowly and treat us all like children.
You come back and put paint on the farm,
standing the trestle where it belongs,
line the cupboards with fresh paper.
Your plump fingers heal Grandpa's eyes,
clouded with boredom, with whiskey;
you scold him for drinking,
pour the bottles down the sink
and wash everything twice.
Your aprons are back in the buffet.
The clock rings the hours.
The cold stays outside.

One night, you told my mother
she was worth something after all.
You hadn't meant to beat her down,
all the time telling her
she would never amount to anything;
telling her it was her fault
she got pregnant, married outside
the church, so worthless,
and where's being a woman get you?
For the first time you told your daughter you loved her,
but it was my dream, only my ears
felt the slight hum.

Why was your lap always a safe place for me?
You screamed at Gramps
and slapped around the kids when they sassed you.
And when I wanted to go out to the barn
you said girls did the dishes
and boys did the chores.
I want to do the chores now,
to throw hay down from the loft
as each cow goes to her own stall, knowing.
I need the ache of familiar muscles.

Ice disappears from my roof as I turn pages.
Strings of limp pheasants hang in a haze.
Cream cans line the walls
behind three of your sons suited for war.
You always turned away from the camera.

Easter Sunday, 1964, you finally stand with Grandpa.
You hate pictures; this is the last one.
We do not eat before church.

I hit my chest as the bell rings,
copy your every gesture,
memorize Latin nonsense for your smile.
My stomach growls, louder than the priest,
louder than the purple splash filling this country church,
covering the prayers in my mouth.
During communion, lines of people
shuffle toward the altar.
Lines deepen in my mother's forehead
as she and I sit back to let them pass.
Lord I am not worthy to receive you ...
She grows absolutely still.
I feel a sadness I do not understand.

Ten children by forty,
your heart stopped at fifty-two.
It was a Sunday. I was a child.
Your grandmother loved you.
She was a good woman.
She's at peace now.
Your lilacs filled the funeral home
for those still living.
Yes, I can say now, I suppose she was.

Tulips in my own yard
keep the sky at a proper distance,
their black stamen centers
punctuate the crimson clarity.
The lilacs are blooming again, Grandma,
letting go their perfume.
I inhale deeply, take it in
and let go.

Nadine Lambert

THE WAKE

She was ninety.
I am twenty-five.
That's why I'm not too sad, but slightly miserable,
high-heeled in her kitchen. Slipping out
of one black shoe at a time, I wiggle my toes
with each stocking foot momentarily relieved
by cool, flat linoleum. I eat

the neighbors' offering of fried chicken
with three kinds of beans (black-eyed, butter,
and crowder), all forced down with sugared tea.
The house is filled with the sound of scraping
forks against styrofoam and the praise of the dead

"… much better off now …
a full Christian life …"
even "… finally met her maker."
I escaped by sneaking a smoke behind the house.

Barefoot in the backyard,
I was as happy
as they said she is,
with her pink dress, folded hands,
and sewed-shut eyes.

Alison Reed

AT THE BEDSIDE OF A DYING GRANDFATHER
WHO ONCE PLAYED THE VIOLIN

Start right in with the proper word
and the steady face, now. No,
say it over. He has not heard—
oh, perhaps he has, in some low
clef beneath the normal tones
of conversation, but I'm sure
he hasn't understood. He drones
so inside his pillow, you're
forced to nearly lie down with him,
to get his words. So say it once more.
He'll give the illusion, a dim
floating smile, that you restore
his senses, in a brief light
remind him of all that he once knew
so well, and that what you say is right—
in other words, he will help you.

Sometimes I think he must be hearing
old songs or parts that take him back
as a child hearing his mother sing
in the rocker that went tick-tack tick-tack.
That's why I said he drones, and why
I think he senses us as if
we were musical forms, high
notes hovering along a cliff.
It may explain, too, the reason
he yanks at the bedclothes—some fiddler
wandered in, a skeleton
carrying a tune, and stranger
than anything we can imagine.
Don't be afraid of him, not now.
Take his hand, like this, Jim,
Like touching a baby. You know how.
Look in his face. Come, say you love him.

Elspeth Cameron Ritchie

FLAGSTONES

Time to plant new bulbs
in my family's backyard.
Last year's bulbs grew bloodless shoots,
drooped to earth, no tulips.

Days shorten, October ends.
My father made this garden
thirty years ago,
laid flagstones in the shade
of the tulip magnolia
where even lilies wouldn't grow.

Stream splits flat from hill.
My brother and I trapped crayfish here.
My mother laughed, offered them for dinner.
We ate poached eggs instead.

Now the water is caught
on bricks and leaves.
Now my parents are divorced.

A creased brown photograph is taped
in my grandfather's nursing home.
Framed by a stockade fence,
a small girl thrusts an ice cream cone,
vanilla on her pout.

I ease my mother's father into his chair,
roll him to the sea of meals,
pat his face free of pudding,
I remember that girl is me.

Last year, my husband tore down the stockade,
snapped old rails against his knees.
A backhoe dug new foundations
cracked cross lilies and flagstones.

The tulip tree died, roots severed.
Concrete and cigarettes block
the muddy paths of worms.
Yellow tinges the azaleas.

I dig anyway, time to plant,
bags of topsoil and bulb food,
iris and daffodils waiting.

The shovel rings on rock.
I strain to pry it up.
My pitchfork outlines, then
levers up a buried flagstone.

My father's flagstones,
bedrock for picnics and jump ropes,
are buried by construction and time.
New growth is blocked.

Again metal clangs slate.
A bed of stone lies six inches deep,
Covered with earth and last year's bulbs;
their roots spread out instead of down.

My grandfather is dying,
my father remarried,
my mother traps poetry,
my brother teaches his son to fish.

I pile up the old stones,
mix in the new dirt,
throw exposed worms back,
plant thirty narcissus bulbs
and clumps of snowdrops.

Norbert Krapf

COMING TO TERMS WITH APRIL SNOW

1

The third spring since we
surrendered him to earth.

Wet snow gathers in the folds
of tender lilac leaves, rises
up the stems of grape hyacinth
glowing purple in the sheen
of this unsettling day.

2

By afternoon pelting rain
has guttered the snow
and driven sparrows
to screech beneath eaves.
I walk from study to
living room and watch
buds drip in the woods.

A puffed-up mocking bird
balancing on a branch
of a black oak raises
and lowers white wingbars
in strangely silent protest.

Even this master of mimicry
cannot recall or compose
song equal to the occasion.

3

After we have gathered
from our various corners
at the supper table,
I soak our irrepressible
daughter, just three,
in lilac-scented suds.

When I strap my watch
back on my wrist
after drying her, she
taps the crystal face,
looks up, and asks

in her sing-song speech:
Was that your Papa's watch?

Not wanting to spill into
end-of-day sentiment, I nod.
He died before I was born?
I wind the watch and nod.
He loves me? I keep
winding and nodding.
Papa, is he in heaven?
Unable to imagine a myth
better than the one I have
always found inadequate,
I pat her and nod again.
Why don't you call him up?

4

How to make the right
connections, Love? How
to match music and words
for the workings of weather
and time and mortality?
And perch on the branch
raising our wingbars
for a flight we hope
will go well as soon
as this weather clears?

Alice Connelly Nagle

THE WHISTLE

It was *Send in the Clowns*.
Gently. November twenty seventh. All four daughters
were home for Thanksgiving, sleeping
downstairs. I was still in bed,
reading in the poor morning light
when he went into the bathroom
to shave.

Everything was familiar. The suction
pull of the medicine chest, the click
of glass when he closed it. Water ran
into the basin,   he sighed & splashed
his face a few times, then the long rhythmic
stroke of the razor, the in-between rinsing.
The bowl gulped down the water. *Ahhhh,*
& he rubbed his face with a peach
towel. I was as alert

as a puppy, teased,
when I heard it. Thirteen months after
losing Mike, the first whistle. There was a time
when he whistled in and out of every door every day,
in that time when Mike was the Prince
and his dad was the Dude and I was Mama-san
with a dishtowel over my shoulder
we called *the rag of life.*

This is what is so
surprising: we are alive
without him.
We are living another lifetime
on the way to our own deaths.
Then, we were children,
young parents, dolls I move around
in the bright, windy castles
I have memorized.

This morning, a soft herald,
the first notes for what will be
another past.

Betsy Barber Bancroft

RESOLUTION
ON THE DEATH OF MY
POET-FATHER

Returning to the earth where he now lies
I take no flowers gathered here and there
For what is fresh before the noontide comes
Lies pale and perishing in twilight air.

To leaves of paper where he poured his soul
I lean to garner blossoms from his scrawl,
To lift each fragrant bloom and drink its breath
And turn its face outward to bless us all.

That mound of earth made precious by his bones
Holds little of the man he was alive,
But old and brittle pages of his words—
His heart's anthologies of life—survive,

A benison, perpetual, to us
Who bore his ashes to their cool retreat,
And rather than lay wreaths upon his skull,
Return to learning poems at his feet.

Susan Luzzaro

TRIBUTE

Blind Bob's Newstand
kept long hours and my father
would walk there, sometimes
twice a day when he heard
the paper was coming out
with my first published poem.
It took weeks to arrive
and you would often see him
walking, his khaki shorts
revealing the tangle
of varicose veins
that climbed his legs,
the blood rising, nevertheless,
in an orderly fashion,
entering now the left ventricle,
now the right. It comforts me
to think of his heart beating then,
you might say, just for me.
When my father was murdered
his blood pooled senselessly
beneath him, his big heart
pumping it farther and father away,
on a journey I can never follow,
on a night I don't dare imagine.
How I wish when he finally
found that poem, he found
at the top some small dedication,
some tribute with his name.
How I wish that out of the grey ash
that is his heart, he could rise
to see this spillage of love
without object, to open
the closed shop of my heart.

Susan Luzzaro

PARADOX

Some say art brings order
to chaos, but what order
can this small poem bring
to the death of my parents—
to their brutal murders
in the dark of their own bedroom.
I notice how words still work
for my neighbors who barricade
themselves with their differences—
"oh it couldn't happen to me,
I have dead bolts on my door,
I don't drink, I take my vitamins
daily." Some have even said
that the lord has a plan.
Psychologists say distancing
is a protective strategy.
Well I say let my neighbors
turn under their wild garlic,
let them cut back the unruly
bramble of berries or pokewood,
in their place they can plant
rows of head lettuce
till kingdom come—theirs
is the wild card.
As for me, I will spread
lemon oil on the table,
slice vegetables into the soup,
invent an order for my children
in which even they no longer believe.
When I asked the police detective
for the thousandth time—"Why my parents?"
He answered exasperatedly—
"Why not your parents?"
Neighbors,—this careful placement
of black marks on white paper
is only the eye of the maelstrom—
life is a found penny.

Peter Cooley

WINTER LIGHT

In Memory: RR

We hear the music raging
Under the lids we have closed.
                    Donald Justice, "For the Suicides of 1962"

Outside my window the hard ground
holds a sparrow to its bones
again today, January 8th.
One-legged he takes the snow, the fog,
sprigs of juniper I laid out
after Christmas, their crushed black stalks,
stiff, upright against the sun,
that vestment he casts off.

* * *

Your last letter was one sheet, torn,
spoke of settling in, wife & children—
suddenly then, how a family of deer,
surprised at the edge of your yard,
broke, a white field opening, opening.

* * *

You had your demons, they had you.
You were proud of them like sons
who reflected your eyes, the pool clearer
each year, the surface deeper, gleaming.
They gave you visions you were a river
of blue sperm, coming forever.
Later you told me nothing they said—
why did I ask?—could be repeated.

* * *

I heard your voice today
standing beside me on the lawn
that summer you drove in suddenly
on the way to a new life & laughed,
my wife laughed, I did, pouring the wine
over my poem I stole your favorite image for:
the white stone from *Revelation*.

* * *

90

"All poets are brothers," you quoted
from Logan repeatedly. I give it back:
We looked enough alike to be each other
or Double, why did you do it?

New snow in the hospital yard
raises the ground up leavened bread
for angels you carved, thrown back
or belly-flat fronting the cold
that afternoon you ran past
the sleeping guard. Angel against angel
against angel. You lie down. You lie.

* * *

Over your name the mass is lifted
over the blessings my mouth closes
too quickly the stained glass
light exposes bones the grey stripped
shaking of branches in fog.
                        I kneel
the altar rail is wind the priest
dips a wafer into his cup
& I go down on it the fog
entering my ribs. Now I am fog entirely.

* * *

In bed I pull the dark up
around my nakedness, my body curling
like Jarrell's ball turret gunner.

I let myself feel myself
thinner, rolling out of myself
through cold air, falling through colder.

I give up my legs, my arms,
my extremities, I annoint myself nothing.
I shatter black water.

* * *

Driving the shoreline home tonight
Lake Michigan scatters, breaks
wave after wave, I watch a cold sun
burn off fog, the whitecaps fall back
washing through sumac, sugar maple,
torches there in fall. Between seasons now
all my words blow past us, spoken
in the winter light. The ground is breaking up.
Even you are getting tired of my song.

Carl Djerassi

"I HAVE NOTHING LEFT TO SAY"

Five years after your death,
My only daughter,
I find this note:

"I have nothing left to say,
So I don't talk.
I have nothing left to do,
So I close up shop."

No date
No address
No signature
Your handwriting.

Written for whom?
Yourself?
To whom it may concern?

Written when?
Days,
Weeks,
Perhaps months
Before your walked into the woods?

If only you'd said these words to me.

Gerald Cable

MORTALITY TABLES

He dreads dying in the supermarket,
tomatoes rolling in the aisle, as in a dream
groping at some final displacement of pain,
searching deep in his pockets
for the fire of oxygen.
But who wants to know when the random static
of death will enter the stethoscope.
It could be with no revelation,
in spite of green tongues in the leaves
and hydrangea
igniting the houses,

a way of escape, leaving everyone else to their
vague sense of tint, as brushed on windows
streaked with raindust, this freedom
unseen before now, rising up
at his feet.
He said three years were too long
and not
long enough. The strenuous pleasure
of running the rapids, the piteous loss of appetite,
closing hours, and church.
A week, a day

the adventure of knowing, or not,
except in the crystal
of mortality tables fogged by his breathing.
Any minute, about ten on a Saturday morning,
the sun burning an earlier haze
from the mountains. He stands, barefoot
on the warm floor, looking
from the window at plumes of white smoke
that thin out and vanish,
leaving the blue sky, as always,
alone and untouched.

David Stringer

BILL IN BED

Bill tells me he is having a crisis of faith.
Tears slide into his beard.

He lives in a hospital bed on the glassed-in
porch of his home. His dog

dozes at the foot of his bed. The TV sends
lively ghosts from the corner.

He tells me he is afraid he is never going
to get well again. I decide

not to cry. I see creases in the skin
of his bald head propped

on the pillow. I wonder if the radiation
caused them. I remember

my father's death, a death I missed.
Bill tells me

late last night a friend said it is
all right to lose faith

but not all of it. I decide not to cry.
I picture the tumor locked

into Bill's brain, tentacles inching into
the wet folds, squeezing,

with pitiless eyes and a beak. Bill says
he envies my trips out west.

I decide not to cry now.

As we talk I stroke Bill's unparalyzed hand.
I rub his foot, but

I'm uncertain about touching his left hand,
still indented where his rings

were removed. The nurse arrives, takes
Bill's blood pressure, gives

him a shot, checks his skin and the response
of his pupils. Sue

joins us, kisses Bill's forehead, tells
the nurse and me she sleeps

joins us, kisses Bill's forehead, tells
the nurse and me she sleeps

here with him, likes to cuddle in bed,
jokes that they make out

heavily when people aren't around. I rise
to leave. Sue asks

the nurse to make room in the bed for her when
she turns Bill over. Sure.

I say it's OK they are married. Sue and the nurse
lift, using some leverage tricks,

relocating the tube leading to the urine bag hooked
on the frame of the bed.

I try to stay out of the way. I'm uncertain
about touching. I am having a crisis

of faith. Sue leans down

to arrange Bill's head on a pillow. His good arm
reaches to circle her neck, holding

her in a fierce headlock of an embrace. I
can not see her face or Bill's.

I am jealous of this broken dying man. I see
now the death I missed.

Gerald Stern

BOB SUMMER'S BODY

I never told this—I saw Bob Summers' body
one last time when they dropped him down the chute
at the crematorium. He turned over twice
and seemed to hang with one hand to the railing
as if he had to sit up once and scream
before he reached the flames. I was half terrified
and half ashamed to see him collapse like that
just two minutes after we had sung for him
and said our pieces. It was impossible
for me to see him starting another destiny
piled up like that, or see him in that furnace
as one who was being consoled or purified.
If only we had wrapped him in his sheet
so he could be prepared; there is such horror
standing before Persephone with a suit on,
the name of the manufacturer in the lining,
the pants too short, or too long. How hard it was
for poor Bob Summers in this life, how he struggled
to be another person. I hope his voice,
which he lost through a stroke in 1971,
was given back to him, wherever he strayed,
the smell of smoke still on him, the fire lighting up
his wonderful eyes again, his hands explaining,
anyone, god or man, moved by his logic,
spirits in particular, saved by the fire and clasping
their hands around their knees, some still worm-bound,
their noses eaten away, their mouths only dust,
nodding and smiling in the plush darkness.

Jack Coulehan

THE SIX-HUNDRED-POUND MAN

Of the six-hundred-pound man on two beds,
nothing remains,
not the bleariness with which he moved his eyes
nor the warm oil curling in his beard.

Though the sheets and plastic bags are gone,
his grunts, his kind acceptance gone,
I see him now, rising in the distance,
an island, mountainous
and hooded with impenetrable vine.

When I awaken to the death
of the six-hundred-pound man
and cannot sleep again,
I paddle to his shore

in search of those flamboyant trees
that flame his flanks,
in search of bougainvillea
blossoming his thighs,
of women who rise to touch him
tenderly with ointment,

in search of healers, singers
who wrestle souls of old bodies
back to bones, back to dirt, and back back
to their beginnings.

As I enter for the first time
this medicine circle,
bearing chickens in honor of the god,
words dancing from my lips,

spirit like the plume of a child's volcano
rises

and then the medicine, the medicine is good
and the tongues, the tongues are dancing
and the fathers, oh! the fathers are dancing

and this worthless and alien body,
this six hundred pound man,
I discover him beautiful.

Jack Coulehan

THE SORROW OF THE WORLD

This is the last he will ever remember
the person he was, Robert Wilson,
a guard who stood in the Museum of Art
beside an entrance to the Classical World,
and clicked the boys and girls who wandered in
and snorted in their sleeves when they saw
marble bodies with their bulging fig leaves.
200, 201 ... His heart stops.
The sentry collapses. A column bites the dust.
The sorrow of the world that worketh death.

When I stand beside the bed of Robert Wilson,
humors pitch and feint like ancient warriors.
He is receiving salt, potassium,
sugar, cefoxitin, and into his throat
a hissing machine pushes oxygen.
Around him, the air is full of oracles
who whisper, "I am taking your blood pressure.
Turning you in bed. Giving you a shot.
I am patting your body with powder.
Do not sink into weariness or suffer
the sorrow of the world that worketh death."

These oracles always tell the truth.
"I am going to shave you. To pull a tube.
To give you the bedpan." I stand by the chair
of this wizened androgynous Greek
whose mouth is unslung, who leans on his tray
like a sentry staring at the past,
who sleeps without dreams, who awakens
to a world without Robert Wilson.
He does not exist. In freezing rain
outside his window, headlights creep—
a phosphorescent army from the sea.

The sentry starts. He says that nothing hurts.
"Bob, it's time to eat breakfast. It's time
for your potty. To walk with your walker."
Someday ... time to go home. With a heart of scars,
this man who was Robert Wilson, who remains
a mystery to himself, girds his loins

98

and stumbles out the door—the temple surrounded—
to meet that phosphorescent army.
And though the oracles whisper the truth,
they never say if anyone survives
the sorrow of the world that worketh death.

Jack Coulehan

SKINWALKERS

In these old buildings
one after another
the deaths accumulate.
Though each is transparent,
it leaves behind
a taste of someone,
a skinwalker.

Elevators are packed,
the halls bustling.
I am surrounded by skinwalkers
who change their appearance
so they look antiseptic
and distracted, like people.

They don't intend to harm.
The walkers want to help,
doing and touching
the things they remember.
Some sip their coffee and smile.
Bishops, some push their poles
like holy croziers.

The skinwalkers mumble,
G'morning, when they jostle
and bump me, so close
the touch of their souls
is a lotion
that clings to my raw hands.

Hardly anyone remembers
the dead can't harm us.
The dead can only make way.
Hardly anyone notices
these faint souls, flickering
with traces of sympathy.

Carolyn Page

TELEPHONE BOOTH

For Dr. Robert L. Green, Jr.

Life is counting up,
counting down.
Numbers hold you steady,
slow you down.
You borrow a truck,
find a phone booth outside
a country store.
Count out your Valiums,
twenty three ... in case,
punch up the number
with cold fingers,
calling Dr. Bob.
Like playing telephone roulette—
would he be in at 10:00,
or gone till Tuesday?
Should you have him paged?
Is death an emergency?

This is a pleasant place—a pleasant
peace once you've decided.
If your caring doctor speaks
through the black plastic
into your eerie euphoria,
you might take it as a sign.

It rings four times before his
nurse answers, transfers you,
and a voice from Durham
talks you back to life.

Janice Townley Moore

UNDERGROUND: AFTER A FRIEND'S ATTEMPT

Like the pills you took, my words don't work.
If there's anything I can do....
I'll be thinking of you....

There are no flowers in your room,
no bouquets of balloons.
Disbelief whispers in all the corners.

Driving home later in the rain
I pass Indian Trail Road
where a man nailed a woman

into a box, buried her underground for days,
a small pipeline surfacing for air.
At least it was for ransom.

I think of Kathy Fiscus caught deep in a well,
for weeks the inevitable circus tainting the site,
hotdog hawkers, flags flying until she died.

I think of all the diggings down,
doctors sweating under the hot lights
to bring up a body.

Linda Parsons

NOT A SUICIDE POEM

The children talk of suicide.
Boys in art class carve
no geometries on oil pastel, but
their bellylike inner arm
with exacto knives.
Girls sit in the dark with candles,
burning the same soft place.
Some tell of making a cut, milking a drop
or two, putting out the flames.
My daughter says, *I would do it with pills,*
just take them all, see black all day.

How do I tell you I've taken
the aspirin, codeine, amoxyl,
stuffed them inside my socks.
How do I say,
Live long.
That the statice I kept from my grandmother's grave
stays and stays, in fact it seems so blue
one minute, so purple the next.
That I nursed you, the nights went on,
I forgot how the world looked. I saw
it differently, as mountains can look,
depending on where you stand, sometimes large,
sometimes not.

James Sallis

TEMPORARY LIFE

This happened some years ago: on March 6, a few days after her thirtieth birthday, my wife took a massive overdose of the medication given her for depression.

We had been married less than a year then, since May. The last months had been difficult ones as I pressed her to seek help and she continually denied needing it. There were sudden rages, long periods of withdrawal, a bottomless sorrow.

Kim was brought to the hospital where I served as chief respiratory therapist. For almost three hours we pumped her stomach, flushed her full of charcoal and Ipecac, resuscitated her. She was having terrible seizures and required huge doses of Dilantin. She had almost stopped breathing. The medication she took, we all knew, often leads to brain damage, kidney shutdown, cardiac dysfunction.

I held the mask over her face, leaned close and spoke to her the whole time as I breathed for her. She remembers none of this. I will never forget it.

At last she was stable and we rolled her along the corridor, out into bright, bright sunshine to the waiting helicopter. Kim rose with a mighty heave into the sky. It was a three-hour drive and I didn't know if she'd be alive when I got there. I had to clean up, see to the girls, pack Kim's things. I looked down and saw charcoal all over my tie, shirt, pants. There was blood, too, not a lot of it, but it was Kim's blood. The director of nurses made me drink a cup of coffee. It kept spilling into the saucer.

***

The first time I wrote about her was in an essay on death published in the *Star-Telegram* not long after we met. There would be others later on —"Standing by Death" as the gulfs between us grew, and finally, when Kim was gone, gone at last after many rehearsals, "Old Story at Airport"—but much about that first essay now seems prophetic.

I watched three people die today, it began. Then went on: It is something I have been doing for a long time now, something one does not want to become good at, but does. One signs off the chart, gathers up equipment, walks away.

On my thirtieth birthday a fist closed inside my father's chest and he fell to the floor. Almost without thought I started CPR, and the world came slowly back to his eyes. But it was a much smaller world than the one he'd left. For almost a year we watched him hunt empty fields, sniffing at the stillness, disability, pills, his days like birds forever suspended in midflight against the morning sky. After numerous rehearsals, after an afternoon spent in a lawnchair in the sun watching me mow the yard, he at last left us.

Tonight, as the moon buoys in and out of clouds, I have lain awake thinking of all the others.

The first I remember is Mr. Sheldon, dying of emphysema. For almost thirty years he had carried in his wallet a tattered pay stub from the week he'd made over a thousand dollars operating heavy equipment, and showed it to me late one night in his room.

Mr. Petrie, a bus driver whose lungs blew up like stiff balloons and burst. The newborns I've worked with for so long now. Debbie. And the other kids—cystics, surgery patients gone sour, Siamese twins, chronic hearts—each with his own private battle pitched, and going on invisibly, above the bed.

An hour or so ago, unable to sleep, I walked to the corner store for a paper. A nearby house stood burned out in the moonlight, car after car reversing or slowing to look at it. For months, walking by, I had watched the woman and the children who lived there, wondering about them, what their lives were like, what things might be important to them.

Lately, they'd not been around very often. I'd see the car in the driveway some days, and once or twice a week old newspapers got gathered from the front yard. I supposed that some great change had occurred in their lives.

So many things crowded into my mind as I walked. I remembered a poem of Edna St. Vincent Millay's: "I shall die, but that is all that I shall do for death." I thought of the knight's wife in *The Seventh Seal* saying to Death: "You are welcome in this house, Sir." Of Dylan Thomas' "Do Not Go Gentle" and "If My Head Hurt a Hair's Foot," a dialogue between mother and fetus. Of Camus, that there is only one imperative: to come to terms with death, after which all things are possible.

Back home, I lay staring at the moon's pale, round face. Clouds the shape of a piano, of South Africa, of a fig, crossed it. Winds nudged at the side of the house. I fell asleep, death's first degree, that daily rehearsal.

***

Six weeks have passed (*I wrote*) since the above words were put down. As often occurs, there was a space between the beginnings of a piece and its end; these words waited in a file until I came back to them. I always do come back, sometimes after moments, sometimes years.

There have been other deaths in these weeks. As I write, a 22-year-old woman daily loses ground in ICU. In the other ICU, for newborns, a 25-week-old baby struggles for life. I stand over him thinking what a sense of loss these children must have, obtaining the world.

Almost daily I walk by the burned-out house.

On the day I watched three people die, I went out for the first time with a woman I had watched across many rooms. She told me of a man she had loved who killed himself. I had no idea, writing of death later that night, how important she would become to me, how in later weeks my days would gather around her troubled face or smile.

It's a warm, windy afternoon and she'll be over soon, after work. I have been defrosting my refrigerator, and something about that —the slaking of ice, unfolding the ice's lie, its whiteness—seems appropriate.

As a child, I fell from a fig tree. The world went away, and I could not breathe. For what seemed a long time I existed in a kind of limbo, not breathing (and so not quite fully alive), senses poised but blank. Like moonlight, like ice, I was white, I was pure, in that moment before the world reclaimed me. I had then, I think, my first sense of how terrible and difficult endings are.

***

When I wrote that, I was living in a garage apartment in Arlington, Texas, not far from the hospital where Kim and I worked; many days, I'd walk over. I spent hours walking all *over* Arlington, hours more watching squirrels out the window, the remainder of my free time writing. I was writing at a fairly speedy clip: a novel in a little over a month, a dozen or so stories and articles, new poems. I'd no expectations of ever being other than alone and had given up dating. I'd just go on writing, working, listening to Mozart and Mahler, walking, running. Martinis at night as I read.

Then Kim came into my life, like a nail into cork.

Everything had always been difficult for her—childhood, previous marriages, parental relations—and as I got to know her (or thought I did), I thought I would be able to make it all easier, I began to *want* to.

We just met incidentally at work, at first. In the halls or cafeteria line, at various nurse's stations, in ICU when we were both assigned there. We began to talk, a little more each time, coming to recognize our common attraction. Then one day I asked her to have lunch with me and, after lunch, walking back to the unit, dinner the next evening. *Yes.* For hours that afternoon, gravity lost any claim it had on me.

I was forty, Kim twenty-nine.

When I picked her up that first evening I was stunned, stunned as I have been ever since, by her beauty, by the life in her eyes, the gentle ease of her body, by the way her mouth shapes itself around words. As we swung out onto I-30 for the drive to Dallas, everything about me—my writing, my books, age, prior marriage, study of French and Russian, longtime work as a musician—came out in a sudden rush. Kim was quiet for a while then. She crossed her legs, tucking her feet under her, and looked off towards Dallas, towards Reunion Tower. "There's nothing to tell you about *me*," she said.

I looked at her and felt something changing inside me: borders or walls going down.

There turned out to be, once we settled in at The Wok, quite a *lot* to tell me. For almost two hours Kim talked about her life. The man she'd loved who killed himself, her first marriage at fifteen, a history of offbeat illnesses going back to infancy; things she treasured and things that broke her heart, her mother's debilitating illness, daughters Carey and Katie; and that all she'd ever wanted was someone to love her, someone *she* could love, someone who wouldn't *change* on her.

When I got home that night, I wrote her a brief note on stationery from DMFA's Bonnard exhibit. In forty years I had never felt these things for anyone, never known *any*thing of this intensity, and I tried to restrain myself: I was afraid.

***

In the one-room apartment to which I retreated from the one we shared, I looked over Arlington, the lights and evening bustle, and I thought: I am again alone, wholly alone, as I was before Kim. I knew early on that there was a deep, irredeemable wound in my wife, some dwelling hurt that might swell and swell till it overcame her. And I knew, I think, that our marriage would not survive that wound.

I waited for her feet on the stairs, for her letters, waited to open the door and find her there. I got up every few minutes and looked down into the parking lot.

***

Today it rained everywhere in the world, Kim. I sat in the new apartment watching it come down, blurring the contours of our world, softening, healing. Earlier I had walked for an hour or more in the park, following Marrow Bone Spring alongside which Indians once lived, now almost dry and choked with rotting vegetation and the detritus (soft-drink cans, cigarette packages, plastic wrappers, paper) of our civilization. Birds and living, stirring things everywhere, except inside me.

Returning, I passed the Confederate cemetery we never visited but meant to, thinking that the first time I wrote about you was in an essay on death and dying.

I've been thinking a lot about pain today.

About the pain in your eyes that morning when you woke on the ventilator and turned them towards me. *I hurt,* you wrote. You had hurt a long time, hurt horribly, and I had never known how much, never suspected.

I've been thinking how something further broke within you with each hospitalization. And of all the pain of these final weeks, when you began to turn your hurt and anger out towards me, preparing to leave, but having to do that first in order to.

I waited on the edge of your life, obscured by your pain and preoccupations, reduced at last to nurse and parent, to movies at two in the morning and morning drinking. We had been so proud, right up to the end, of our sexuality together; and when that went, when you could focus only on *your* need, I knew it was over.

I've also been thinking of your seizures in ER, those great shudders as though death were already violating you horribly. About the scars and bruises that riddled your body for weeks afterwards.

But finally there's no moral to a near-death, Kim, just as there's not to this rain, to a morning walk along a spring, or to terrible, difficult endings. They happen and we survive them, finally. We go on.

Gradually you stopped caring. Clothes were removed and thrown on the floor where they stayed. The bed remained unmade. I cooked all meals, did all cleaning. You put makeup on only when we went out, and instead of brushing your teeth, ate toothpaste. Then you lost all taste for food and for days ate nothing. I found lipstick on the gin bottle's mouth. When I came home you were always on the couch facedown, half-nude.

Now you are elsewhere, in some other house, one not burned-out perhaps, and I have my own pain and terrible anger to deal with, to survive.

Your first weekend out of ICU I visited, sitting with you for hours on plastic chairs beside heaped ashtrays at the end of the hall, pigeons looking in at us from beyond locked windows. The following weekend they gave you an overnight pass and we spent it in restaurants, bars, a cheap motel room, holding one another mostly, looking into one another's eyes and talking, trying to rekindle kindness, concern, love.

I think about how we felt that weekend, Kim, how you could hardly speak from having had the tube in your throat, about the way your back hurt and the sadness and surrender that's never since left your eyes. Maybe it was always there.

It goes on raining.

***

Returning to the house after it was all over, that first part of it, ER, court, telling the girls, to hurriedly pack things for you, hoping you'd need them.

Breakfast dishes were piled on the counter, drawers and cabinets stood open. A saucer with the birthday cake Melba brought you was on the table. A few bites had been eaten; much of the rest was smeared across the table's surface and edge. A fork lay on the floor alongside, crusted with icing. There were pill wrappers everywhere.

With even greater dread I walked to the bedroom. Peaceful and orderly here, just a blanket pulled onto the floor, phone on the bed, your clothes spread about on bureau and chair. It doesn't look at all like a place someone's life almost ended. There's no real sign of the pressures, of the crushing pain and turmoil, you went through just hours ago here.

How could anything so terrible, so devastating, I think, leave so little wreckage in its wake?

***

Damaged though she was, you have to understand this, Kim made me part of humanity again. Taught me to feel, to care deeply, to turn loose and give up myself. And so in her months of need I flooded her with letters, poems, stories, notes. I thought words could fix her, words could repair the damage, bridge the gulfs opening between us. I've always believed too much in words.

And much as I did, *just* as I did, all of you are waiting for the expository lump, for the part of the movie where some eccentric genius comes on to explain it all away: to tell us why things have got to be the way they are, and how, with employ of his rare understanding and arcane science, they will be set back in order by movie's end.

As we went from facility to facility, from crisis to crisis, each one more bleak and damning than the last, *I* waited for explanations, for magic pills or words, for some god (wearing a white labcoat, of course) to descend from the cyclorama and tell us what to do. I knew better, of course. But I *loved* her, you see: that's what this is all about.

So you won't find explanations and a tidy case history here, because I don't know; no one knows. All you can expect from this accounting is a scrapbook, a collage, bits and pieces—because that is what our life together was.

Somehow Kim never learned to act, only to react. Her entire life was a passing parade of improvisations, of momentary coping in which truth, often in the same conversation, took on quite different masks. Speech and action grew ever more dichotomous, and her focus, her attention, was tugged a hundred ways at once. I managed to keep her up, keep her afloat, for a while, but when *my* energies were expended, we both almost went under.

Sartre tells us that life is the reworking of a destiny by a freedom. For Kim, all her life, there was only a destiny. She couldn't break through to the freedom, couldn't find it, couldn't believe in it.

***

It's four in the morning and the untidy pile of manuscript beside me is almost done with now. Beer cans litter the apartment. I am playing country music because that, too, is part of Kim, part of our life together. A thick folder of her letters and notes, of mine to her, of souvenirs retrieved from unlikely places, cardboard boxes and the back corners of drawers, lies on the floor beside me. There's no desk or table in the new apartment and I'm sitting on the foot of the bed with an endtable pulled up to me, typewriter and dim lamp on that. This is how I've lived my life: with these departures and partial retrievals, alone with words in new apartments in many early mornings.

***

This all happened years ago.

In *this* early morning, in my bare apartment, in Texas half-light with the smell of magnolia and tomorrow's rain lofting in from outside, I take out an old manuscript and read it through, making changes as I go, adding words or phrases, deleting whole paragraphs: *this* manuscript.

I have gone on to another life, and from these calmer ports am trying again, as I tried then through storms of sentiment and anger, to understand.

Day puts itself together outside my window, finding me not at all surprised that I don't understand much better than before. And while anger and pain remain, sadly I can recall now little of the joy or good times, little of that love I felt so strongly, save what I've put down here—reason enough surely, to send this story, after all this time, into the world.

Richard G. Beyer

TO MARJORIE—REMEMBERING

Death had crossed my mind
had left his ugly mark upon my skin
and pointed out the bottles on the shelf,
yet could not touch that part of me released
within this room and free
to live
as long as you remember.

from "First Day Of the Rest Of My Life"
by Marjorie Lees Linn, Alabama Poet, 1930-1979

How do I recall thee? Let me count the memories.
I remember our first face-to-face in New Orleans,
Our bus-ride with Polly to the Bluff Park Art Show,
The downtown Birmingham bistro ... between courses
You told me bone-marrow cancer and two years at most,
Downing pitchers of stingers at some little place
In an all-night rain that mixed well with my tears ...
The poetry conventions, your readings in Montgomery
And Memphis, Jesse Stuart in Kentucky, how I called
You from Madison to say that we were both winners;
After fifteen years I still know your phone number.
A grain of salt in an ocean of pepper, you stood
Tall in a balcony to hear Dr. King preach the word,
Shone to become a Worker Sister For The Holy Spirit.
Then, later, the small-cell carcinoma of the lungs,
A riverboat on the Mississippi ... our toes wiggling
In warm Arkansas sands, weekend writers' workshops
in Florence, all those times we came to be with you
To hold back the dying years—your legacy of poetry,
And every word of every sentence you ever said to me.

Roger Granet

THE EMERGENCY ROOM

Once in February
behind unnecessary lights and sirens
the attendants wheeled in the
dead black lady who looked
more grey or white and said:

"You gotta pronounce her, doc."

She must have been
dead since December.

Supine and frozen
emptied of fluids, she was
pulled from the heatless building
when the landlord in his
fur lined topcoat and warm wool scarf
came to claim the overdue rent.

And they told me again:

"You gotta pronounce her, doc."

As I tried to pull her
paper thin lids across
her vacant eyes, I wondered
who and why she was and did she
have grandchildren like my parents
until I walked away held in a fragment of a dream
denying the last lifeless call:

"You gotta pronounce her, doc."

Frank Finale

LAST VISIT

"Squeeze my hand if your hear," we repeated
in that room of living corpses where only
the tubes had intercourse with their bodies.
The living debris of old age: this one
wailing through the night, another delirious
in her prayers of pain, that one with mouth and eyes
open, a plant overlooking the traffic (arteries
of the city, cells of cars flowing on
Riverside Drive). Stories below, a valley of tracks
and traffic; beyond, an arching of stones, swellings
of dirt—last names, flowers. "Squeeze my hand,"
she heard and was made to dream the relatives
over again, before she chose her world
and forever closed her eyes and ears to us.

Pamela Wampler

PERENNIAL

I have repotted the pink geraniums and placed
them on the porch, their petals clustered

like sleeping moths. The week of your death
I gutted the backyard, turned it inside out,

stomped on a shovel with boots you had bought me,
hurled earth and worms. I buried bulbs—

cool and white as knuckles—along the garage,
daring anything to grow. How could you have

dreamed what you did? You opened your eyes,
spoke of buds rupturing into clots of color

so beautiful no one could see them and die.
Roses, rhododendrons, delphiniums. Everywhere,

a contagion of flower and flush. How could
you have? As if there were no tumor rooted

inside, no profusion of cells, no paralysis.
As if you believed in the perennial promise.

Elspeth Cameron Ritchie

SPRING LETTUCE

When the March wind tossed sandy Maryland,
When the osprey began to steal sticks,
When jellyfish floated in, their wombs red,
We planted the first black seeds.

The city was closed, rain leashing
The hospital in tethers of traffic.
Patients played cards, smoked, dreamed.
I stayed late, dictating charts.

Radishes burst first, tearing up to the sun.
Timidly the lettuce peeked to spy on
The fanfarewell of the geese, and duck at
Shotgun shells raking from dead blinds.

Mad men and women flew in from Europe,
Lashed to gurneys, legs twitching,
Minds aswarm, families left, souls beaten.
We helped them up, switched their meds.

Time to plant feathery dill and fetid cilantro,
But the purple basil failed of cold.
Starflowers thrust through the antique grass.
Tractors flung open the furrows.

A man put a plastic bag over his head and died
In a froth of vomit. We could not revive him.
Police came. Cameras flashed.
Patients cried. I clamped down. Work to do.

White and red radishes fill the fridge.
Time for tomatoes, tamped down with dung.
Tears finally came, as the cages went
Around the stalks. How could you suicide in spring?

The inquest ended. No negligence.
Patients found their clothes, called their wives.
Volleyballs pounded the office windows.
A nurse announced. Baby showers.

Now the ospreys tend their eggs
In the locust leaning over the tide.
Underneath sound the thwocks of croquet balls.
We dug the sailboat from the sand.

A woman with AIDS lost her unborn child.
She asked me whether he would go to heaven
Or hell, since he was tainted. I replied,
Heaven, I think. She, too, wants to die.

A hundred head of lettuce extrude.
Spinach has gone to seed. Girls glide
On the beach. I read Freud.
Black men plant tobacco by hand.

Time for me to leave the ward.
Cocaine addicts revolve through the doors.
I feed the staff lettuce and catnip.
Turkey vultures roost in the barn.

The baby jellyfish gather offshore.
Boundaries of ward and garden fade.
Worms swarm in both. I weed and fertilize.
Sails fly, frantically, through the river.

Rebecca McClanahan

HATCHING

Seventy years later and she still smells it in her dreams. She is my aunt, my father's oldest sister, and she tells me this over lunch at an uptown department store in her midwestern city where I have come to visit, hungry for something I am afraid will get lost. Last month she had a triple-bypass. Under her designer pantsuit, she is stitched from breastbone to navel and, again, from groin to ankle where they stripped the vein that would feed her heart. It's not the family tree I seek, not the official line a genealogist is paid to trace. What I need are the small moments, the details, the stories aborted that never found their climax, their denouement. Rag-tags of faded dresses, like pieces my grandmother salvaged and stitched together for quilts. Maybe if I listen hard enough, the scraps will come together. And if the quilt is not beautiful, at least it will be warm, something to throw around my shoulders late at night.

The smell in her dreams is the smell of warm eggs from an incubator that was kept in her bedroom, the room she shared with four sisters. The eggs were in a covered tray with a lightbulb hung above for warmth. They were turned once a day. Over the weeks, one by one the chicks hatched. Usually the girls were asleep when this happened. Sometime in the night an egg would break, a wet chick nudge its head through the shell. Hens are born with thousands of tiny germ cells, each one a potential egg. And each of my aunts was born with 400,000 ova. When the girls got older, they probably all bled at the same time each month. That is what happens, scientists say, when women live together. Five daughters swimming under the same moon. Imagine. No wonder my grandfather often slept under the stars after a day of haying.

Two days ago, I visited my father and took a walk with him. "My warranty's run out," he said, laughing but not really laughing. His heart operation six years ago was more serious than my aunt's, and the plastic valve was guaranteed only for five years. Walking with him, I tried hard not to think about this, so hard that I *did* forget for a minute and walked too fast, until I heard my father's valve clicking. The love and fear rose in my throat, decades of words rising that I should have spoken, but didn't.

My aunt is seventy-seven years old but still beautiful and somewhat vain. She wears a scarf at her neck to hide the wrinkles. Once she was a model and she is still tall and graceful. "Always wear shoes that match your stockings and skirt," she says. "That is the key." If my father had been a woman, he would have been my aunt. Maybe this is why I have come; she is as close as I can get to knowing him. I see my father's chin in her chin, his nervous hands in the flutter of her hands straightening a pleat or refolding the napkin, his eyes in her eyes when she looks away, unable to stay grounded in the moment. I do the same thing. Even as she speaks— now she's finished with the incubator and is onto the caul—I am jotting it all in my brain. The moment is never enough for me. I am never wholly there. I justify this unattractive trait with the fact that I am a writer. Every experience is material, I tell myself.

The waiter has brought our chicken salad, served on lettuce ruffled like a doily. My aunt has become very talkative and I take advantage of it. "I don't know how much of this is true," she says like a little boy relishing a naughty joke he's been warned not to repeat, so of course I lean forward. "Your grandma had a sister. Aunt Ceel. She was born in a veil." My aunt says veil but I translate it as caul because I have learned more from books than from life and this is what books call the membrane that wraps the heads of some babies. I should use my aunt's word. It is more beautiful and more mysterious. "So she had powers," my aunt continues. "Plus she was the seventh daughter of a seventh daughter, so she could see things other people couldn't. That's how your grandma first knew she would marry your grandpa. Grandma and Ceel were sitting together in the outhouse, a two-seater. Grandma was sixteen, Ceel much younger, maybe ten or eleven. Suddenly Ceel said that a man was on the road and he was the man your grandma would marry."

As it turned out, my future grandfather *was* the stranger on that road, arriving with a team of horses. It strikes me as ludicrous that this is how my pristine father was engendered, that the romance between my grandparents began in an outhouse, foreseen in the crystal of a young girl's eyes, a great-aunt I would never know. I don't say this to my aunt because I am afraid she will take it wrong. There is something solemn in her expression. Perhaps to her also, this moment is more than this moment. We aren't just an elderly aunt and a fortyish niece eating chicken salad in a department store restaurant; something is being written here. *All these bits,* she seems to say. *They matter. Don't let the pieces die.*

This is my justification for prying. Because of course it finally comes around to sex, and the discussion of sex across generations is always prying. I don't ask for the information directly. It starts as a research question, generic, something an interviewer on a talk show might ask. "I heard you and Grandma were like midwives, that you helped other farm women with their babies." This is what my father once told me and it seems a harmless question, but by the time she finishes answering, I will know more than I ever wanted to.

Because it wasn't quite like that. I should have guessed. How could my father have known what went on in the birthing room? He was a young man, out in the fields with my grandfather and the other sons, but already plotting his escape from the farm. Later he would father nine children, two of whom would die in the womb and one as an infant. Six of us would live, but he would not be present at our births. It was not his fault. In those days, men simply weren't present. They paced in waiting rooms, walking the edges, the perimeters that marked the women's place. My father did the best he could, but the closest he ever got to the blood of it was when my mother was pregnant with my sister and almost hemorrhaged to death. He didn't know I was watching, but I was eleven and curious and afraid he was holding something back from me, that maybe my mother was dead, not safe in a hospital miles away. So I stood at the bathroom door and watched him kneel beside the tub, sloshing her blood-drenched nightgown in the water which was quickly staining to pink.

This is what I'm remembering as my aunt begins the story. "No," she says. "I only helped with one birth. Jack's." Jack is her brother, two years younger than my father. My aunt was seventeen and still living on the farm, the year before she left for the city and a job. Grandma's labor started earlier than expected, earlier and faster, too fast for the family doctor to get there. I am trying to imagine this—watching your own mother give birth, delivering your own brother. There are lines that we draw and this is one I have trouble leaping. I have come close, but not that close. I was present at the birth of my nephew. I held my sister's hands and looked into her wild eyes and calmed her when she screamed that this was a bad idea, that she wasn't going to finish this, that the baby was tearing her apart, was killing her. But a doctor was there, wheeling around on a low stool, taking charge. There was a mirror on the opposite wall and I could look if I wanted to, but I didn't.

My aunt says she doesn't remember much, just helping Grandma onto the dining room table and hearing the screams and seeing the blood, all that blood. Maybe my aunt's head was so filled with hate there was no room for storing the memory. "Hate for Dad," she says, for she had decided at the moment Jack was born that this was all her father's fault, that she hated men and that she would never have children. Never.

"But we knew nothing back then," she says, and suddenly it spills out, something even women who might *think it* will never admit aloud—that her two children, the parents of those smiling grandchildren whose pictures line her bookshelves—were accidents. I have suspected this all along, for in this, my aunt and I are the same: we like our lives well ordered and under control. You can see this in the careful way we dress, the schedules we keep, our early to bed, early to rise, one-a-day-vitamin mentality. Which is probably why I never had children. Sometimes, mostly in dreams, my body mourns what never was—those 400,000 ova floating unfinished—but most of the time I live in my head, not my body. This is my father in me, not my mother. And it is my aunt. If my aunt had been me, she would have been childless. And if I had been my aunt, married early in the days before The Pill, I would have been the one with two accidents. I would have been the one laid out on that same dining room table where three years before she had watched her mother give birth.

Yes, this is the real story, the one that finally breaks it all open, that hatches the fear inside my head: fifty-seven years ago in Illinois there was a blizzard. This is not exactly the way she tells it, but I am doing the math in my head as she speaks. She was barely twenty, married less than a year and living out her pregnancy. Because, short of killing yourself, there is no way out of this contract. The baby *will* come. She was visiting her parents and because of the blizzard, her husband could not get to her. "Or wouldn't," she says, after all these years still not sure. The doctor had been notified, but it was doubtful he would make it. When the contractions started, Grandma helped her onto the table. For two nights and three days she was in labor. Outside the dining room, Grandpa walked the floors, stomping and cursing, knowing that if no one else arrived, he would have to hold his daughter down. He had never been this close to the birthing room before and if he hadn't thought his daughter might die, he wouldn't have been this close now.

At the last minute the doctor did arrive with ether, but he couldn't give her much. Grandma couldn't hold my aunt down by herself, so Grandpa was forced to help. The doctor finally pulled the baby out of her. It took eleven stitches to sew her up. "I felt every one," she says. Her father was holding her head, his rough farmer hands tight on her temples. When it was over she looked up to him and, "as hateful as ever I said anything," she says, and her teeth clench on the memory, "I said 'You did this to Mother too.'" Later Grandma told her the dining room had looked as if a hog had been butchered there.

When my aunt finishes the story, her eyes are lit with pain and I sense without her saying it, that she never forgave her father. Not to his face. Not while he was alive. Knowing my aunt (because I know myself and I am like her) she probably also never forgave herself for what she said. And she probably never spoke her love, even when it pushed to the surface, even forty years later when it was *he* who lay helpless, attached to an oxygen tank. I decide at this moment that when lunch is over I will call my father, wake him from his nap if necessary, and say the words.

The waiter brings the change and lays it at my aunt's elbow. We stand to leave, then suddenly she sits down again and, as if she doesn't want our time together to end on a minor key, here comes a last remembrance, too small and ragged to be called a story. "One year at the beginning of the war five of us came home for Christmas." (That would be five of my grandparents's nine grown children, accompanied by their spouses and families. By then, both my aunt's children would have arrived safely on this earth.) "The day before Christmas, Dad butchered a hog." She says this as if it were a miracle, something accomplished at great sacrifice and indeed, for those lean times, it was. "He gave us each a tub of lard and some pork. A real treat. We lived on it for months." She begins to laugh and cry at the same time and her brother, my father and my grandfather, her father, the one she loved but never until this moment forgave, both sit down at the table with us. This is when I know that in forty years, long after my aunt is dead, I will carry her inside me. Like a snowball that starts small at the top of a hill and barrels down, growing larger with each roll, I will collect these memories and when I am her age and rolling towards death, I will roll faster, heavier with her stories, carrying the weight of all she has known, her grief and shame which is my own, and perhaps if I am lucky, the joy.

Sue Walker

GLIDERMAN

Always when we drove up
You would be there,
Swinging in your glider,
Waiting for me...

You were too old to work,
But I never asked your age
Or questioned what you used to do.
It was enough that you were Grandpapa
And waiting...

Somedays we'd play checkers
Though you played hard
And seldom let me win,
But on those rare occasions
When I did, you laughed
For I would preen like the peacock
Out back, the one you took my picture with,
For I was more splendid, you said, than he.

In the back room
(Where the basket of apples
Perfumed the air that day you died)
Was the safe you let me unlock...
Whispering the combination in my ear.
I'd have let twenty robbers
Slit my throat before I told
Those numbers, Our secret.

They told you not to climb
Those steps to church that Sunday morning;
Your heart won't take it,
The doctor said,
And you laughed again;
What a way to go.

And you did too—
Leaving your old heart
At the altar
With the collection.

Robert Bixby

NASCENCE

In me
a desire to own
a pearl taken
from a man's lung
in autopsy

revulsion
as the lab technician
turned it in his
gloved fingers

then desire
to possess
that dark pearl

to touch
to peer inside

Conrad Rosenberg

DOCTOR IN THE HOUSE

Supine on cocoa-brown carpet,
lips parted, waiting,
heart beat the hoped for climax.

Mouth joined to mouth,
nostrils squeezed shut,
no surrogate breath escapes.

Palm flat on breast,
no soft nippled breast
but bone hard sternum,
no tender touch
but jolting thrust.

Warm lips return to chilled,
frothed with salty foam;
spit, wipe, breathe.

I, a pendulum, head, chest,
head, chest, puffing, pressing,
breathless, aching.

"Anybody——know——CPR——
four——five——six——
Good——you take——chest——
ten——eleven——I'll take——mouth——
fourteen——fifteen"

I search the neck for a pulse,
no artery responds;
pupils dark, dilated; no light
will ever again shrink them.
Police, oxygen, ambulance arrive.

She moves towards me;
carries his coat.
"Is he dead?"
"They're still trying,"
a non-answer, too soon for truth.

Down the stairs, very weary,
scoops of soap and water
to rinse my mouth,
the taste of the taste stays.

Kenneth Frost

UNTIL I THINK

It's a strange thing to say
I am going to die
is a problem
in applied math.

The bidding on the stock exchange
sounds like Gregorian
over the radio,
so does Grand Central, late.

No need to count
how many scuttle,
weave and advance
across the almost open plain

like prizefighters boxing a dream
they have of mine
as I sit on the head of things
not things until I think.

My shadow almost floats
into my hand
wanting to
point something out.

Susan A. Katz

COLLISION
(To Don)

Einstein said that death dissolves us,
spreads us like a mist
back into the sea; I understand

   the theory in my head,
that we are all a part of something bigger
than ourselves; that nothing starts or stops,
just for an instant moves a bit apart
from all the rest; but in that instant

   you and I collide, and know the need
of boundaries on the skin that fingers
might define: explain

   to what I call my heart,
thrown back into the soup of time,
how I will bear
the parting pain.

Susan A. Katz

CALLING THE ANGELS

No, it is not all
vanity my son. My end
is your beginning.

I shall never be
stone-asleep, a sterile mute.
Silence is all song.

Hear next year's crickets
still in their eggs, serenade
all future autumns.
        —Menke Katz (1906-1991)
        "Song," *A CHAIR FOR ELIJAH*

I.

At dusk I watched the slaughter
of the light; imagined how it died
beneath the fist of night, breathless
and bloody; this morning sunshine rolls around
the lawn like laughter, hugs the trunks
of trees, finger paints the leaves and I find
I disbelieve in darkness.

How can resurrection be
routine? How is it that we do not mourn
beyond our own small death of sleep; wake,
to clasp the promise of forever,
inherent in the morning, that we know
a few short hours will unkeep?

II.

You taught us what there is to know of joy;
something whole that can be held
within an open hand; you taught, that sighs
escape the heavens, are the distant voices
of the angels singing, and you

were intimate with angels, knew
the words to tempt them

to the table, called them
and they came, their merriment an echo
within the aftermath of glasses clinking
in an endless litany of toasts: "L'Chaim!
L'Chaim! To Life!"—we chanted
and their voices adding
to our own filled up the room.

III.

She was your lover; slept beside you naked
took you in to sleep and silence; kept,
for those few short hours, the words
at bay so that you could rise refreshed
to embrace them;

they were your lovers too; each word quivered
like a virgin's breast beneath your mind's
caress; seducer, and seduced by their innocence,
their lust, their raw need for you to bring
them to release and how you stroked
their passion into flame upon the page.

Inspiration was the substance of dust,
of weeds, of childhood dreams that burst
beneath the bombs of war; until your images
undid the gore and the shattered land
grew green again and dead men walked;
Aunt Beilke talked again, "the head
off death;" Rachel, the cow, gave cream;
"Yoodl the alley dancer" danced lively
"for a crust of bread;" mothers tended
to their children's needs, all
the seeds of Michalishek bloomed
in the soil of your remembering.

IV.

Indeed, light does not die; things come together
not in endings but beginnings; you knew that,
always; meant to tell us how darkness strokes
the thighs of light until they spread welcoming
the seeds of morning.

Menke dead? Impossible! You visit me
in dreams and call the angels to my bed;
you said you had no time to die, your poems
holding you hard against life and so you bargained
with the angels, not for years, but days; a basket

full, a small unhurried row of hours, one day
of minutes and they gave you
every one; calling to you as you slept,
calling you, home;

and how we smile to know
not even angels dared
to keep you, Menke, from loving words
into one last poem.

Joan New

JOURNEYING ABROAD

What is it like, this journey
Out of the flesh? If one journey
Is about like any other, then I know
You take your time; perhaps a bus
On an English motorway through pastures
And apple orchards of Kent, Canterbury
Cathedral rising above the plain.
As you settle back, you put away history
And literature, feel yourself moving
Further from knowing. You smile, remembering
A donkey that grazed by the castle wall.
Nearby, we spread our lunch of bread and cheese;
You fed the donkey a piece of yours,
And held its head in both hands, in love
With its dim eyes, their distant stare.

At Dover you queue at the docks
To make passage across the channel.
You say goodbye to the surprising cliffs,
To England, to all but the gulls—it seems
They follow the ferry halfway to Calais.
On the other side your bus continues
Through the farms of France. Without fence
Or hedge, green fields stretch endlessly,
Though now and then rows of manicured graves
Enclosed in white fences interrupt
The eye. You remember a child's grave
In a field back home, and how, year
After year, the spring plow turned
Furrows around the iron fence; how
By summer the tall corn leaves
And tassles hid the lonely grave.

I begin to guess your destination,
Not this place of death and fertile earth,
Nor Paris either. Forgetting the Louvre,
The Musée d'Orsay, even the Orangerie,
You'll take a train to Vernon,
Hire a taxi to Giverny.

You'll stroll Monet's paths, lean for awhile
On his Japanese bridge, or rest
On a garden bench among the flowering beds
Before you vanish, forever into light.

Madeline Tiger

POEMS FROM IOS
for my son Homer

I. THE AGES OF WOMEN

Caves gave way to whitewashed houses
of stone, and in front of the small doors
gardens — of stone flowers!
Bleached earthbone in striations
on cragledges, facing the sea.
We know the centuries taken by the civilization
of this village, the vertical effort, but
we can't even guess the ages of the women.

II. WHAT MADE THE POET SING HERE

The gods lived for thousands of years.
Zeus made love for a three-hundred year night.
But only the nine years of the Great War
were counted and counted as
particularly significant
among all things. That's what made the poet
sing about everything under the sun.

III. IOS, 1980

Oft of one wide expanse had I been told
That deep-browed Homer ruled as his demesne
John Keats

On a hill piled high on hills of stones
on stone, glinted and crumbled in sun,
you can hear—from the ground:
mule bells and bird chirps, early morning ... noon,
where barely visible lizards run, more birds, flies ...
Notice the scent of anise, sting of nettleweed, wild
wheat of mountains without trees, walls
and walls and walls of stone
carried up and laid by hundreds, thousands
of men crisscrossing, terracing the mountain,

marking and shifting and falling and decorating the
mountain. A lizard turns, green to brown. We sit still.

We left old Ianni at his fig tree where he'd grafted
four new strains; we left him in his fields of grape,
wheat, fig, stone, and we climbed
quickly up the first hill after the third bend
in the road to Theodoti. We've been told
no donkeys go today to "Homer's tomb" and hikers lose
their way, so we'll never see the "one plain stone"
that's often claimed to mark him. But here where we are
on a rocky hill, looking over the harbor, with the white
village houses clustered in that distance—
breaking bread, dipping it in yogurt and honey,
drinking apricot juice, we satisfy ourselves
with tastes and sounds and wind, and with the scene.
Serene, we feel breezes on our arms, welcome in the heat;
we chase flies, languorously gazing at the hills,
the same for ages, and the peaceful Aegean.

My son is reading modern mysteries by Dashiell Hammett,
and I'm reading Book IV in which
the butchering begins, the poet telling how the blood ran
beside the clear water under this perfect sky.

The Homer who is here repeats a question, Why
does the one poet get so much credit
if so many told the stories? I can only say again
how he collected myths and tales from people
in the villages, on dry hillsides, in valleys
of olive and fig and apricot trees, from farmers and
stone carriers who fixed the hills, he gathered stories
blind, remembering every name and the many passions—
of love, wounds, deaths, the violations done
to corpses, that wild grief witnessing, and the parallel
conduct of the gods, the jealous and costly actions of
the gods, each by name, each taking sides. And somewhere
deep   walking these hills   brow furrowed   he
composed. Sometimes his decision must have been
to stop—maybe in the evenings—and sing.

"If he couldn't see, how could he tell the sea
was aqua and how did he know mica and how
did he find his way?"

Isn't it amazing. He composed all the stories
and carried them over all these hills and
terraces and villages—and to other islands
with unknown terrain, with worse than nettles
or wheat stalk stubble, probably on steep mule
trails, even at night and in the heat.
Across these crags and carefully poised walls
of boulders and the stone chips piling.
They must have echoed his stories.
These are the herbs he smelled.
This is the honey he tasted.
These birds are like the birds singing 3000 years ago.
The faces we've seen are like the faces turning
to hear him, and spreading his name. He knew these
mule bells and fields, where the Christians later
built churches, he knew the hands that built these walls
like the hands building tourist hotels today,
letting the fields go fallow and paving the roads.
Hands like these took him
when he went farther into darkness, and carried him over
a hill just like this hill
and put his ashes under a stone.

We have to believe it's true if they say the place they marked
is too far to walk, even though we've planned this visit
so long, knowing we'll never come back, much as we travel.
Well, they don't know if the poet's grave is pure truth,
anyway … Let's say some god—Apollo, the god of song—
had us stop here, like some "watchers," from this hill.
This must have been his style, when "darkness covered his
eyes" in the beginning and his mind was lit with chronicles
that he could sing, of men and arms. Stopping high,
in air, with sea smell and the feel of sun, and the sound
of birds, of the land. In the end
it must have been the same, the song in the dark

and the same Apollo directly above us now
bringing us here to learn
the terrain…lizards, bees, wind;
and to answer questions, and know "thalassa blé"
and pick daisies that grow in the roofless room of
an old stone cottage, half rebuilt, and write this down,
and remember … Maybe he's not buried in this earth at all,
all the better! Think of him! Homer.

IV. ABOUT WHAT THEY DO ON HORA, THE FIRST VILLAGE VISIBLE
ON IOS, THE ISLAND WHERE HOMER IS SAID TO BE BURIED

They planted stone flowers in front of the houses of
Hora, where the women in the doorways seemed to be
held, watching the port, really too far away to see
much arriving; but the dark habit of watching may be
a tradition most unforgettable on an island where
the gardens are stony and the steep steps forbidding
of rambling, the best entertainment after all those
ups and downs being to be seated and leaning and
watching for sailors whether any are ever forthcoming or not. The catch is the catch isn't
worth much between them on the island.
The market is for tourists.

The other commodity and sales-pitch on Ios is a death-
place, its promise. One of the seven where Homer the poet
is supposedly resting (or maybe it's seven birth-places
and just this one grave, the story keeps changing.)

But those women in black shawls would never be watching
for pilgrims. They don't know the path and they couldn't
be bothered to look for Ianna: The one man with a donkey
is (*you'll hear three days after you get there
and eat fresh fish in the little restaurant and
answer some questions and request water in the half-
lit, still-under-construction, unlocked motel room,
and try to go sunbathing over the sand dunes
among American campers and German families and
schoolboys in wrestling positions, and feel rather
restless, abandoned of mission*) terribly busy
building motels now, on the south shore of the island,
so he couldn't be tour guide,not this month,
not this season, to take you to the burial place,
and no sense your trying to walk there
unguided—the path is unmarked, and the terrain
gets too rugged. Not even the villagers go toward
the center of Ios. Most people here feel secure
in range of the bay, preferably facing the water.

It wouldn't have been the same for a blind man,
and not for a singer, not for the one

who carried so many stories in his head.
He would never have needed to see things to know them.

May he rest in peace.
And may those women of Hora, in their dark shawls, also
have reward for their vigils.

IOS

(from the port, 4/26/80)

On this island where the mountains show their age,
no groves protecting them in green veils,
a thin road twists up through the wind-carved rock.
Hora, the village on the first hill, gleams
across the bay: Those white walls appear
so stark on this island
where the mountains show their age.
Day after day the women scrub the walls,
barefaced to Apollo and Mnemosyne,
they dream a thin road twists through.
The wind-carved rock and ravaged ledges
crumble: Men reconstruct—stone on stone
propped with the rooting fig tree of this island.
The mountains show their age.
Facing the sea, lined, in their dark shawls
the women lean like little mountains
watching the thin road twist up
through wind-carved rock. Gnarled stones
edge a walk the men keep clean:
Shards of quartz could run rampage
on this island where the mountains show their age.

A thin road twists up through the wind-carved rock.

David Ignatow

FOR MY DAUGHTER

When I die choose a star
and name it after me
that you may know
I have not abandoned
or forgotten you.
You were such a star to me,
following you through birth
and childhood, my hand
in your hand.
        When I die
choose a star and name it
after me so that I may shine
down on you, until you join
me in darkness and silence
together.

Peter Cooley

FOR ALISSA

This is a poem for my daughter,
her of the topaz eye reflecting mine
eight years into the world.
Women have told me my eyes are like a statue's,
unmoving, cold. Hers never stop dancing.

Nor does her little body
lost to a plié or the dark woods
in the midst of Brothers Grimm
surrender its sharp grip
on the ground under it, spinning.
Nor on the wind over her always lifting.

Who from her mother was ripped
before her time and clung to Death
three days until he fell.
Who cocks her head like a bear cub
at my approach, moving too fast
that I should touch her with my expectation.

Who in a night season
seven years back
when I lay in terror of myself
cried out and drew me to her
hours while I walked her.
That tiny head pressed to my shoulder
downed with hair fine as cowslip
or the soft, white fire of milkweed
spilling over my skin—
and lifted these wings here
nubby, oracular, stubborn,
which brought me to morning,
nudging their small way upward.

Peter Cooley

THE LAST GIFT

Tonight my mother, dinner over,
alone or with the widows
she names friends,
walks the shingle of gulf water,
the twilight violet on her rings.
Far from my father,
the old house in the North,
she is barefoot, halfway through her seventies,
and the water is emerald and then clear
this mid-December as she stoops
to claim a shark tooth, a sand dollar.

The voice which walked above me
by the cold waters of Lake Huron
resinous with pine and parted them
to take me in, who named the stars,
the roaring at the Royal Oak Zoo,
the first seedling in the garden
streaked with frost and sang the night asleep,
rests now within her finally.
What last word did it bend to give me
in the garden by the fishpond?
Was it forsythia which at that moment fell?
What name did she give me for the rock?
What kind of luminescence did she spell into my hand?

Vivian Smallwood

THE PARTICIPANT

I am a part of something big.
Dust that is now my dust was blown
Through the corridors of the pyramids
Before the final stone was placed.
My blood has raced with the Amazon
And surged in the tides of the Yellow Sea.
My bones were sketched when the world was new
And etched on the ocean floor.

Everything everywhere touches me.
The smallest beetle is my affair,
And the oldest man, and the youngest child.
When pink flamingos feed at dawn
In the shrinking marshes of Bangladesh
I too am fed. When the polar bear
Claws at the bullet in her flesh,
And her young ones crouch in the growing chill,
I am not quite what I used to be,
I am less than I was before.

Just where I stand in the grand design
Whatever the grand design may be,
I do not know and I cannot guess,
But I give and take with a careful hand,
And I watch the world with an anxious eye,
For I share in the life of all who live
And the death of all who die.

Vivian Smallwood

THE DENIAL

You are not here. The stone that bears your name
Is only stone, carved by a foolish hand
In ignorance or jest, a thing of shame
Propped on a hillside in a wasted land.
Whatever lies at length beneath this clay
Is not the flesh and bone that I hold dear.
I touch the starveling weed and turn away.
You are not here. You never have been here.
Though others climb this hill with measured pace
and stoop to read your name and cry aloud,
I shall not look in this unlikely place
For one so young and beautiful and proud.
   I turn my back upon this marble lie.
   You are not dead. I will not let you die.

Vivian Smallwood

THE WAKE

After a while they will go away
With their trays of food and their pleasant faces.
After a while I can wash the vases
And close the door that is still ajar.

What do they think that doors are for?
Maybe something needs shutting out,
Maybe something needs shutting in,
Something that they don't know about
      And haven't the right to know.
Whatever it is, it is up to me
To lift the latch or to turn the key,
      To hold it or let it go.

Nothing but kindness brings them here,
Nothing but kindness makes them stay.
I tell myself how kind they are
But I watch their faces, I watch the clock.
      I know what a door is for.

E.P. Bollier

ALL HALLOW'S EVE

31 October 1980

This then is the use of memory: that love endure.
For this I keep private vigil still
this one night of the year,
All Hallow's Eve, when ghosts must wake
to walk the familiar places the living haunt.
Born with them, you too must come again
to the garden where I wait

and where once we watched another moon
your only birthday here.
Your own ghosts came that night,
but happy ghosts of a childhood Hallowe'en
when Brother and Sister and you
followed Mother in Father's second-best suit,
a scarecrow stuffed out with straw,

across frozen fields to kitchen lights
where neighbors awaited your trick or treat.
Listening, I heard that child in your voice,
felt her warm hand in mine,
and saw in your shadowy face
turning slowly toward me her eyes
offering her world and self with love.

So tonight I become your memories:
again the scent of honeysuckle lures
you and that swarm of bees to the same spot,
a brief entanglement with curls,
and rescue leaves your head cropped as a boy's,
and again you play doctor and nurse,
your wailing patient your favorite cat,

its tummy shaved for the knife
dropped at Mother's sharp angry shout,
and hiding behind the shed you cry and cry—
and later cry to see Brother laid so stiff
in the parlor where lights are never lit
and watch with Sister your parents' eyes
to learn for the first time how real ghosts are.

So tonight I welcome again,
not only the sweet-voiced wife of twenty-four years,
or the child of six, but the high school girl,
the coed dreaming of a New York career,
the young woman I kissed in the rain
and made love to once under the Cape Cod sun.

Welcome, and with you your world
led by the brother too early lost,
the grandmother who let you help hanging the wash,
the father who kept buying fish
his wife would not cook nor his children eat,
and now even the mother who wept at your grave.
O dear familiar ghost,
let all who in our memory live
join us tonight once more in love.

Joan Vannorsdall Schroeder

PARACHUTES

He lay listening to the carpenters sawing outside his door and knew that he was going to die by nightfall.

"It's my coffin they're building, isn't it?" he asked the fat nurse.

"What? No coffins in this place. They're fixing the walk rail. It fell down yesterday. Remember that?" She sat down heavily on the edge of his bed and hoisted a puffy foot up high enough to adjust the laces of her white shoes.

This girl was new; no name-tag rode high on her huge breast. Who was she, he wondered. How did she get so fat? Her fingers were like cased sausages, or full cow teats. He laughed thinking about her fingers dripping milk on his bed.

"That's funny? Somebody could've gotten hurt bad on that rail." The fat girl stood up and tugged on her uniform, which had ridden up over her massive hips. "Doesn't it get to you, that you can't remember your own name sometimes? It would me, having everybody think I was crazy, or like a baby again." She grunted with the effort of tucking the top sheet beneath the mattress.

"Made out of maple. Tiger or bird's eye. Is it?" Anders had always admired maple and, lately, dreamed often of lying in a fine wood coffin. He could make pictures from the grain of maple. He guessed there would be nothing more to do than that after he died, while he was waiting for God to point him in one direction or the other.

The fat girl's arms jiggled as she cranked up his bed. "You're going to have to speak straight with me if we're going to get on together. Breakfast will be around soon." He watched her walk to the door of his room, heard her thighs swishing together. She stopped, read his name plate beside the door. "Anders McKenzie—that's like a fairy tale or something." She left his room humming tonelessly, only the high notes reaching the old man's hearing. She left behind a good scent, and he strained to remember where it came from. A whitecap mushroom, perhaps, or a spadeful of dirt after rain.

Anders watched the traffic pass on the four-lane highway outside his window. Last summer he had seen men working to widen the twisted, pitted road, which had once carried wagons into town and now bore the burden of commuters' impatience. The flow of busyness that had nothing to do with him now. Today he was going to die, and not one of the people driving those cars knew that. It seemed to him that someone should know. Someone—one of the men driving to work, maybe, or that man's wife taking their children to school—should feel the urge to turn into the driveway of the Stoneleigh Nursing Home and ask for him by name.

The heat came on below the drapes, causing them to flare out from the window like a woman's skirt caught by wind. He watched them change from light to dark and back to light as the air moved them rhythmically through bands of sun. When he shut

143

his eyes he could still see the drapes fluttering gently above the whish of warm air; he thought he heard a woman sigh happily, a soft Ahhhh escaping slowly from her throat.

He could not die alone. Who would come to be with him? It scared Anders that he could bring no face to mind. His cousin only came Sundays, and sometimes not then if his wife wanted to ride into the city. He did not want Gerald here today, Anders decided; he was too much like Anders himself. After years tending cows and on the tractor, alone, Gerald just didn't have much to say to people. Sundays when he came he sat in the orange chair twisting his hands up in a ball, watching the door like he was waiting for some bell to ring and dismiss him.

It should be a woman, Anders decided, to come sit with him while he waited to die. Some woman, who would come from her bright kitchen, where she would have been washing out coffee cups stained with her own lipstick. She might not be especially pretty, but would be fresh-looking, and maybe her clothes would smell of being hung in hot sun to dry. She would come in the heavy front doors of the building, not hesitating which way to turn as she passed through the lobby.

She would be wearing high heels with good leather soles that would sound right moving across the shining linoleum floor. She'd be wearing a simple cotton dress, full-skirted, a bit too tight around the waist. Her hair would be fixed neatly beneath a hat the color of a cockscomb, and maybe she'd have a net veil pulled down over her eyes.

She would come directly to his room and pull the orange chair right up next to his bed. "I'm here," she would say. "Anders McKenzie, I'm here."

She might talk about the weather, about the asparagus pushing up at the garden's edge, and then some more about the weather. (Anders loved weather, how it changed days around. This woman would know that.) She would go on and on about church choir and her mother's surgeries and the babies being born—"I can't believe my own are grown so fast!"—and there would be no end to her flow of words, ever.

Anders opened his eyes. The drapes lay flat against the spotted windows. He pulled his blanket over his chest and stared at the wall.

It was hung with pictures. Not of people, but of land, glued onto cardboard in thick layers. Anders had taken them from the *National Geographic* magazines that had appeared in his mailbox every month except two from 1942 to last year. Not once had he ordered the magazine, but it came, and each December the mailman brought a gift card announcing another year's subscription. Always the giver's name was absent; the blank line puzzled and delighted Anders.

At first he had cut out only familiar scenes, drawn to the birdseye views of ridged mountains like those he knew. But as the issues began to accumulate beneath the kitchen stairs, the flatland farms, with their true corners and stripes of color, began to be beautiful to Anders, whose modest travels had stopped some time ago. And then the hot colors of the desert, and layered jungle green, and even the stark blue glacial views caught his eye, until Anders found himself with one entire kitchen wall papered with the world.

As suddenly as the sunny yellow magazines had started, they stopped. When Christmas came last year and he found no card, Anders thought he had simply thrown it away, or put it someplace odd as he did more and more often. He spent New Year's Eve searching the house, turning over drawers full of receipts, used-up calendar leaves, and yellowed horoscopes which he clipped from the weekly paper. But there was no card, and by Twelfth-day Anders knew that there would be no more *National Geographic*. He wished then he could know who for so many years had thought of him at Christmas, and, more, why there no longer did.

It was the end of February, a time that always left Anders wondering what to do with himself, when he began to sort the *National Geographics* into piles. Decades of Januaries were tied together with baling twine, then laid close by February bundles. He thought that he would recycle the magazines: start all over with them and imagine that each was coming to him new again.

It was from an August issue near the top of the stack that he cut the picture of the Brazilian rain forest. It had some people in it, but that was all right. They were children, a half-circle of them, and they stood open-mouthed watching the land being cleared: trees bulldozed, then stacked and burned, the exposed earth (which Anders thought must be rich beyond imagining from centuries of leaf fall) torn up, seeded, and then smoothed over with Johnson grass so that beef cattle could get fat.

He read the caption out loud: "American interests are buying thousands of acres of Amazon tributary land each year so that their hunger for beef can be sated. The Burger King chain is the world's largest consumer of South American beef."

"And here we are in America getting paid not to raise cattle," he said to Ike, the collie bitch nursing her puppies in the corner of the room. "Something's way wrong there." He cut out the two-page spread and smeared mucilage on the back. Then, having decided on the perfect spot for his picture—up in the corner, next to a picture of a granite prairie schoolhouse—he reached over the top of the stepladder to fix it on the wall.

It was the puppies that kept Anders from dying that day. Like their mother, they saw Anders fall off the ladder and heard his hip shatter in the socket as he hit the cracked linoleum floor. They wondered at the way he lay there, as still as their runt brother had lain before he was taken away and thrown down the hill out back. And they cried and yelped when their mother let herself out the screen door and ran down the driveway, her teats leaking milk in the dust.

That was what Anders's cousin Gerald heard the moment he shut off his truck. It made his neck prickle to see the largest puppy splaylegged at the screen door, yowling for his mother. He knew that what waited for him on the other side of the door was not going to be pretty.

When Gerald told Anders what the doctors were saying—that Anders's bones were just old, and would never come together well enough for him to walk freely—he began to cry. Gerald cried because he knew his wife would never allow Anders to live in the spare bedroom and be a burden to her; there was no use in asking. And Gerald knew that in the Stoneleigh Nursing Home, confined in a bed in a shut-up room, Anders would set his sights on dying.

In the hall the whining saw fell silent; Anders could hear the tools clinking into the workmen's boxes. "That's it," a man said. "Let's get out of here."

His gut lurched. They were done with it. Where would they store the coffin while he died? Oh, but someone would have to smooth the edges, he thought, and varnish it. He wanted nothing fancy, but his coffin must at least be finished.

He would tell the fat girl about that, ask her if she would see to the coffin's finishing. Despite her size and quick tongue, he liked her. She said what was on her mind, straight-on. She seemed less in a hurry than the others and less skittish, as if she had no one waiting for her elsewhere and was not afraid of stink and need.

His sister Norah had been like that. Not so fat as this girl, but thick-waisted and trunk-legged. She had been happiest out of the house, doing broad-stroke things like swinging the scythe and splitting firewood. But she was best beside a laboring animal, willing to sit for hours, patiently letting the animal work and then, when the time was right for it, helping just enough. "When you have your own baby, you'll not be able to do this well anymore," their father had told Norah. "You'll hurt along with the animal and lose your nerve. And then you'll do something foolish, like pull a calf too soon."

What had happened to Norah? Anders had to work very hard just to remember her face, and that face was so young. When had she left home, and where had she gone? Norah had disappeared through a hole in his memory. It was horrible how he could lose someone like that; no one could know how that hurt. It should not be some strange woman who leaves her yellow kitchen to be with him today, wearing good shoes and a full-skirted dress. It should be Norah. Anders began to cry, his tears tracking in the dry furrows that ran down his face.

"Ah, look, it's the laundry truck this morning! Clean linens for you, Anders!" The thin, skittery girl was there with his breakfast tray. "Here you are, hon, you'll feel better when you eat something," she said. "We always do perk up after breakfast, don't we?"

Anders ignored her. He watched the slow progress of the canvas laundry cart as the wheels caught on the cracks between the concrete slabs. It was wonderful how patient the white-shirted man was: how he stopped to turn the wheels straight each time they went awry, as carefully as if he had a baby nestled in the cart.

"Over here, hon, look over here. Your coffee is getting cold." The small girl skittered from dresser to serving tray to bathroom, checking this or that and not once looking at Anders. She was like a mouse, he thought, like a mouse running from the shine of the kitchen light late at night. An apron-string tail trailed her as she moved about his room, setting things in order, nesting for him. Women loved to make nests: places of shelter. This one might like cheese, but all he had was oatmeal.

"Here, this is for you." Anders held his bowl out to the woman, who turned and looked full-face at him for the first time, her mouth wide open. "What? Your breakfast?" she said.

"Here, this is for you." Anders held his bowl out to the woman, who turned and looked full-face at him for the first time, her mouth wide open. "What? Your breakfast?" she said.

"You look hungry. Eat from my bowl." Anders's hand shook with the effort of holding the heavy dish. She made no move to help him with it, and left the room on shoes that squeaked angrily down the hall.

So no one would eat this breakfast, then, Anders thought. A morning meal meant nothing to someone who was going to die before dinner came around.

"Look how strong it is! This will hold anyone! Good wood!" It was the voice of Mrs. Cochran, whose room was across the hall. She was a busy-minded woman, watching the comings and goings in the hallway from her wheelchair and grabbing attention as best she could. Was she talking about his coffin?

"Not anyone—it's mine!" He called out to her. "They made it for me!"

"Like hell, like hell! You don't even get out of your bed, old man. You don't need it!" Mrs. Cochran's wheelchair bumped the wall angrily as she swerved into his room. "Kee-rist, McKenzie. You're just like the rest of 'em: kee-razy!" Sitting there with her yellow hair sticking up from her shriveled head, her dress pulled up in front showing mottled legs, Mrs. Cochran made Anders feel glad he had never married.

"That's my coffin out in the hall, the wooden one. It's mine," Anders said.

Mrs. Cochran startled, wheeled over to Anders' bed. "Coffin? Nobody's coffin is in the hall. I didn't see any coffin."

"They built it for me," Anders said. "It's maple, isn't it?"

The old woman propelled her chair backwards, keeping her eyes on Anders. "Kee-rist. You're thinking about dying—you keep on thinking like that and that's just what'll happen to you. Don't talk to *me* about it." She began to cry. "A hell of a way to start the day, old man."

When the fat nurse came to push Mrs. Cochran down the hall for television, she hushed the woman and winked at Anders. He noticed that she had a large red bandanna stuffed in her uniform pocket. "Take my tray?" he asked. She nodded and told him she would come back when she could.

He rolled over to watch out the window. It was May, windy, and the hoisting rope flapped crazily against the metal flagpole. Lining the front walk, the daffodils bent backwards in the west wind. Sun shone off large puddles in the driveway like bits of glass. On the farm it was the sort of day that had thrown dirt in his eyes and tied his wispy hair in knots, the kind of day that had filled his lungs like balloons and tugged at his moorings. So hard to remember the feel and smell of such a day. He no longer had the energy for it. Anders began to cry.

There was the laundry boy again, this time carrying in what looked to Anders like lengths of velvet. He carried them straight-armed, careful to keep the edges out of the puddles. For the coffin, Anders thought, to line it. So he would lie on green velvet.

Who would come to be with him today? He could not wait alone.

When the fat nurse bent down to get his breakfast tray, Anders saw that she had tucked the red bandanna into the front of her uniform, tinging her vast bosom with pink.

"You didn't eat," she said. "You need to eat."

"I'm going to die today," he said. "No need."

"There's no sense in thinking that," she said. "You're not."

"I saw the green velvet coming in," he said.

"The drapes," she answered. "For the social hall."

"For my coffin," he said. "Are you helping to line it?"

She pulled out the bandanna and blew her nose noisily. "No," she said. "There's no coffin. I told you that before breakfast."

Anders reached for her hand. "Will you be sure that it's finished by tonight? Someone needs to do that for me."

The girl did not flinch from his touch. She sat on his bed, her body like an efficient potbellied stove. "You're not going to die today," she said.

"Soon," Anders said. Her warmth was delicious.

She sat very still, thinking. "Sometime," she said. "Maybe soon."

Down the hall a quavery voice called "Nurse! Nurse! Come!" but the large woman didn't move from Anders's bed. Anders closed his eyes, comforted by her smell and her warmth. The rhythm of her breathing lulled him.

But she had no name. What was her name?

Hidden in the corner stall, he can hear the restless noises of the cows, their night peace disturbed. He has followed her to the barn, seen her bulky shape climb the ladder to the loft. Though he cannot see her now, he can hear movement above him in the hay.

Other nights he has seen her leave the house, watched her climb out onto the roof and use the maple tree outside her window as a staircase to the ground. Because she seems not to care about who sees her, he thinks there is nothing very wrong about her doing this. Often she will stop at the verge of the yard and look back at the house, as if she is daring someone to throw open the door and call her back in. Then she walks down the dirt road, jumps the ditch, and disappears into the field that runs along the river. He has never seen her come back, but she must, because she is always there for breakfast in the morning.

But this night, late in the summer, he has followed her, because he is twelve years old and can no longer bear not knowing where she spends her nights.

He is ready to climb the ladder when the noises start. First they are soft, spaced, and then more insistent. The cries come closer together, pushed from her gut; they start low and rise up high in the air until they are hopeless wails.

He does not want to hear, wishes he were in his bed dreaming simple dreams. He claps his hands over his ears, and still the noise works its way into him. He begins to cry, and buries his face in the straw. Next to him the brown mare dances nervously and kicks the side of the stall hard. The jolt travels the length of his body.

The silence that follows is more terrible than her hurting noises. She is dead, he thinks, she is lying there dead and she is alone. His shame is unbearable; he cannot move beneath the weight of it. The moon moves light across his back, marking time.

Then their father is there with a lantern and it is shining in Norah's face, blotchy and hardset. There is blood on her nightgown and on her hands and on the packed dirt floor. Between them something very small lies wrapped in a towel, and there is blood on that too.

"Give it to me," he says.

She shakes her head. "It's mine. I'll bury it."

"It's a terrible thing you've done," he says.

"It's not," she says. "It happened."

Her father snorts. "It's yours, then." His eyes look terrible in the tossed shadows. Not until he leaves the barn does she bend to pick up the towel.

Three days later, Norah left her room. She took her father's Swiss knife and her mother's watch and the money she had earned selling eggs, and no one spoke her name again.

"Look! Out the window!" Anders's bed shifted as the heavy nurse turned for a better view. It was so much easier to keep his eyes closed, but the vitality of the woman's voice made it impossible for him to do that.

With one hand laid on top of his two, she pointed to the laundry cart. It lay on its side, the load of dirty linen spilling out onto the pavement. The white sheets and pillowcases whipped in the breeze and glistened in the spring sun. The delivery man, who had this time misjudged the cracks in the concrete, stooped to right his cart.

Then from the south came huge swells of wind which pushed the righted canvas cart out toward the busy highway and sent the man's hat along after it. White sheets scattered across the lawn. A few caught in the branches of the maple trees which separated Stoneleigh from the plowed fields to the north; the fabric of the snared sheets flapped frantically. Others scuttered along the ground, earthbound.

But it was the two sheets which had grabbed the wind at just the right moment that caught the eyes of Anders and the heavy nurse. They rose high into the blue sky like parachutes and swelled proudly. Over Stoneleigh, across the fresh-plowed field, above houses and factories and schools and mares and cows at pasture the white sheets flew. If they fell to earth, Anders and the woman never knew it, as they sat together wondering at the surprise of what they had just seen.

Elspeth Cameron Ritchie

PARATROOPER
FORT BRAGG, NORTH CAROLINA

I am lonely and cold.
No wartime. No Vietnam.
Peacetime is empty here in
Fayetteville, home of The Airborne.

If only I could parachute in
Somewhere real. Fight with my unit.
Get my combat badge, be a hero.
Make Mom be proud, stop drinking.

Instead we rehearse how to land,
Shiver in the November cold
Of pine-ridden North Carolina.
Will I break my leg tonight?

Two C-130's crouch on the strip.
Two hours more until we board.
A message from my current girl
Tacked on the barracks door.

Can't call till we're back
In the dawn. Is it "Dear John"?
Is she pregnant? Or broke?
Do I care? Not tonight.

My father, a colonel,
Jumped until he crashed
Into a camouflaged jeep.
Now a wheelchair is home.

My mother switched to vodka then,
My brother went to med school,
I ran off to jump school.
On weekends I also drink.

I pack my chute, tighten straps.
This year three jumpers died.
I'm out of smokes. Bum one.
What are lungs compared to legs?

My squad buddies have wives.
They fight. Babies squall.
I just want a woman.
Tomorrow night, it's Bottom's Up.

Women there don't wed.
Dollar bills fly instead.
My roommate bedded a dancer.
Two shots cured him.

My doctor brother is staid.
Disapproves of cigarettes,
And me. He hasn't jumped.
Coward. Do you love me?

I try so hard to match
You and Dad. I've quit cocaine,
Won my stripes. I jump.
What else makes a man? My M-16?

Time to load. We file aboard
in order. The plane is cold.
I clip to the static line.
Dad's voice calls to me.

I can not hear him
With the gibbering wind
In my ears. The Jumpmaster
Calls, "Jump!" I do.

Marge Piercy

POP-SICLE

Martina had a mama, Anna-Lisa
and a papa and a house on the corner
of the block with a birch tree
and Herbie the Hamster.
Herbie let her carry him in her blouse
and never bit her, although
his claws were pins sticking her.

When her papa yelled, Herbie would
wake too and scrabble in his cage.
His beady eyes looked at her without
a moment's anger and never swelled
with tears like her mama's.
Papa would pull on her and
then Mama would pull on her.

Then her mama took her to grandma.
A week after they moved into
mama's old room, Herbie died. It was
winter: Mama put him in a box
in the freezer till the ground thawed.
Mama got a job in a doctor's office.
They moved to a yellow brick building.

Anna-Lisa got sick and lost the job
They lived with her mother's boyfriend
Carl and then back to sour grandma
and then to a new boyfriend Jerry.
Herbie goes along in his box.
Spring has come and gone and come
and gone four times, but Martina

will not give Herbie to the embrace
of somebody else's earth. He is
her lost love, her cropped roots
as they move from one man's apartment
to another man's house. They are not
fathers. Martina glares at the men from
slitted eyes. Herbie's still frozen.

Sandra A. Engel

MAKING OF IT WHAT I CAN

Eight years ago on the sunny Sunday afternoon before Thanksgiving, my mother took the *New Hampshire Sunday News* with her into the garage and with the garage doors closed, turned the ignition on and ran the engine of her Torino. It had been her habit to fill the gas tank Friday after work so as to have gasoline for the weekend and the following week. When my brother found her, just a half hour too late, the gas gauge was down only one-eighth of a tank, and the car had stalled. The house had been cleaned, the bills paid, and all the potbound African violets watered. "Sorry you had to see this," her note read. My father had died just over a year earlier, and the past month had been their wedding anniversary, the anniversary of her father's death, and her fifty-sixth birthday. The same doctors who a few years earlier had concluded with her that she was fine but needed to be more assertive had a phrase for it: "anniversary syndrome." The newspapers called it "self-inflicted carbon-monoxide poisoning."

I am not sure I have figured out what I finally want to call it. I understand why she did it, and sometimes I don't understand why, just as at the time it was a surprise, and it wasn't a surprise at all. When my brother told me the news long-distance, I just sat down. I hadn't expected it and certainly would not have predicted it, but it did make immediate sense. Then I understood what she called her sinusitis, her explanation for always sounding froggy on the phone. She had never been a woman who especially liked pets, but she had become fond of my housecat Rudder during my visits, and I had offered the cat—or any pet she'd like—for her birthday. "No," she said. "A lot can happen," and she told me she didn't want responsibility.

I am finally beginning to understand her suicide now, I think, not because I am eight years older or because I think I know my mother better (although both may be true), but because I have learned something about how language works—how we use it and how it uses us. And I find what understanding I do despite my recurrent feeling that I am looking for language for an act possibly completely irrational and perhaps for which there is no language: the suicide of my *mother*, for God's sake. The giver of my life took her own. What else need I know?

As much as I can.

I once saw my mother's high school yearbook. The picture was not of my mother as I knew her, but of a younger, dark-haired version of the woman with the silver-blonde bouffant. She was in the Future Homemakers of America for two years, a Glee Club member for four.

That is all I know about my mother's early life except that she was the oldest girl of seven children and after high school, she worked for a while as a bookkeeper. I know she married my father (and in fact had another suitor, Joe Somebody) in 1946, and eventually, they had my brother and me. We were, we were told, wanted children.

From where I was, their marriage seemed all right, but then ours was a house where, if we were to argue, we were to close the doors and windows. I have no idea what—or how much—I was not privy to. I know my mother was not a helpless woman; she had a job after her children went to school, and she balanced the checkbook. She drove.

My mother was the daughter of a farmer and too proud and stubborn to take the Librium the doctor prescribed for her during menopause. I remember her sewing lace on a doll's dress, or playing solitaire hour after hour at the dining room table and looking out the bay window as she did. I remember her trimming the hedge inside the backyard stockade fence, and later watching the clothes rock and fall in the washing machine. Summer afternoons she used to spend in the backyard, talking, my brother and I used to say, to her pansies.

What she saw in those flower faces, I don't know, and I certainly can't say I ever heard her speak to them despite all the time she spent tending them. It might have been well if she had, although I suspect they might not have been enough to sustain her.

My mother gave me language, but her language could not save her.

I remember her listening—at the dinner table, during the ride home from dancing school—but I cannot remember having what might be called a conversation with her. What there was instead were aphorisms and admonitions: "It hurts to be beautiful," "Straighten up and fly right," "Use your head for something other than a hat rack." She made sure I wore clean underwear when we went for a ride, and she also told me that if I wanted to go to college, the first in my family to do so, she and my father would find a way to pay for it. She was also in charge of punishment, punishment that usually consisted of a quick swat on the behind, or, for major offenses, being confined to my room with no one to talk to.

She was the woman who left at the foot of my bed a book rather than tell me the facts of life, and she was the woman who regularly went through my suitcase whenever I came home from college. Once she found my birth control pills, and while she never mentioned them directly, she did make a point of mentioning the assorted ills I would be prey to if I *were* to take such things. There was something furtive about the woman, but not obviously furtive; I was her daughter, and I accepted it. That was who my mother was. Aside from the few women I remember she knew when I was little, I don't remember her having any friends. She was the kind of woman who talked to the neighbors over the hedge and kept to herself.

Aside from her suicide note, the only letters she wrote were thank-you notes. Although I can remember her reading to me *The Little Engine That Could* and *Make Way for Ducklings*, the only book I knew her to own, we found after her funeral, *How To Find A Mate.*

By understanding what I can of her life, I begin to make sense of her death. It feels as though I understand as memory begets memory. One thing I remember about my mother leads to another, but I end finally with a too-tidy version of her, and sometimes what I remember strikes me as too much of a piece for a person to actually have been. I am a student of literature, after all, and what I know strikes me, I'm afraid, as being more art than life. But I take heart, then, from the fact that I'm still unsure, that I still have questions: Why, for example, did she never sing after four years in the Glee Club? Although I never knew her to go to church, how does the fact that she was brought up an Episcopalian figure in? How would all the things I don't know about her fit in, or change how I see her death if I knew them?

I don't know.

Sometimes it seems to me that my mother's suicide was the logical conclusion to her life. Yes. But from where I am, it seems she had reasons to live as well. She had her children, her plants, her home. She had her hands, those hands I remember the feel of even though I cannot remember her actually touching me: hands that were always red and rough despite the lotion she regularly applied. They were hands that did things, hands that could do things other than start the car in the closed garage.

I have my mother's hands; my first two fingers lean outward, the ring finger inward. But I also have, I think, what my mother did not, especially towards the end of her life; I have the hand that language is, a hand that forms and re-forms again and again. This language makes; this language yields choices. My mother, I imagine, finally could not see things for or name them as other than what they seemed to her. Her language gave her certainty—and finally only certainty. Such a life without a generative language must be a life without possibility, I think, because to have language, the kind of language I mean, means always to begin.

To have this kind of language, I think, is for me to have hope, hope despite my recognition of the impossibility of absolute certainty. My hope, though, is not easy; I will never know for sure what to make of her death, but knowing what I do know of her, I will make what I can of it—and so, whatever understanding I have, if only for now, is at least for now. Perhaps it is that every story is necessarily in some way incomplete—but a story must be told, though, for whatever understanding I have, such as it may be, comes only in the telling.

Cynthia Lelos

SWEET PARSLEY

All five foot ten and one half inches
of my father, his black hair, thick nails, even
smoke-stained teeth, mauve scar on brown chest,
sixty-two years of his
life, reduced
to one 11x11x11 inch cardboard box
handed to me ceremoniously
by the white-gloved undertaker.
My father, condensed
to an unmarked, unadorned box
brimming with bone-slivered ash.

I board my skiff, drift across the lake
and with head curved back,
the sun warming my father's remains,
I stretch my hand out   far
as it can reach   and cast
the flecks that were my father
into the cool waiting water,
gray dissolving already
into blue gray lake. He is slipping

through my fingers, disappearing, shadows
of ashen dust left behind.

I gather the last handfuls of my father,
cupping him in my palms,
saving him
until I reach the shore.
I walk to my herb garden
past the rosemary, the summer savory, beyond
the thyme, and lay my father's remaining life
to rest
in a soft, fragrant bed
of sweet parsley.

i**//**ness

"Don't leave because I'm not done with you, we're only starting; I need you in the world with me..."

Alice Jones
"Ottawa, March 1986"

Mary Oliver

UNIVERSITY HOSPITAL, BOSTON

The trees on the hospital lawn
are lush and thriving. They too
are getting the best of care,
like you, and the anonymous many,
in the clean rooms high above this city,
where day and night the doctors keep
arriving, where intricate machines
chart with cool devotion
the murmur of the blood,
the slow patching-up of bone,
the despair of the mind.

When I come to visit and we walk out
into the light of a summer day,
we sit under the trees—
buckeyes, a sycamore and one
black walnut brooding
high over a hedge of lilacs
as old as the red-brick building
behind them, the original
hospital built before the Civil War.
We sit on the lawn together, holding hands
while you tell me: you are better.

How many young men, I wonder,
came here, wheeled on cots off the slow trains
from the red and hideous battlefields
to lie all summer in the small and stuffy chambers
while doctors did what they could, longing
for tools still unimagined, medicines still unfound,
wisdoms still unguessed at, and how many died
staring at the leaves of the trees, blind
to the terrible effort around them to keep them alive?
I look into your eyes

which are sometimes green and sometimes gray,
and sometimes full of humor, but often not,
and tell myself, you are better,
because my life without you would be
a place of parched and broken trees.
Later, walking the corridors down to the street,
I turn and step inside an empty room.

Yesterday someone was here with a gasping face.
Now the bed is made all new,
the machines have been rolled away. The silence
continues, deep and neutral,
as I stand there, loving you.

Susan Jacobson

GOING HOME

Matt, listen to me.
I am going to help you
if you will let me.
I am going to touch you.

He is nineteen and has brown hair and eyes,
 a strong tall body and two shattered legs.
He is gasping, choking off most of the screams,
his eyes rolled up into his head.

No-o-! he screams, lifting his hands.
Despite the Hoffman devices,
the metal spikes driven into bone fragments
and joined on the outside by rods,
the open wounds packed with gauze,
he arches his body until
he is resting on top of his head.
The muscles in his legs are spasming.
His wounds have just been debrided—
scraped clean—and for the first time,
the only time, the pain and his fear
are beyond his ability to control.
Don't touch me.

Just your face, Matt.
Listen to me, let me help you.
(Oh God, help this child, comfort him.)
My thumbs stroke hard
from the corners of his eyes
across to their outer edges
and reach the hollows at his temples
where my index and middle fingers press
in a steady circular motion.

Breathe, Matt, breathe slowly,
in through the nose, out through the mouth,
in, one, two, three ... Out ... slowly.
Slowly, Matt, good. (Father, have mercy on us.)
My fingers find the pressure points,
the little hollows along the hairline,

161

pressing them, stroking circles,
move down to the hollow above
the bridge of the nose, down ...
Another spasm hits and I lose him.

Matt, breathe, listen to me:
Don't fight the pain: let it happen.
Walk straight into the pain
and you will come through it
and it will be behind you.
Breathe, Matt. Walk into the pain.
Let it happen to you.
My thumbs stroke the dark circles
under his eyes, the muscles of the cheeks ...

He is sweating. That is good.
Matt's face is my whole world.
His breathing is mine.
I feel that his mouth is dry,
ask for swabs and clean the dessicated tongue.
Sweat is standing on my face,
running down my sides. I can
no longer lean over the guard rail,
let it down, putting
my right knee on the bed:
he gasps, but doesn't scream.
Breathe, Matt, in, one, two ...
(Fill me so that I may fill him.
My fingers find the hollow
at the tip of the nose, beneath it,
in his chin, press the earlobes.

He is breathing through his nose now,
his teeth unclenched.
We have been through waves of pain
as cyclical as a woman's labor.
The morphine which couldn't work
before is working now. He says,
I feel another pain.
It is not so bad as before,
three, four, five.

Suddenly, it is over.
Matt is relaxed, a little stoned,
almost asleep, his face dry and rosey.

His mother and father move to the bedside,
an RN and the supervisor are behind me:
I hadn't seen them there.
The resident, delayed in the OR,
comes in with more morphine
which isn't needed now.
Over an hour has passed
imploded into one moment.
I walk out of the room
into the too-bright nursing station.
It is time to go to the place
where I live—
I have already been home tonight.

Paul Martin

THE DELICATE BOAT
(A Prayer for Fritz)

The stillness of morning.
Through the open windows
only the dove's soft weeping as I wash my brother's face
and prepare to shave him.
He lies back in the pillow
and closes his eyes
and I look at his broken body
and see, in his sunken chest and the deep pelvis,
in the high arch of his hips
and the raised curved ribs, the slender,
delicate boat, so perfectly crafted,
waiting.
Along its sides the silent waters
are lapping.
Christ, all he could, he has done.
Let the waters rise,
let them rise and lift him
drift him free of this troubled shore.

Ruth Brinton

I OWN THIS TRUTH

This body
with her cover
easily cut,
torn,
abraded,
burned,
with her ridiculous
needs to eat,
to sneeze,
to sweat, push out
waste, stay warm,
her constant
vulnerability
to viruses, bacteria
and trauma, colds and cramps
and winter flu.
And yet this body usually
can get me where I need
to go; she walks,
she talks, she gazes
out the window and reports,

"Blue sky and sun. Three wisps of cloud
crossing under white, daylight moon.
Squirrel running the fence,
bird feeder empty and laurel hedge
needs a trim. Apricot tree starting
to drop leaves, toes are cold" and this pencil,
warm in my hand, moves by fits
and starts of thought,
the locomotion making manifest
possession of the scene outside
the window, the eyes that bring it in,
the hands translating scene to symbol,
physical to metaphor, this solid body
I call home, this body serving me,
body I serve, coming into her own
by gathering a body of the details

eyes and ears, fingers, tongue collect,
body of perception, knowledge, memory,
kaleidoscope arrangements I own,
abandon, own again—words I learn,
forget, then find again when need compels
and re-claim as my own.

Marian Steele

TRAUMA CLINIC

Code Purple, as in bruises.
Casts covered with graffiti,
once blinding white, now grayish,
with only a bluish foot or hand extruded.
A maze of crutches crisscrosses the aisles.
A welter of wheelchairs,
powered by sullen attendants,
or miraculously motorized and mobile,
their inhabitants of color.
The signs are bilingual, "No fumar ..."
All stare unseeing at the complex-patterned linoleum floor,
except when casting surreptitious glances
at nearby stone-clad limbs—
encased injuries probably exceeding in severity
their own.
Somnolent, for the names being called
are never their own,
they dream of walking, maybe even flying.

Berwyn Moore

RECOVERY ROOM

Something like a huge hand
presses against my chest
to keep me from rising.
Voices cluster above me,
slow and wet, my own voice
sludging heavily through water.
No one hears me.
A large shadow moves quickly,
scattering angles of cold blue light,
leans so close a sleeve
scrapes across my cheek.
I reach for a hand,
but my arms do not move.
I smell metal,
antiseptic and dull,
and the pale blue walls fold in,
arc over my head.

Darkness swallows the air
and I somersault through a cave,
toes knicking the cold stone,
and I think: this must be death,
one long, dizzying fall,
the body hurling itself in painless suspension,
fingers curling against the pull of spin,
histories spiraling toward a single point,
a blue light, unreachable, illuminating nothing.

I rise to a circle of yellow light,
trees dripping with rain,
hickory, sweetgum, delicate ash,
bark graced with lichen,
leaves spreading like open hands,
the air humming with morning cicadas,
and there, standing in the spray of new light,
a fawn, waiting to enter.
I feel a tugging on my foot.
Someone has come to claim me.

James Snydal

LIVING IN AMERICA

It is true fortitude to stand firm against
All shocks of fate, when cowards faint and die
In fear to suffer more calamity.
From *The Roman Actor*
by Philip Massinger (1626)

1

Accident

I carry Hemingway's memoirs and stroll down
a familiar sidewalk. Repairmen are working close.
This is summer: lawns are green again.
On Saturday and Sunday, I will hold
a party to honor the season. Now, though, I walk
to look for work. Seven stories up,
someone kicks an angle iron off
a narrow and wobbling plank. It strikes my skull.

Thousands of miles from bullrings, thousands of miles
from a worthy death, someone dials for help.
My brain splatters the grass. Ambulance wheels
rush toward me. I bleed on blooming flowers.
Months later, I rest in a hospital bed.
I believe that, soon, I shall be less weary.

2

Sleeping In A Hospital Bed

A dead friend talks to me.
He says this building is run by Sears.
He had stayed here after his accident.
He says that I should leave
to save my life.
They had made him run
all over these halls for a living.
Now, they are making me go
everywhere by myself

in a wheelchair during the days.
He tells me I should leave.

3

Remembering What Had Been

One of the bosses from my last job comes
to see me. His mother had told him of my health
crisis. A local paper had said my story.
I'm sorry to hear him, having lost that job:
I'd sold sandwiches for a living, but
had broken rules.

        My wife and I once
had problems, so I'd started seeing a girl
from work. The bosses said I wasn't supposed to.
I met her for drinks. I met her mother and father.
I met her husband. I even staged a party.
I lost my job. Now, a boss is with me.

After he leaves, I try to build a mental
model of the city I am living in.
I remember my daily sandwich routes,
my favorite stops, even my customers.

I wish the woman who used to be my wife would visit.

4

Having Things Wrong

One week when I wake up,
I think I am my dad.
He's lived a long life, building a fortune
making his business.
Doctors tell me I am wrong,
I'm not my father,
I am myself.

I don't believe them.
I telephone the woman who used to be

my wife. She's busy working: her line is unhooked.
I call my sister because the doctors bother me.

She is glad I'm calling, but then
gets angry.
She says that I am wrong.
She says I'm not my dad.
She says I am myself.

I don't know what is going on.
I get warm under my covers.

5

Hospital Roommates

I hardly know who Ivan is.
A fishing boat he ran
went down. He almost drowned.
His brain was hurt forever.

When doctors send him away,
they fill his bed with Tom,
who'd jumped from the third story of a building
but lived.
Doctors labor for months
to make Tom's body work a little,
then send him to a mental institution.
I am still in bed.
I hear him holler, then scream.
No nurse will go with him.

6

All The Time

Each day, I see the same hills
sitting in the same window.
Each night, I spill coffee on the same
floor. Someone always cleans the floor.

Evenings, I gulp two glasses
of coffee and sip some Seven Up.
I believe that I shall be less weary.
Because I always make loud burps
when taking phenobarbital,

I call those little white pills great
burp-it-all. I wet my bed
so an orchestra I dream can play.

7

Recovering

I sleep in a tidy bed, yet dream
I am breakfasting on a shady hill
in Hiroshima. The atomic bomb
is going to drop today. I wake.
Doctors tell me not to worry.

I sleep again. White
light seems everywhere.
A doctor sits at her desk
and writes letters. Glass
from windows shreds her skin.
People start to walk,
but vomit, then die in parks.
With their eyebrows burnt away
and eyes melted, they stink.
Pus oozes down drains at a corner.
From under my comfortable quilt,
I think I see daylight darken
with dust. There is wind.
Flowers from a dress
burn onto a wall. Poles
from lights fall along
with raindrops as big as marbles.

I wake. My gums begin to bleed
less. I brush my teeth and talk
with a lady. She says she nurses to make
a living. Somebody else is a nurse
to be of use. I argue with each
over the hospital's work. They say
it does its job. Snow is falling.

I visit with the woman who used to be
my wife. I balance on my legs
for hours, alive in America.

Peter Viereck

AT MY HOSPITAL WINDOW
(for Joseph Brodsky)

*Sick people ... need a literature of their own.... A critical illness
is one of our momentous experiences; yet I haven't seen a single
nonfiction book that does it justice.*
Anatole Broyard, *N.Y. Times Books,* April 1, 1990.

The sublime as the artistic conquest of the horrible.
Nietzsche

PART ONE

1. *Sacred Wood*

Land of shy kindnesses and embarrassing stains.
Land of appraising stares and starched white stance.
Like cameras that reverse their glance
To photograph their cameraman's
Own face, own smirked disgrace,
These thousand hungry hospital windows graze
On us as if our nerves were grass.
Here the Boojum Snark of the childhood to which we regress
Is the Conquerer Germ. Its hunters, face muffled with gauze,
Are the surgeons. You'd never guess
They're really white blood cells in surgeon-white togas.
With gaze of Argus,
These phagocyte cops—in their bogus
Biped disguise—
Are gumshoeing after our cargoes
Of germ in blood's archipelagoes.
As sunlessly pale as a fungus,
We breathe the air-conditioned poison gas
Of progress. In such Freudian vertigoes,
Disinfectants are stern superegoes.
    And our ids? They're the rats, down where the garbage goes.

* * *

Land—no, cocoon—where butterflies unhinge
(Regressing into caterpillars) wings.
Land of droll metaphors: doc says of gut,

173

"You've got a garden hose I've got to cut."
Snip snip—he solves me like a Gordian knot.
When he claims I look young, is gut's inmost decay
My Picture of Dorian Grey?
Come praise—more than "the dignity of man"—
The faced indignity; go clear-eyed down.
When even charm and status face the deadpan
Smirk of the bedpan, indignity
Is the great leveler.
Outside our lair,
That surreal clown, Mr. Reality,
Taunts "loss"—the word's my leitmotif today.
I've seen lost beauty; the patina went away
Not altogether.
I've seen lost awe; the wonder went astray
Not too far to regather.
In the sacred wood of losers, still some tatter
Of loved-enough loss must stay.
"All's illusion"—still some there is really there.
… And yet what's there, no matter what its form,
Crashes. "So be it." Share
Leftovers; dregs matter; some ashes
    Warm.

2. *Sacroiliac*

Must we blubber at death (what a dowdy gaffe)
Or counterclown instead?
Uneasy (it only hurts when we laugh)
Lies the clown that wears a head.
All patients have jitters—O isn't that why
Our cocktails are bitters, our whiskey is wry?
"O.R." (I looked it up) means "owner's risk" and / or
"Operation room": court of last appeal
("Doc, what odds I'll live till April")
When odds appal.
Hospital: a nation. Where the buildings inhabit the people.
Where tender-loving-Medi-care reigns papal.
Where, when I sleep, my nurse-spy-pal
Wakes me to give me my sleeping pill.
Hospital: a campus the fund raisers propel.
Where Pain is dean in regal purple
And Angst his flunky prof and I their flunking pupil.

I complain? Yet I scorn—all the more when the lines are mine—
    Confessional verse's professional moan.

* * *

Enough fluff. Only elementals hone
Simultaneously brow and sacroiliac zone.
Elementals hurl the elements;
Flesh is the beach their hone-waves drench
With sea's—with bloodstream's—undulance.
Waves and moonrays, back and forth.
Rays work waves as tongue works tooth.
Armor for continuities:
Rays as frail as gold-thread gowns,
Stored in old trunks for granddaughters by crones:
Stored powers, veiled as frailties.
Far voice (seeping through from worlds more unreal, more true):
"Don't tease elementals—nobody paws
Buzzsaws. Tide can't be shushed."
Oh yes it can: my tideproof window screen
As earplug. Here I'm stashed
Soundproof inside when the hone-waves pound.
Sick, safely sick, in walls a gut-length thick
And fever-tall, by anesthesias guarded,
I'd "bet my life" (a harmless cliché I don't really mean)
That I'll never again hear tide.
       Far voice: "Bet recorded."

    3. *Sacre de Printemps*

Just once
To be one with the dew on the leaf, with the sun's
Autograph on the dew.—
No! Too "nature" simper. Too
Poesie. Outside my window's
Real-world prose,
What aresenic-colored plague resumes its tour,
What verdant saboteur?
The blithe metastasis of May
Is spreading the recidivist gangrene
Called "spring," its tumors flowering.
Their sweet pus lures, they bud and preen;
Wing'd pimps reel round the brew.
Bees poke each flower, as they're gened to do.

175

But bees can't hump my sickroom's rose bouquet
(Its chastity belt is the window screen)
Telegraphed by true friends too important to come.
I'm a vase for a poppy of rosier bloom,
My blood its sap, my meat its loam.
A shot of morphine its opium,
     Its garden the surgery room.

    4. Sacrilege

Above the border that's the neck's,
Senility stages less bloody a bout:
An optic test. *Fiat lux* or *fiat nox*?
My eye scans fadeless CAT-scans of my eye;
Says fader to fadeless, "Do I flunk or sneak by?"
Says metal to jelly, "Prognosis: lights out.
Cataracts gone amok."
Comes nurse; one hand holds my water mug,
The other a vacuum cleaner *de luxe*
To vacuum the mess on my rug
From the "previous tenant," now cinders in morgue;
Fiat Electrolux.
Nurse—water—to toast who got toasted. No, stop!
Those dentures he'd lost and got furnaced without,
they're bobbing—stop pouring—like crabs down and up
(Clack clack) in the water jug.
At once I recognize Grim Jack
The Reaper's style of joke,
Half merry jig, half crying jag,
With *humeur noire* his pet gag.
Straight down like the sun at the equinox,
His scythe gleams overhead. My neck's
Already feeling the first teasing nicks.
"Judge Reaper," I shout, "when your gavel knocks,
Why is your verdict on plea bargains 'nix'?
From hospitals to hospices, Old Nick's
Scythe connects.
Yet gentle sorceries, found in no almanacs,
Rhyme's whispering web, mild garden nooks,
The on-target quip, the just gibe, the human-scale knacks,
Shapeliness (in thought or in carved onyx)
Defuse your nukes.
I've hide-and-seek burrows you'll never annex,
A poise that no longer panics."

—"Your exorcist-spells of slant-rhyme knickknacks
Are duds," death cackles. "To hide from my *nox*
(Since Thanatos' mother is night-goddess NYX)
Is SACRILEGE. Here I come. Ready or—
Not."
I need help quick—I invoke on the spot
My anti-death "her":
"You life-core of ocean, creatrix long hidden,
Half soother of storm, half stormy harridan,
      Don't let your clown-priest down."

5. Sanctuary

Enter (what price santuary?) a new kind of showdown.
Invoking my her, I've unleashed from history's den
Surf's very first hone-hug of dune.
Just when I'd fled from tragedy into farce
(And wanted to bask there like fops in cafés)
What's this unwanted tidal fuss?
I fear it, I trust her, I can't refuse;
Elementals return and claim their sacrifice.
She's all the world's seas, I'm suddenly all the world's surface.
Out of control; my lines not mine; all's cleft or cliff, her fierce
Full emptiness or penisula's counterforce.
Revise that; not "or" but "and"; in my new cycle's phase,
Her seas *and* my shores—O nothing less—suffice.
Polarities: sparring face to face
Without bodies—till lusts fuse foes.
Are we pipe dreams of opposite fictions, embodied only as pairs?
Ta-TUM-ing—into existence—each other, my iams and hers?
Whole continents, pounded by seesawing pistons,
Their mist in the distance a fading oasis,
Are crumbling between us. Only the spray's
Shapliness stays.
Strength isn't hard lone rocks that surf erases
But fragile intertwining laces,
These sand-probed bays, these salt-probed beaches:
Both reshaped by what they're shaping,
Each the player and the plaything,
Neither wholly sea or land.
Fleshed mutualness, each reached by what it reaches,
Shares Holy Land.
These my shares and these my riches
      Till the third Fate's fatal shears.

6. *Sacred Ode*

Right now as I talk, are her seas, are my shores
Straitjackets we burst when we sleepwalk?
Straitjackets? The hospital really a loony
Bin for the love-curs'd?
We inmates acting out hang-ups as "therapy theater"?
Asleep, let's escape—let's clamer toward Luna—
Let's eke real-life theater from farce
By love's sheer force.
Done! Like champagne corks our souls pop up with a fizz.
Safe till we wake into prose, right now do we teeter
On tightropes of moon-pull as if they were stairs?
No! No to such a romantical saga.
Once more my fantasies totter
Toward poesie-mush unawares.
We lovers, we shores and seas, neither godly nor gaga,
We're down-to-earth matter, true poetry's meter,
The resonance of my odes, the undulance of her doze,
Oneness from twos.
Ashamed—O they cloy—of woe-is-me hospital blues,
I'm starting an ode of stark joy
To her whose cavernous darkness lights my dark:
"Life-code of surf-sob, hear your landlocked landfish;
Will you shield me from the Reaper till I finish?"
　　　　Her voice (or is it my echo?) answers, "Finish!"

*　*　*

And when my ode's ripened, when reap-time is due,
What then?
Then it's you, you-my-her, I'll be reaped into.
Beached mapless from sea lap, still panting for water,
I'll then be scythed home to the foam
Your famous giddy daughter blossomed from.
Sea older than goddesses: grandma of algae,
Globe's first fecundity
Midwifed by silver [1]
Forceps of Luna.
Then I, a twitch of that primal shiver,
Will join all your flotsam, all bobbing in chorus,
My ode your metronome's sonorus quiver.
(Wheel of Fortuna, spin slow till I end my rhyme.)

Then I'll "step twice in the same river,"
Ebbing my time-wheel backward in time
From my lungfish-ancestor's beachhead to birth's first arena.
　　　Then, vulva of Unda Marina, sway me the tide of the dead.

PART TWO

7. *Sacred Code*

All my life is a search: to hear—to decipher—her source.
I track her Morse through the inland lurch
Of sea in seed's underground bells.
"Depth" and "death" sound alike; how infer
Which undertow counter-tracks me from afar?
(Near is the morgue's crematorium-belch, getting rid
Of its diet in hiccups of red.)
No message emergent; I've eavesdropped in vain
On the musical migraine of shells,
Gull's cryptic cacophony, salmon's steep road
To *Liebestod.* —Suddenly
I hear her. I hear her far breakers, resurgent
(Or is it the morgue belching nearer?).
She's throbbing throb-throbbing a message most urgent
　　　In a code I cannot read.

8. *Unsacrosanct*

Can abstract set up shop behind shingles
Announcing, "I'm really concrete"?
Can ideas dance on physical sandals
With metaphysical feet?
Though your seas pulse a touchable sonance,
They can be deconstructed by savants
As a trope my need carved from air.
Though waves tinkle cymbals, they're really tide's symbols,
Not meat but metaphor.
Your vitality has no resemblance
To vita. Your there is un-there.
—And yet (refuting what I've said so far)
Your un-there of pheromones sends the old signals,
those brine-stings of senses in gene-mingle seasons,
　　　That nose-eye-ear tangle, the musk of brute fur.

* * *

179

Land can't escape, you're its breath, you're its broth.
Stealing your froth, I too brew a spell;
My sound waves, they too can compel.
            (Compel? There's an Eden earliness,
            As if song were invented this morning,
            When kindred sounds of unkindred meaning
            Meet in rhyme's assignation motel.
            They embrace in a balcony-scene duet
            Of three. The third is the poet.)
Ignore my parenthetic ego trip—
But not our complicity: flesh-tuners both, dear sea trope.
I tuning with ink, you with bath;
I micro—you macro—musician.
You scan me with brine tweak; with rhyme beep I scan
You right back.—Or reversed? Which first?
Who whom? And did "will be" or "was"
Make creation's first skyrocket zoom?
We earth bums, we flukes of a rogue gene's birth,
It's we who hatched Big Bang. [2]
The bang was a hearerless boom, the world a scam,
Not even a trickster to blame,
Till nested in conscious "I am."
Creation? Brow's spasms outwomb
All merely cosmic merely immortal loins.
Parental world-sea, you're my oversized
Baby, anthropomorphized by these very lines.
And now that you're lessened, unsacrosanct, down from
      "*l'amor*
Che move il sole" to sunny wee loans
Of warmth on my windowpane lens,
I love you not less but touchably-humanly more—
        While on his scythe my waiting reaper leans.

9. *Safe Inland*

Hospital. Back from my sea trip (*if* that's where I've been).
Spring's rampage is back at my window screen.
Last night some kind of solitary Reaper
(That phrase, a quaint Wordsworthian sound)
Haunted my trip. It's good to reap grain. Why did I scream?
It's good I woke up, safe inland and undrowned—
Except that there's no inland and there's seaweed in my hair.
The breakers the breakers, they're far off, not here—
Except that some arms reach far.

Well, back to work; now I'll finish—
What was it I told her I'd finish?
And who was "her"? And where
Did I lay my glasses? Age's memories blur.
More about ocean—it's one big briny tear,
Fed by the tears our tightwad eye-banks owe
The dead and are slow to shed.
Will finny bill collectors gouge from our dunned sockets
Our salt debts?
Unda marina, rocked by moon's penumbra,
     Cradle my slumber when breakers break over my head."

* * *

A visiting bore once disrupted
(*Flagrante delicto*) a doped poet's hug of the muse.
I, pain-killer-drugged, have my own Xanadus,
Daily cut short by some do-gooder's "have a good day."
Then how may I salvage hopes unharvested?
Ormolu or-mo-lu—there's my answer to loss.
The sound of the word—look it up if you must—is its gloss
(In both senses of "gloss"). Its rhythm, more vibrant than gongs,
Relumes our loss's obtunded bronze
With gold—well, almost gold—of ormolu.
Interruption: now brine (or more illusion, mere rain?)
Is pelting me. Bard crowned with seaweed, not laurel,
I'm summoned by seas crowned with treacherous coral. Who
Crossed the bleak tundra of my windowpane?
I'm a pond-skimming pebble no brakes can encumber.
I'm ringed by Marina's rotunda; pelt harder.
I'm nearing—to drown or reach haven?—her harbor.
No answer? I'm hurtling too headlong to hamper.
     Unda, where's to, where to?

10. *Sacerdotal*

Overhead next day from a goodhearted underpaid nurse's aide:
"Wet again. Like he vanishes somewheres for secret swims.
Between you and I, he got them so vexed
They morphined him to stop his—can geezers that old have wet
dreams?
It figures the drugs are what grew
Sea guck on his scalp—that's science for you.
     I declare, what'll they think of next?

181

* * *

After the needle jabbed my hide,
I levitated from the operating slab and prophesied,
"Gadgets have wronged the elementals—beware.
You all are retractable breaths of salt air.
The gills of the sea, they'll re-inhale the soul of the land,
Leaving it blank-eyed. Mind will end."
… Puffed up with this Cassandra venture,
I hear—clack clack—a new tormenter,
My cindered predecessor's missing denture,
Chortling, "I nip your heels when your hubris tugs.
The moths are at your sacerdotal togs.
Gold was brow's goal, gut's rot has made it dross."
      Watch me shape shapely silver from gold's loss.

    11. *Sacrament*

Days passed. Am now sealed from all the blurs I forgot.
I've safe daydreams if not "a good day." But:
Where stillborn futures are kept, where "almost" is stowed,
There's some one I owe an ode. Blurred belovéd, accept—
As an inept lover's caress—
Unfinishedness. Invent
A new Sacrament, the sharing of leftovers,
The unholy Communion of the unfulfilled.
… Once I willed to go down clear-eyed.
Now my bleary eyes are glued
To spring's window. Have a good
Bye. Where's sea? My only tide
Is my catheter bag and my I.V. pouch:
My two ebb-flow machines.
Plugged into gimmicks of expensive ouch,
      I squint gray cataracts at what regreens.

             (1988-1992)

NOTES

1. S. Lem: "Life should start only in aqueous solutions of certain chemical compounds....the frequent but gentle produced by the tital ebb and flow, caused by the moon, hastened the protobiogenesis in these solutions."

2.   "The universe needs us in order to exist.... Has the universe required the future observer to empower past genesis? ... The observer is as essential to the creation of the universe as the universe is to the creation of the observer."

John Archibald Weaver, cosmologist.

Henry Langhorne

LOOK FOR MARTINS

The tubes in my body still hurt
Doctors frown at my chart
A swollen novel of failure
Blood drips through
My plastic link with life
Voices fade from blurred faces
Floating over the cold rail

If my arms were free
I would open the window
And let the smell escape
I would walk outside
Sprinkle fresh dirt on my feet
Stand under the live oak
Wait for the purple martin

Sue Saniel Elkind

IN THE WOODS

I leave the hospital room
walk to the woods
in the rain
where wet leaves fall
into other leaves
where he loved to talk—
this man, my son.

Now he lies still
not yet waking to
wave upon wave of light;
not yet coming back to us.

I want to hear the doctor
say he'll be fine.
I want to call Rabbi Jacob
hear him recite, without stumbling,
the twenty-third psalm backward.
I want him to tell me
my son will be fine.

I want to see his man-boy face shine
like a face card.
I want to see his joy again
like an arc of light
dazzling
as he watches his first born
take her first step.

I stop, kneel
in these leaves
and pray.

Sue Saniel Elkind

I WANT TO KNOW WHY

Every time I'm sick
I feel like a child
caught committing a misdeed.
I'm the one in pain,
yet I am the little girl
on trial before her father:
for having stolen her sister's watch,
for having killed her own chick by drowning,
the young woman who returned from her prom,
the sun her escort, dress torn, dignity, too,
the young woman whose father lined up three
liquor bottles in her room like soldiers
before a firing squad, bottles he found
on the front lawn after a party.
(It wasn't her fault someone brought liquor.)
Why now, when I'm an old woman, do I feel guilty
because I didn't make dinner for my husband,
who understands, but becomes my father,
and once again I'm on trial. Once again
I'm naked as when I was born, naked
as an old lady's gums, naked as I plead
understand
        please
          love me.

Tina Marie Conway

MY MOTHER AS A CHILD

I row my mother as a child across
the lake. Pixie haircut, fist tucked
under chin, she dangles

toes in water. In another time,
she could be aristocracy, an artist's
model: parasol overhead, cradling

a porcelain doll. Now ribs like
frets hug her cotton gown, leggings
torn and puckered

at her ankles. The sun above us
round and yellow, a hot coal
on my back.

Only I know what is in store—one
breast lost to cancer, forceps scar
her first born—and the weight

of memory keeps both oars circling.
My mother offers her hand, lean
and quaint. In my roomy palm

she places a history unimagined
for herself. A thick breeze prods
us close to shore.

Mary R. DeMaine

SIX DAYS

Thursday

One instant, she snaps the x-ray
onto her light box. The next,
my head feels like it has been
slammed into a brick wall.
On display is my right breast
immobilized, illuminated, invaded
by a sinister black arrow, its
point focusing on a small spot
just behind the squashed nipple.
She measures for another x-ray.
Informs me I must embrace that
tortuous machine a second time.
The pain sucks my breath from me,
but I am too numb to cry out.
Somewhere in the deepest recess
of my mind, a dirge begins: is,
isnot, is, isnot, is, isnot, is....

Friday

My restlessness wakes him early.
He turns over and nuzzles his
face against my neck, expecting
me to roll on him as I always
do when I rouse him before dawn.
Seeing I'm not moving, he circles
the nipple of my left breast
with the palm of his hand, asks
how it went with the doctor, no
doubt assuming I want to talk
first. I breathe slowly, deeply.
Prepare to tell him that which
I had skillfully avoided last
night by going to bed before he
came home from his meeting.
I say, as calmly as I can,
the radiologist found a spot

on the x-ray. He kisses my
breasts and laughs. For years,
we have shared the same joke.
Whenever I go to the doctor
for a routine check-up, I come
home insisting I have some
exotic illness that will
require abstinence from my
share of the housework,
days of special pampering.
He takes my face in his hands
and begins to gently kiss me,
but my agitation tells him
I am not teasing this time.
We lie for a long time crying.

Saturday

Yester-
day lies
buried
in
night-
mares.
Today,
I will
keep a
tight
rein
on my
mind.
There
will be
no acci-
dental
straying
into
the
dark
abyss
of my
imagin-
ation

where
terror
skulks
hungry
for a
chance
to
tear
any
 hope
it
finds
into
shreds.

Sunday

Today is my mother's family reunion.
All my aunts, uncles, cousins; my
cousins' children and their children's
children have filled the park pavilion.

I am determined to talk with each one
of them, even the babies, before day's
end. I want to reminisce about my
childhood. To remember everything.

I tell my cousin Marlys' children about
the day she coaxed me into their pig barn
and one of the sows bolted, ran between
my legs, took me for a piggyback ride.

I'm chiding her for being a stinker when
my sister Fran reminds me of the day I
coaxed her to the top of a tree and left her
there, unable to get down by herself.

My cousin Doris informs everyone she
got a spanking and was sent to bed for a
whole afternoon after I'd talked her
into going swimming in a mud puddle.

Aunt Vollie tells the kids about the
day I got my sister, Carol, to ride
her trike down a flight of stairs after
I'd already ironed both of my hands.

Of course, my mother reminds me
I had to be tied to my bed at night
so I wouldn't crawl out of my crib,
sneak out the window, into the street.

We all laugh as the stories continue
and when tears gather in my eyes and
they think it's from laughing, I
refuse to spoil their day with truth.

Monday

There is a path worn through my house
around the living room down into the basement
into the upstairs around my desk
where correspondence deadlines so important last week
no longer have any relevance
I pace and watch the hands on the clock
dragging their way around and around
the telephone rings every hour I pick it up
tell him I haven't heard from the doctor
he's getting upset demanding I call her to find out
I keep putting it off I know I will regret this when
it comes time to get through the night
but I cannot bring myself to pick up the telephone
and call her

Tuesday

I call the doctor's office.
She hasn't come back from
the weekend yet. I explain.
The receptionist promises
she will call today, not when
though....

I wait, pacing over the same
path as the day before, examining
and re-examining everything.
At last the call comes. The
doctor says she understands
I've had quite a scare. Her
voice has the casual sound of
someone who has seen hundreds
of women with breast cancer.

Mary R. DeMaine

She tells me the radiologist says
it's a protein deposit. She's sorry
if I was unnecessarily worried.
I want to tell her exactly what I've
been through, but I can't. I'm too
too busy repeating, thank you.

Michael Dennis Browne

YOU WON'T REMEMBER THIS

for Peter and Mary and Nellie

1.

You lift your arms to your head,
which looks so dark, then turn
to lie on your side, the fluid
swilling in your abdomen.
The radiologist says:

"Anything dark is liquid,
anything white is muscle,
anything gray is bone."

These like the moon pictures,
wavering, grainy, the lens
lurching, and again you turn;
that shadowy bulb is your head,
those snow streaks your muscles,
those blurred tundras your bones.

  you won't remember this

At ten days
you look lonely.
You seem between countries.

You look at me briefly,
not with interest.
You give no sign.

I toss you shreds of song
to where you lie,
down in the cradle canyon,
looking up.

Remote to you my moon
drifts over the rim.

You lie,
looking up.

  you won't remember this

You don't want to go
to day-care today; you weep,
you cling to my leg,

193

you roll your eyes:
oh no on no; all the sorrows
of my mother in my daughter.

   you won't remember this

I hear a moaning from upstairs;
slowly you descend—*whooo whooo whooo*—
over your head the nibbled blanket;
on the last tread trip, topple
—*oops! ooops!* —
and I gather up my ghost.

   you won't remember this

Yesterday you set up a stall on a table,
invited us to buy. "How much is *this?*" we asked.
"About ten hundred," you said, frowning
at a pair of plastic feet.

Daily you bring us gifts with a shy face
and watch us while we open them—
say a box with a wooden lid and in it
your yellow hairbrush, scraps of paper or card
with your green and blue coloring on them—
they're maps, you say, of the ocean, the sky.
Sometimes pictures we've cut out for you
that now you give back, wide-eyed
at our delight in getting them from you.
Daily you assemble such treasures and appear.

   you won't remember this

2

Cresting the stony hill, the edge of England,
   and there was the sea,
the holiday town our parents brought us to
   when I was fourteen.
I found the dunes where we'd tumbled,
   swam in those waves again,
the breakers forever rolling in
   from the new world.
Such a boy I was then, all aware
   of myself in the waves
but now the salted element itself
   and look, so many the swimmers.

At the country pub, sitting
   on the same stone wall

but now with Peter, six, and still
    the leafy pulse of wood doves—
Hoo HOO Hoo, Hoo HOO Hoo—
    I wonder how I could want them back,
who are done with the human.
    Let them go.
Hoo HOO Hoo. Hoo HOO Hoo.

Heading home, we'd drive the moth-thick dark,
    wind-burned and dreamy,
both of them leading us in songs,
    easeful baritone, meticulous soprano,
and we'd chorus on,
    the waves, the doves, the gulls, the hedgerows
flashing inside us
    as we slid toward sleep.

And here my mother's little notebook now,
    its English addresses and numbers,
("Is it alphabetical, darling?" I asked her.
    "*Alphabetical?*"),
her late-night wartime notes to my father,
    (at last we're sleeping),
some of my father's letters to her,
    some to *his* father:
"As I walk the streets of the City—*your* city—
    when I hear old tunes, oh! in so many other ways
which my poor pen cannot describe,
    I think of you constantly."

Love beyond naming, what will we keep
    when we've let go of all remembering,
what can we know when we've relinquished
    all rooms, all limbs, all breathing?
Gardens of daughters, and sons we've tended
    and must leave, remember?
Lips and foreheads we will still want to kiss
    when we've no mouths for kissing,
remember?

3

Night. Night light. Now you are sleeping,
far from our own childhoods, deep in yours.
Nothing, loves, to remember,
no day, no street, no sky,
only rooms scribbled on water,

voices chasing voices down corridors
of seas, all the old cargoes
rolling. Unless we become as you,
we won't enter.

In such a sleep as this,
when all day is forgotten and runs
like a river under the skull, dividing
and tumbling up a million tributaries,
when the air is all words and leaves,
the garages adrift, the old barns wandering,
and even the careful stones are unstrung,
then, mother, then, father, go into
the dream with them, where the grief
we are separate is not known, till even
Abraham is understood, who would have
let go his son.

As you laugh, children, as you cry out
in your sleep, as you are blind,
as you are ghosts to the day
(though I love the days),
as the tongue has nothing to tell,
slumped like a beast on straw,
as the wine of the crushed days
spills and the ripe clocks burst,
releasing their seeds to the air,
then like climbers roped by the silks
of sleep, fragrant with the dreams
and forgetting of those mists,
we wander together.
Unless we become as you, we won't enter,
who have forgotten what the world will be,
to swim with you that dark unmaking
where the new life forms.

4

Someone should tell the dreamer to rise.
A day's begun that needs you; stir the fire.
Sleepers for sure, and soon, will need you,
swaying or stumbling down the stairs.
Hoo HOO Hoo. Hoo HOO Hoo.
Liquid, muscle, bone. Hold them.
Go with them into the day.

Gerald Stern

THE SACRED SPINE

It will always be invisible, it will
have hair on it, but that will be false,
and skin, but that will be stretched over
the branches like a sweater dipped in alum.
It will hang from the mouth
like a piece of paper or a large caterpillar.
It will twist over doubly
like a ravenous birch.
It will lie rigid.
It will scream out,
trying to find a position.
It will turn in pain,
trying to escape, trying to release
itself, trying to live again
without fear and exhaustion,
trying to float once more, trying to rest, trying to rise
in the fine dust and the feathers,
in the wet leaves and the grass and the flowers,
on the bleached wood and the pillows and the warm air
and the weeds and the water.

Joyce Odam

THE ADDICTION

I have survived one day without you.
I am strong.

Today the sun is real.
The wind is not rising.
The cries of the crow are sharp
and my ears are deep.
I do not hunger for you and this
surprises me.
Whatever name you were
I do not speak.

I make one tally
on the calendar.

Susana Gomes

ADDICTED

I am not like I was before. For many years I had suspected that experience, not time was the herald of change. I was right.

It is hard for me to believe that this difference in myself is really there. And to anyone else, this thing that has happened to me is just another unfortunate incident.

Maybe it was. But I understand it differently.

I remember laying on something very hard, like a sidewalk. Momentarily, I thought I was dead. I wasn't sure of anything. I would be surrounded by darkness, then be astonished by beautiful colors. But I was alive. My lungs were expanding and collapsing. The air they sucked was arctic cold.

Soft pink light that gave the impression of being florescent, made it hard for me to open my eyes. Between my lashes I saw a beautiful girl. She had smooth skin the color of ivory. Her eyes were large and black; shaped like a bird's. I think I was still asleep when I saw her. There were other faces too, but when I try to remember, they're only shadows.

My head hurt. My stomach hurt. My hands and feet hurt but I couldn't do anything about any of it. I was angry, guilty, ashamed and relieved all at once. I was being swirled in a whirlpool of emotion. Emotions that were similar in potency to those I had experienced the night before.

Daryl was supposed to be at my house at eight, but he was late again. I waited in the living room for him. My mother was there. She was planted in front of the TV set. Her sagging eyes were barely aware of the images flickering before them. Occasionally she managed to blink when the light became too intense.

My mother was a sad person. She had not had much of a life—stupid people seldom do—and therefore did not have much to inspire her children. My mother was nice, but she was not intelligent. She was a lazy person. She figured that nothing bad would ever happen to her, but rotten things happen to her all the time; she's just too drunk to notice.

When I heard loud, raunchy music coming closer to my house, I knew it was Daryl. He pulled in my driveway and stopped a foot before running me over. I saw him laughing behind the wheel. He was stoned. I knew because when I sat next to him, I saw his eyes ... they were sparkling. His eyes only sparkled when he was on heroin.

We arrived at Kevin's house late. The people there were already partying. The music was really loud, but no one was dancing. Daryl and I went directly to Kevin's room. And the evening began.

The only drug I did was acid. I'm not stupid, so I stayed away from the smack Daryl did. Those tracks crawling up his arms were obvious and ugly.

Acid is clean. You can sit in the dirtiest place imaginable and it will be as clean as a hospital when you take a drop. Pure and clean, like fresh snow. Dirt and filth are afraid of the good, clean sensations acid brings. The drug sweeps over my vision like a paintbrush, and the bacteria runs from the surface of everything I see.

Sex while on acid is stupefying. Sex is better when you don't feel dirty. After his first high, Daryl would get anxious and moody. That was our signal. I reached for him as he untied his arm. This made him smile. It had been difficult to make him smile lately, but this aspect of our relationship was one he especially enjoyed. As for me, making love to Daryl stoned was one of the few things I still liked doing with him.

After, I slept a little. But it wasn't a deep, pleasant nap. I dreamed unsettling dreams. They were short and sweaty dreams of a woman calling me and a man leading me to her. She was hazy, but I got the impression that she was beautiful. She had a calmness—a serenity—that I was not familiar with. But the man was different. He wasn't fuzzy, as much as he was bright and changing, like snow on the TV. These dreams were short but disturbing enough to make me try to stay awake.

With eyes still clouded with sleep, I noticed the ceiling. It was changing. My acid wasn't working anymore. Panic set in. I knew I needed more drug. I could feel the goodness leaving me. I was being depressurized, like air escaping a pop can. I was empty.

I scrambled through my bag. It was near the bottom. Trembling I held my vice in my hands and was relieved. Pretty little gelatin capsules with paradise on the inside. To simply hold it, to have the material object in my hands calmed me. My shaking stopped as my anticipation grew.

I dropped more acid.

I waited.

I dropped more and waited again. And I dropped more. The familiar feelings did not come. My drug wasn't having any affect. The ceiling wasn't getting clean. It was turning black and rotting with bacteria. It ate away at the plaster and left a black, running saliva behind. This mucous was thick and quick moving. It gleamed like oil, or a snake's eye. It was a long stream of oily, black eyes, chained together, and it was moving toward me. In a matter of minutes, it had reached the floor.

Screaming, I hid under the blanket. I wanted to run, to hide, to get away from the dirt; but I was immobile. All the energy I could muster was consumed in voicing my fear and clinging to the blanket. I warned Daryl to get up and run. I wanted him to get away from the germ spit.

It took him a few hysterical seconds to get up, but when he did, he brought me back to my senses. He shook and slapped me back to reality, then tried to comfort me in a numb embrace. He said everything would be OK, but Daryl was unconvincing.

When I looked for it, the saliva was gone from the walls; so was the bacteria. I looked around the room trying to find where it had gone. I saw a thin trail of it leading from the ceiling, down the wall, across the carpet and up the bed. The trail was alive and moving.

It slithered its way across the bedclothes and Daryl's protective body to my navel. The filth had gotten inside of me! My belly button was acting as a funnel for the evil dirt. Oily eyes were running in my veins instead of blood. I watched as all my beautiful crimson blood was devoured by the satanic germ thing.

I could feel the oily bacteria inside my body. It had already entered my heart; it had polluted my lungs and was travelling to my brain. The vision of my brain being eaten like the ceiling had been eaten flashed before me. My brain would be nothing but a slimy, decaying peach-like mess covered in black when the germs had done their thing. Then the black would go away and I would have no brains left.

I was afraid, but still sensible. On my way out of the room, I tripped on Daryl. He woke up. I locked myself in the bathroom. Moments later, Daryl was pounding on the door: "Jesus! Cathy! What are ya doing? Get outta there ... Hey ... Hey ... Will somebody help me get this bitch outta the john ?..." He sounded cruel and hard to me.

The scissors looked clean and sterile as I aimed them toward my stomach. My plan was to make cuts in my veins so the bacteria would pour out, leaving my brain safe. The blades bit my flesh and some song from a tea bag commercial filled my head. Slicing my stomach was surprisingly easy, like cutting into a cream pie. There was no pain and the saliva poured out thickly. The next incisions were easier.

Someone had broken down the door. Daryl held me, tried to stop the blood; he couldn't believe what I had done. Someone called 911, but before the ambulance came, I had passed out.

Lying in the hospital beginning to come to, I realized that my buzz had worn off; that was why I could feel my stomach. I heard someone mention surgery and someone else painkillers, but I really didn't pay attention to that world. I felt like lead, but I longed to fly in all the emptiness I had discovered inside of me. There was a bright light inside my head. It came from behind this door. On the inside there was a beautiful man, a man from my dreams. He was clear this time, not like the bird-eyed woman. He was young and wore a robe that looked like a toga. I thought I knew who he was but then his face changed and I didn't recognize him. For a moment I thought I had seen God, but then laughed at myself. So I ignored the light and the changing man and let myself drift to the darkness where I wanted to fly.

The more I walked into the darkness, the more lonely I felt. Occasionally I would see people I once knew, or images I recognized; but they were all unclear, as if I were seeing them through an ice cube.

And the light was always after me. It was hot and blinding. I wanted to kill it, but there was a voice telling me the light wasn't something to be afraid of. By now I was running.

The light was always after me. I would try to hide, but it always snuck up on me. It was something I couldn't get away from. Every so often, I would get far enough ahead of it, that I would be in complete darkness for a while. I would be at peace, resting, but the chase was never over. The light, I knew, would not let me go until it had captured me, enveloped me in its brightness and clarity.

When I didn't expect it, the light suddenly disappeared. I was left alone in all the dark emptiness inside of myself. At first I thought it was good. I was alone, with nothing to fear. I could simply exist and be happy. But it didn't stay good for very long. I grew to despise the darkness. It offered me nothing. The emptiness I thought I had longed for was what I grew to hate. And then the light came back.

It snuck up on me and before I knew it, the light turned a hidden corner and the shock of it sent me flying through the door. The voice I had heard before was back. It was my mother's voice, unbearably loud. She sat next to me in a clean hospital room calling my name. There were doctors and Daryl there too. I wanted to smile, but didn't have the energy, or the temperament really. Going through the door made me mad in a way, for I now understand what I had not wanted to accept.

But the pain of understanding does go away. And the more I think about it, the easier it is to accept; happiness and freedom—are not always compatible. I was not free. I was trapped in the narrowness of my future. I was trapped by a pleasure I didn't understand. I was not happy. I think I am happy now, because I believe I am free from that part of myself which oppressed me before.

I don't need Daryl anymore, or acid. My pain is gone, like it's been healed by a giant band aid. The light was saying a lot to me as I ran from it. It was saying: Look Around. Reality is going to be waiting for you, no matter what, and some things are worse than reality.

Kathryn Roach

GENERATIONS

Mary can remember the first time she was drunk when the kids came home from school, and then the times blurred one into the other.

The children grew used to her friendly greeting. They stood back and judged just what it was they could expect from her. Sometimes it was tears and apologies, sometimes money.

"Go to the store," she would say. "Buy yourself some candy. When you get back I'll have dinner ready."

And when they came back with their brown bags twisted at the neck, she would more often than not be sound asleep in her double bed.

She tries to remember. Sometimes she believes it was just a few times. Sometimes she knows it was her whole life with them. Now when they come home to visit she thinks they see a dried out old woman. Sober.

"You could get something better," says her daughter, Sandy.

"They know me there," she says.

"Why don't you sell this place?" says her son.

She starts by trying to name their teachers from kindergarten. She knows that some years she didn't meet those teachers. She goes through the photo albums and report cards, memorizing names and grades, reconstructing their childhoods. When they ask, she has the names on the tip of her tongue, and they are surprised when she can remember things they have forgotten. She has organized the letters she wrote to her own mother.

Her sister, Edie handed them to her after the funeral. "I don't know what you'll do with these," she said. "Burn them I guess."

She reads things in the letters she believes someone else lived. Jerry broke his arm in the third grade. Sandy never missed a day of school for three years. She shakes her head and smiles. She'd remember to tell them the next time they came to visit.

She worked nights; the kids got themselves off to school. They received boxes of clothes from Edie. Some of the clothes had never been worn. Almost brand new, she had written.

There is one long memory of sitting at the kitchen table, writing letters to her mother. She would pour a little bourbon in a glass and put the bottle back in the cupboard each time, and by the time the letter was finished, she had enough courage to walk it out to the mail box.

She'd run away from home in 1950. Her mother wrote only once to tell her there was no need for her to write. She had two kids real fast and then the freak accident on the ship came, and Frank was gone, and the checks started coming in the mail. The next thing she knew she was holding a bundle of her letters to her mother. Her mother had saved them. They were all opened; she must have read them. Then she stopped drinking, quit her job at night, got the job at Sprouse Reitz, but the children were gone. They sent letters and visited once or twice a year. She read her letters and then began to write to her children about what it was she had found.

You were top scholars, she wrote; I'm so proud of you. The dress Edie sent fit just right, and you wore it to your first dance. You looked so grown up. I must have cried.

Her hands had stopped shaking and she began to walk in the early evenings. One afternoon she calculated her age. Sixteen when she left home. Nineteen when Frank died. Yesterday, she must have turned fifty-six. She wrote everything down on the back of the fliers that were rolled in the door or on the inside of shopping bags. Not much changed from one day to the next. Someone would bring back a pair of pants that had split in the crotch; once the store was robbed.

***

Sandy slits open the letter with the brass letter opener.

"I turned fifty-six, just yesterday. Remember the yellow dress?"

She tucks the letter safely into her desk drawer. There is a whole line of them now in different pastels of stationary, blue to yellow, then pink. She knows her mother is trying to make up the time, but with each letter the old wound feels exposed.

***

Jerry's girl friend, Pat opens the letters, tells him how proud his mother is. He can't bear to see his mother's writing, so small and neat now, and he remembers the time she was unable to sign her name so anyone could read it on his basketball health form. He'd torn it up, decided not to play.

When two or three letters have come he sits down and prints a few words back. "Got the new job, have taken up tennis, Yours truly." He leaves the envelope for days and only the fear that another letter will arrive drives him to put the note in the mail.

***

My name is Mary Anderson. I was born in 1934. My father committed suicide the year I was born. I ran away from home to marry Frank. He joined the Navy when I told him I was pregnant again. "The benefits are fabulous," he said.

She licks the end of her pencil, a habit of her mother's. She sharpens it frequently. There is a pile of shavings on the table. She goes under the sink for another paper sack. She always asks for paper at the grocery store. The pencil marks are dark and broad against the rough surface of the sack. She tears down one side and tears off the bottom. She spreads the inside of the sack out on the table and begins in the top corner. She writes clear across the top of the sack, right up to each edge and slides the sack along, then clear back to the beginning.

***

We lived in a small apartment on Elm street. I've forgotten the name of the city. It was close to the naval base. When the Admiral came to the door, I was holding Sandy in one arm, Jerry was on the floor with a toy truck. Hamburger, mixed with egg and onion, was on the counter. The heat from the oven made the kitchen warm. He didn't stay long. I molded the hamburger into the loaf pan and set the timer. I scrubbed four potatoes and put them into the oven. That night I sat down and wrote the first letter to my mother.

(Tape first letter here.) She writes a note to herself along the margin, and marks it with a star.

***

"I'm almost forty years old," says Jerry. The phone line is twisted around his hand. "We moved into that house when I was six. You were almost five." He waits. Pat is setting the table. Her belly is round and lies on the table as she reaches across it. He hopes he can resolve this before the baby is born. "We moved so I could walk to school. That's what it says."

"Ask her about the car," says Pat. She sits at the counter.

"I thought I'd call her tonight," he says into the phone. He turns his back. "Read me the whole thing."

Pat takes a casserole out of the oven and sets it on the table.

"I'll call you." He hangs up the phone, and turns back. "She's quit her job so she can remember," he says, and sits down. He eats all that is on his plate. He hasn't tasted a thing. "It would be easier if she could forget."

Pat held each side of her stomach. She is past trying to make him forgive. They have been together for six years. She is the one who decided it was time to have a baby. She made the choice, knowing that he might leave her.

"That glassy stare of adoration," he says, and puts down his fork, and glares at his empty plate. He goes to the cupboard and takes down the bottle of Scotch. For a moment he stops, then pours the cool yellow, his little piece of silence, into a glass. It is just at that moment that Pat decides to leave, and when he comes home the next day she is gone and has taken the things she has bought for the baby.

***

Pat stands at the door of the bungalow. She knocks and the screen door bangs against the frame. It has taken her two days driving and one night in a dingy motel to get here. Her nerves are smothered in tiredness, her back aches; she puts one hand on the small of her back, the other on her stomach and is standing like this when the door opens.

"Mary?" she says. "Mary Anderson?"

"Yes," says the woman. "I'm Mary Anderson."

"I'm a friend of Jerry's."

"Jerry?" She opens the door wider and brushes back her hair.

The house is sparsely furnished. The couch is worn. There is no clutter or dust. Doilies are laid out on the arms of the chairs and the braided rug lies between the lines of the floor boards. Pat sits on the couch, leans her head back and closes her eyes. The room shifts and when she opens her eyes, a cup of tea steams on the coffee table in front of her. Mary is not who Pat had expected. She is trim and wears sweat pants and a blue T-shirt with a pocket.

"I called Jerry," Mary says. She sets her tan walking shoes on the floor and pulls on her socks.

"I'm sorry," says Pat. Her own mother is much older, could be this woman's mother. Pat was born when her mother was thirty-six, the same age as Pat now, having her first baby. When she is Mary's age, her child will be twenty. She juggles the numbers as Mary ties her shoes.

"I'll be gone for an hour. It takes that long now. You can put your things in the bedroom. It'll give you time to settle," says Mary. She doesn't look back or close the door. The screen door bangs as she leaves, then she is back again with Pat's suitcase. "I spotted this in your car." She doesn't look up as she sets the suitcase inside the door.

Pat takes her suitcase to the bedroom. There are sections of letters taped to different parts of Jerry's old room. Above a baseball trophy is a piece that says Jerry was on the all-star team when he was fourteen, and growing so fast these days. Pat lies on the bed and slips off her shoes. Tears come to her eyes. She lays her wrist on her forehead to block out the light. She feels the first movement of the baby. More than a tickle this time. She smiles and cries at the same time.

***

Sandy has learned that Pat has gone to visit her mother. She sits at her desk at work and can't believe that she is jealous of the visit, of the baby. She'd made her decision four years ago about men and babies. She'd given up on relationships and directed her energies into her work. It has paid off. Miles from her mother, miles from her past, she has become an advertising executive. Her book is full of accounts. She has been the top sales person in the company two years in a row. She has money to burn.

"Why aren't the walls high enough?" she whispers to herself.

She remembers going to school sick with a fever. How she had to lie down in the sick room while the secretary called her mother. No answer. The school nurse sat on the edge of the bed and talked to her. She'd laid a cool cloth on her forehead and washed her hands and straightened her clothes. "You are a very pretty little girl," said the nurse. Sandy had gone to her many times after school and sat while she put away her papers. And the letter says, "I'm so proud of you for having had perfect attendance."

Sandy folds the letter and puts it in the drawer. She has a new idea that will sell ads, and makes the first call.

***

Frank was the youngest of ten children. His parents expected him to stay and take care of them. When he fell in love with Mary, it was strong enough to break him out.

They packed the car on his graduation night, skipped the dance, and headed west. He'd worked in grocery stores since he was twelve, bought his own car at sixteen, paid cash, and he had enough money and experience to get out of the town that had always seen him as the hardest working kid they ever saw and smart too. His parents were old before he was born and poor as dirt. He'd found a girl whose mother was hard as a rock and as religious as God Himself. They broke the ten commandments that night and swore an oath never to look back.

***

Jerry planned his own way out. A four year scholarship out of town was all that he needed. As soon as he knew what he was going to do he'd stopped talking to his sister. She watched and followed his path a year later. They showed up for Christmas vacations for two years at the same time and talked about little things, knowing that they would never be caught there again for more than a few days. Then the letters started coming, relentlessly and full of lies. Jerry knew Pat was right; if he didn't love his mother, he couldn't hate her so much.

***

Jeremy Haskins-Anderson is born January 10th, weighing in at seven pounds, four ounces. He is cuddled in the arms of his mother. His cheek is still moist from her milk. His eyes are opaque. He must have done something wonderful. Those who stand over him, raise their heads and laugh. In that moment, they would do anything for him.

Leo Connellan

ORIGINS

Mother, Father told me you were
like an impossible lily
that does not need earth or drink
and lives forever in my mind
without ever wilting.

The whole New England town was with him
perpetuating your image
for my boyhood heart suffered enough losing you
to Forever at age Seven,
dumped from manhood's dawn
into my middle thirties believing
you were beyond my grasp.

Father never once broke the ribbon on
the packaged secret through to the end of his own life
he loved you that much.

Mother, I never saw you clearly
until during a visit home a friend
slipped her tongue through the long sealed
tight lips of the town code.

Unanswered pieces of my whole life
my senses instinct into place
from way back in the dark storage room of my recall.

As for the town, they wanted me to always
see you as an Angel floating where
religions tell me you wait for me.

Always now you will be exactly as Father described you
to me but now I can see you.

Love you far deeper for being no longer vague,
a perfect someone I could never deserve.

One has to feel flesh, now rotted in the earth
which bore and I know loved me.

Now to Father, I know you have already moved close,
coffins burst into each other's arms again,
as you did the night you made me, now

at last wrap your lover to you for always
and keep him whose love and loyalty to you
never faltered.

The only way I can thank Father, Mother,
is I have put away the bottle.

Jack Coulehan

DEEP IMAGES

In memory of a young man with AIDS

When I open your door
the blinds are drawn
and you sit by the hospital sink
so long, so quietly,
your beard is an open shack
stacked with logs, branches, dried leaves
and deep nests.

Your eyes the deep image of tulips
at the end of the season
their yellow tongues droop, their tasty organs
bend in the sun.

Behind your shack
a wet weather stream
flows from a stone enclosure,
and at twilight
deer come. They are not afraid to drink,
though their warm loins brush the hair of your chest,
because to them
your hair is rhododendron,
your body is a wild hill
cobbled in rocks and moss and covered in leaves.

In your room the spigot runs,
and these deep images of deer
reflected in your sink
are children, those children you will never,
never see.

Elspeth Cameron Ritchie

AIDS

My sperm encapsulates skulls.
My tears may kill.
Will I live to learn
if I've poisoned my new son?

The zoo of my body busted its gates.
Parasites burrow my open lungs,
the virus inches through my nerves.
Cancer blotches my skin. Purple
boils erupt. I am Job.

Yet, it was a night
sweet as Cleopatra's asp,
his skin a camellia.
We courted like crowned cranes,
frolicked like sea lions, howled as caged wolves.

If he were not dead, would I hate him?

My sight strobes in decreasing shades of pale.
My mind lies beige, limp, sticky.
When the doctor asks, I pretend to subtract.

Friends venture toward my infected bed.
They do not touch my blotched hand.
My wife used to love me. Now,
she enters in yellow gown and gloves.
My mother fears my drool.

I smell the hospital shop carnations.
I would like to sweep in a green rotten canoe
toward the Atlantic,
drown in peace.
Salt grass would hug my empty skin.

In the hospital buzzing with white coats
bugs swarm in my lungs.
Asleep I drown, awake I gasp.
A catfish stranded,
I wait for needles
and creeping snake death.

Where is the garden?

Elspeth Cameron Ritchie

TEARING THROUGH THE MOON

The hurricane rears:
clouds puff with anger,
shield stars from my red city.

Indoors, I interview
patients with AIDS.

Wind sucks at Washington streets,
licks skirts on flame-lipped girls,
gropes at monuments,
crack houses, Congress.

I ask about lymph nodes,
risk factors, depression;
correlate results into papers,
pie charts, presentations.

My own dread roars,
tears at the moon.

My patients have slept with tainted men,
shot retrovirus in scarred veins,
breathed through diseased placentas.

I too have been reckless,
roamed orange city streets,
kissed men in tight pants.

They got trapped
in the henbane of desire.

Wrapped in leaves of death,
they watch for signs,
eat AZT, spray on pentamidine.

I too watch and fear,
insert IV's and start CPR.
After a handshake I wash.
Hands itch. I wash again.

I am no cold planet.
My palm trees bend.

The monsoon batters. Islands of
brittle coral sweep away.

My patients go out into the storm;
clouds blanket the inflamed moon.
Tears heat my skin.

Should I quit?
Stay behind locked doors?

No, I will live through the seasons.
That needle stick innocent—
my blood still tests negative.

Jack Coulehan

ANESTHESIA

At night the landlord lets them in.
They open a valve behind my bed
and fill the room with anesthesia.
Though I'm dead to the world,
I remember them vaguely,
as if they were ruthless children
lurking in a long vacant lot.
They work on my body. When I awake
my body is different,
arms shorter, fingers older.
The things they put inside me rattle.
Now nothing will stop a massive attack.
Nothing can help me now.
Nothing can close the valve in my heart
they opened—Love,
love pours through the valve,
love hemorrahages from my nose,
pours from my vagina,
a red river of love pours from my soul.
Nothing can fill the emptiness that's left
after they open my body up
and dry my soul, and replace it with gravel.
Now nothing but love can fill me.
Nothing but love. Love is what the world needs,
what I need, Love love love
is pouring out of me.
Tell them to stop.
Tell them to stop the anesthesia.
Doctor, tell them, tell them to love me.

Colleen Connors

YOU WILL LEARN LESSONS

The dense thicket of dreams is upon you now.

And you will come to understand that every tree is a surgeon
who can make or break you,
like a flower
breathing gaseous air.

What the anesthesiologists don't know
may already have killed you.

Mary Jo Bang

ANOTHER SURGERY

Another surgery.
I should be prepared by now;
we have done this so often.
I have always said: *Yes Doctor, No Doctor,*
and signed away my rights
on the dotted line,
never once asking:
Where did you study?
How sharp is that scalpel blade?
How many times have you performed this procedure?
Have the patients survived?
Still, I forever watch to see
if your hand is steady.

These walls are rather bare.
Who does your decor?
There is nothing in these frames—
where is that engraved evidence
of your unarguable expertise?
And why don't you ever warn me
about the post-operative pain?

It's time.
Open the mouth wide.
You admire my teeth, the tidy line
of the incisors.
But this isn't why we are here.
Swallow the taste of ether,
anesthetic of my childhood,
enter the blue-green sleep.
When I wake, you will pat my hand,
pass me the specimen—that warm souvenir—
words, floating in a blood-tinged bath.

Anna Rabinowitz

TOP KNOT

Because life is short she learned how to live with things, took them in as if they were waifs at her doorstep and offered them haven.

I found her in the master bedroom divested of props—her fitted dress, the turban that covered her skull. And it was O.K.—a split second jolt, then a quick accommodation.

She looked better, I thought. Her robe fell far enough from her body to conceal how thin she'd become. Her head looked strange but interesting, divided like the map of an irregular landscape—half a dozen territories exposed without modification by the shrill sunlight that plunged into the room—each area a different color—a deep pink over her left eye, pale off-white above the nape of her neck, gray over the temples, even a few islands of skin echoing the marmoreal tones of her face. The boundaries swelled slightly as if cord had been laced under her skull in strategic places, the way markers or dividers are set up between borders.

And crowning the hairless expanse, rising from the modest ridge of her brows, a mound, a top knot of skin the surgeon had gathered, shaped, and stitched into a bun.

Out of frustration, she said, and ingenuity.

Since she imagined he had always wanted to model in clay or stone, what else to do but use the materials at hand?

Robert Mezey

LITTLE POEM:

Thick spriglets of mistletoe
Asthmatic laughter
Even disease is beautiful
When the eyes are open.

Vivian Shipley

IT HURTS TO BURN

I.

My words are naked
their meaning bare and bald
as my skull, a moon glowing
in all my negatives
like a button of bone
where sockets stare
black holes to thread.

Figure 1. My head
a textbook pose of an arteriogram
how to make the femoral stick
without knowing who is being entered
or when a clot might break loose
and stop sound.
Such books are useless.

A light hungry as the sun
broke into an egg splattering
ceiling when the thin plastic
tube entered my groin
inched the dye through an artery
stopping at the tumor's base.
X-rays did not picture
sweat beaded like mercury
exploding on my skin.

II.

I marvel at what people do to stay alive
While brushing my skull
brackets opened, would not close
releasing images that should not be shared;
cooked, the eyeball
like an egg white in boiling water
becomes irreversibly opaque. I wonder
if that is true but no research
need be conducted. Such answers
like pain or torture produce nothing.
Experiments do show that cats, monkeys
die if pressure is applied.

The force that cracks a skull
cannot be determined in advance.
Palming two walnut shells
leaving kernels intact
practices technique
doesn't duplicate the human brain.

III.

Glasses half rimmed bent over
and the news was good:
Only half my head would be removed.
Hair grows back,
even on heads of the dead.
Strapped spread eagle, my legs
twitched as the seizure
my tongue backed into my throat.
Pleasure, pain rest on a knife;
orgasms and seconds preceding a tumor fit
are indistinguishable on the edge.
Street lamps must be globed to shine.
Shaved scalp curls off, an orange
peeling to fruit, a baseball
or the moon
pulling tide
like a hospital sheet
eased over the eyes.

John M. Brand

CHILDREN OF DARKNESS

From Lao-Tzu, to the Christian community:
Are you capable of not knowing anything?

From Nietzsche, to the Christian community:
I want, once and for all, not to know many things.

So my sermon was to begin, here in the fields of the Lord in northeastern Colorado. Seedtime. Behold the seed a man buries and which, while he sleeps, springs and grows up, "he knoweth not how." (Mark 4:26,27). Here the lesson would begin, for even pious country people forget their roots, forget that even disciples see "through a glass darkly." Even hardy country people lose nerve and crave signs, reducing faith to certainty. A curse, I would call such certainty. "Light is to shed," I would say. "What happens to eyes that never close? 'Blind guides,' Jesus called smug religious leaders, impervious to 'your Father who is in secret' and 'who sees in secret.' " I meant to preach the very secrecy of God and hail "that seed planted in the obscure womb of Mary and born in obscure Bethlehem." Does my elation show? It should, for once again Word had led me to the right word: "obscure." In my etymology—it's called ORIGINS—"obscure" is rooted in a word meaning "a barn, where the light tends to be dim." Lo the dark Child who, "like the womb of Mary, opens at night...."

Here ended the lesson.

I never got that sermon to the pulpit.

It used to be said that God puts his Word into servants' mouths. I now wonder. Who shut me up? Put me down? I don't know. Wonder, wrote Emily Dickinson,

is not precisely knowing
and not precisely knowing not

What I know is that somebody buried me.

Here's what happened ...

A tumor in the middle of my head, long hidden, made itself manifest. Had the tumor been planted there? Planted or not, it had grown in secret and made itself felt only when exerting enough pressure on my acoustic nerve to affect my hearing. Then came appointments, tests, X-rays.... I wrote in my journal: "Now all my death-talk is being called: 'With a mighty voice, he utters mighty trifles.' I am told this tumor is 'way up there?' Up is different from down? Either way, this my life is hid—I am being 'made in secret, intricately wrought in the depths of the earth.' "

Burial. Son of a funeral director, blighted early with the odor of death, I had after prolonged spiritual struggle finally seen death die. In, with, above and around it another Power was forming me. The old word for this experience is "Calling." For while

221

sanding caskets at a Dallas casket factory, down among what were called the "Iron-works," I crammed my reading of THE BROTHERS KARAMAZOV into coffee and lunchbreaks. Its epigraph reads, "Yet unless a grain of wheat falls into the earth and dies, it remains alone; but if it dies it bears much fruit." My heart felt more than strangely warmed. I left the casket factory for seminary.

Burials come and go. I learned that surgery would be necessary, that it would be a delicate and high-risk procedure, that if my surgeon blundered around my brainstem I would stroke out, and that, even if successful, the operation could leave me with partial facial paralysis and the loss of speech, and / or vertigo lasting up to ninety days if not a lifetime. And now that I had been told what to expect, in short, the worst, would I help bring it into being? Such is the nature of the witness, namely his helping bring into being that to which he testifies. Hadn't I, as a young withering Southern Presbyterian, once written, "I believe in Death?" If I came again to believe in death, would I then give birth to it? Had I already, in the form of my tumor?

Burial.

I kept busy with my family, friends in the parish, and with my teaching, weeding beds and baking bread, and, of course, thinking. Recurring to me was something I'd decided some time back, that a broken loaf belongs on the coffin of the Christian. HOC EST CORPUS MEAM: this is my body, I break too, I open at night. Yet this solidarity between my life—or death—and that of Christ I found presumptuous to make—"too certain"—in spite of my sermons about our sharing in his dying and rising, making His Body and each of us a house of bread where some One is born. This same reluctance to correlate my ordeal with that of Christ occurred when I read these tantalizing lines of Peguy:

> Such a perfect bond links the last of members to the crowned Chief that the last among the sick, in his bed, is admitted to imitate the suffering itself of Jesus on the Cross. The last among the sick in his bed literally imitates, effectively imitates the Passion itself of Jesus, and of the other saints and martyrs.

Why this reluctance, as if I were still a member of Death?

Two nights before surgery I dreamed my surgeons had opened not my head but my chest, and there in that dripping cavity strange hands kneaded dough. Next morning the dream escaped me, routed by my fears of surgery, vertigo especially; I saw myself as Ixion, bound forever to a revolving wheel. Could I endure? Would I want to? Would some Power intercede for me "with sighs too deep for words," saying Yes?

Surgery, the shedding of blood, is also a shedding of light. Surgery is deep sleep, a thick darkness. Through anaesthesia senses are numbed, the heart slowed, and one is made nil, a nullity, a stone, a sleepy hollow.

I'm told that on awakening I told my wife I felt "sore." But instead of feeling pain I heard music. Amid the expected vertigo and in spite of the total loss of hearing in one ear I heard music. Permeating my reeling brain were old hymns, some of which had never been my favorites, all of which I heard in their entirety, stanza-by-stanza and word-by-word. A doctor friend told me, "Your surgeon pricked your hymn center." Maybe so. The music I heard was hot, a surging heat, deep heat floating a corpse. The music of the spheres? The singing of the morning stars together? Sound, song, dance, it rode the crest of what Joyce Cary said "goes on going on." For how long had my own ears closed off this music? Into what ripe Night, or Whose, had I been lowered? "We are God's field," the Apostle wrote, and I grew music.

Beneath the sounds you hear is the sound I hear, the shrill in the ear that now hears nothing else. Beneath what you hear is what I hear, beneath which is ...

Not music.

I don't hear music.

It came to pass. I neither lament its leaving nor try to bring it back. It didn't have to come.

Maybe it left because, as Hölderlin said, "Mankind cannot stand too long the abundance of gods." Or left so I would not consider it my own. Maybe it left so I would open to still another Deep, the earlier one. The Deep to which I refer is the red dream I let slip, where not my head but my chest had been hollowed out, and in which someone kneaded dough.... "If I make my bed in hell, behold, thou art there." What I can't talk easily about but must, is what I call the underhandedness of God. "I will praise thee; for I am fearfully and wonderfully made."

Margaret Robison

FIVE MONTHS AFTER MY STROKE

Five months after my stroke, and strawberry
apples fill the apple tree
growing by the river.
Five months after my stroke, and bees
hum in the oriental bamboo
that flowers on the riverbank.

"I cannot hold hope out to you," the neurologist said,
standing at the foot of my hospital bed
in which I'd lain for weeks, paralyzed,
unable to move my left arm, my leg.
"You should begin to think about a nursing home,"
my other doctor said. Sober. Grim.

All that day I struggled
with their words, with my body.
By midnight I sat clinging
to the bed bars. Upright.
Triumphant.

Now I've rolled my wheelchair to the open door.
And look—there's wind on the river today.
Wind in the trees. Wind
shaking the leaves of the oriental bamboo
shaking the sumac. The lilac. The beech.
Knocking the ripe apples together.

Margaret Robison

APRAXIA
(June 14, 1989. Mercy Hospital.)

Cars and trucks come and go
along the highway and the trees
are wet. The grass wet too,
and the drenched sky
is a blur of grey. Blackbirds fly,
lyrical and decisive
in their dip and sweep. And so
I search this day for music to unlock
my damaged speech, some
rhythm I can ride
like birds' wings ride the wind. Or words
like wheels turning my brain—motion
of language. Creation: In the beginning
was   In the beginning was   In the
beginning was
the word.

The word.

Pat Schneider

FRIEND

For Margaret Robison

I run to you across a field
and we are falling together
toward soft grasses. Cows
stand quiet at the edges
of our vision and you
read me a poem under an old tree
in Wildwood Cemetery.
I cry, "it is a masterpiece."
You touch a finger to the grass,
bring up a green inchworm, try
to tell me a mystery.

I can't remember what it was
you wanted to tell me
with that short green life
measuring its way along
your finger on a summer
afternoon but I remember
sitting stunned in the aftermath
of your voice reading:

> There are signs ...
> A rusty bucket filled with rain ...

My heart is full of your stories.
The black boy fallen to the iron fence
his poor small chest pierced
by that cruel decoration.
The courthouse burning. Your
mother's marigolds. You
on your knees scrubbing your floor
because that act alone sufficed
on the night your mother died.
Your wide brimmed hat
your father's funeral . The tree
gone. Remembered. Gone.
An uncle lost in a burning house
a ball lost in the bamboo
the painting in the trash can
the story in your room, your
mother crying on your bed.

I am running toward you
across a high hill field
and there are grasses soft enough
to receive us if we fall
and all your stories are like
treasures a child might carry
in her pocket on the way to school
secret, and hidden, and perfect
while the morning dew still sits
in the crotch of the pokeberry leaf
and the berries hang blue and beautiful
and my Casto Creek is laughing
over Ozark stones. Like that.

Today, your words slow
in the aftermath of stroke,
you say, "If I die before you do,
tell them not to let me suffer.
Tell them when to let me die."

We sit quietly. I nod my head.
You do not know I run to you
and the grasses are soft
to receive us if we fall
and the cows stand gentle
at the edge of the field
and my pockets are full of your stories.

Gerry Sloan

RELEARNING TO SPEAK

This is how it's done:
purse your lips for 'him',
retract the tongue for 'her',
say 'ah' when this grows

painful, the glottis valve
releasing air barely above
a whisper. You have to learn
to speak again, the tongue

a healed amnesiac, avoiding
the syllables that might betray
true feeling. When you turn
the larynx off, it stirs

against your palate like
the sea inside a shell,
inundating consciousness:
hrrrrr ... a verbal raft

you drift on in this
hopelessness of moonlight,
dark destination
of married lovers.

Judith Skillman

AFTER WITNESSING A SEIZURE

The victim's persona shifts, as if by plain
a mother must mean not ugly
but ineffably sane and fabulously alive.

You told me there are, embedded in the skin,
strident ganglia like those
that won't grow back

around your scar. But, I might have said,
the disparate will never live together,
marry like cousins,

or come back months later
to reclaim the flesh
like a surrogate baby

spread out in the cradle
of mother's other arm.
A white presupposing rip

like the one a snake makes to reap the gift
of its own stuffing, did someone say
remember not to let her swallow her own tongue?

So it comes back to the peculiarity
of resonance, the fussing objectivity
a spectator culls from observing

or
cat got your bird way back
in the medieval hope of a past, herb bread
wadded on the lip of consciousness,

there must be one ancestor,
one fugitive uncle whose singular reluctance
to disclose the facts

caused her to be angry. I remember them
encasing her head in a helmet, wrapping her
in a plaid blanket, helping her

into a wooden chair.

Robert Noreault

CASE HISTORY

I had to get beyond the mind, the thought
I'd loved with where the cancer was too much.

Sal Cetrano

READ BEFORE CLOSING

Accept a ticking malignancy behind all things.
Accept that you will clutch in your arms
at least one too precious life
exploded for untimely confession.
Accept disappointment, the sheer face you battle,
the mountaintop revealing only cloud.
Expect delay, reversals, wrong choices.
Expect to leave your skull, dispute your being,
cry a pool in which to see yourself.
Admit to the labels you have chosen,
the ether of words you breathe.
See how they have braided soft convictions hard.
Delusion fashions its skin about the maimed
circuits, the wilderness of twitching wire,
the graypink flower of concentric flesh,
igniting old portraits in the mirror.
Choose the one that you would have for keeps.
The balance of life is preparation:
editing refusals, resolving unspoken desires,
trolling for unscheduled joys.
With each survival, death begins again.

Herb Kitson

IN THE HOSPITAL SHOP

It's ten below and the sun
is a fibrous lump within a breast of cloud.
Ice crystals, like strange patterns of cells
gone wild, lie frozen under x-rays of light.

It seems wrong to leave a warm bed
in orthopedic weather when limbs stiffen
and snap beneath too much weight,
to rise in the dark and creep
before breakfast to the hospital
where you'll be injected with artificial sleep
as I wait to hear the surgery results.

Inside the hospital shop, coffee is brewed.
The cook chops bacon into strips. Eggs
sizzle like burnt-out stars.
The natural I can understand,
like the man who took up his bed and walked
or the woman whose blood, reminded of its birthright,
became whole.

Alice Jones

OTTAWA, MARCH, 1986

In the small darkened room
rows of exposures are set
against flat white lights.
A motor hums and the x-rays rotate
stopping with a ratchety sound.
The chief of the flock of men
in white coats shows me
the opaque white bones
that hold lung fields
that should be all black,
and the large white shape
that is my brother's heart.
They wonder at its size
say it's out of proportion
for even so large a man.
I question the grey fluff
that is everywhere, clouding
his breathing, filling the pan
by his bed with blood. I ask—
pneumonia, aspiration, shock lung?
They don't know.
I say his oxygen is falling.
They say they'll intubate.
I ask when.
They say now.
I ask for five minutes to talk
knowing these may be the last words
we speak. I walk to the dark
but gleaming cubicle
where he lies half-naked on his side,
shaking and cringing with coughs
that rattle the metal bed,
squeeze his eyes shut,
drip sputum and blood from his mouth
into the aluminum basin.
Here, I touch his damp arm,
I've come to say something.

I forgot how it happens,
the feeling that when you put your foot down
the earth might not be there.
This is the amnesia of one
who has presided over deaths of others.
The phone call came at work between patients.
My sister-in-law explained he was being moved
to the ICU. She said I'd better come.

In the airplane to New York then Ottawa
I sat awake all night, my sudden bursts of tears
surprising other passengers. They drank and smoked,
played cards, watched some movie, snored. I look out
the window for five hours first at snow on the Rockies,
then plains, then it was too dark to see anything
but clusters of lights and guess how the land lay.
I passed where our home had been—some hills
on a river, near farmland, in grey winter haze.
I remembered summer there, humid Ohio greenness,
large shedding trees: elm, beech, sassafrass,
sycamore. The sky outside the little double window
turned grey. I thought there is no one to pray to,
but there are always rituals, and who knows really,
I pictured his body lying sick and hurt and thought
of his breath going in and out. If I can concentrate,
he'll breath until I get there. I think very hard
about fever lowering, about healing, and watch the sky
turn pink and know the molecules warming up, resonating,
connect me to him.

You can't die. That's all. You can't.
I'll hit you if you do.
I'll lock you out of my room forever.
I'll kill you.
Let him be alive. Heal.

I imagined we were twins.
Everything in common
shared chromosomes
similar height and color
everything but gender
still twins
my one year older brother
third love

after disappointment
by the other two.
The grown-ups
bailed out early
leaving two
bewildered children
silent in our
single rooms
tapping signals
on the common wall.

Arriving, passing customs,
no one was there to meet me.
This is not a good sign.
After half an hour
my sister-in-law came and
I knew from her face he wasn't dead.
She dawdled, did errands, then went home
where my mother was cleaning up,
which is all she knows to do
in a crisis—throw things out and wash.
We drove to the hospital,
parked in a huge lot
under a construction crane,
walked the half mile to the lobby,
up the escalator following the signs
in French and English,
down the long white linoleum halls
with bright primary colors
which fool no one .
In the ICU waiting room
we pick up the beige phone
which is answered in French
by nurses who say wait.
And we wait.

Then we go in.
He's in the corner bed
with IVs and
the fire-engine red
crash cart near by.
He says hello,
recognizes me
even with the new short hair

he'd never seen.
He lay there and coughed
after bronchoscopy
redfaced and unshaven,
a large white mammal
beached on white sheets.
Over the hour I talk
with nurses who say
no he's not on pressors,
yes he's on oxygen,
PO2 of 70 and falling,
temperature of 40°
not falling,
antibiotics—
gentamycin and septra.
I call the chief surgeon
who bruskly arrives and says
"we don't know what the hell
is going on. There's gram negative
sepsis from somewhere,
fever not breaking for days
and now his lungs
are whiting out
and liver and kidney tests
don't look so good.
Multi-system failure.
We're doing everything
we can." I can tell
from the apologetic
lift of the eyebrows,
they think he's dying.
They're saying they're sorry
beforehand, so I'll know
how hard they tried
and not be angry.
I listen to all the rationales
about tubing him and
ventilation and I translate
this for the family.
No one else sees what it means.
They watch my face
to know how scared to be.
They nod at the explanations

that on the machine
he'll be sedated, feel less pain.
I go in and tell him
what is about to happen.
I tell him it's all right.
I tell him I'll be there.
I tell him I love him
and start to leave the room.
He mumbles something,
I go back and ask and he says
"I love you too."
We have never, in 37 years,
said this.

    In the upstairs room
    with the dormer window
    children curled up
    whispering, grew louder
    until our mother
    came to say hush.

In an hour I come back.
He is breathing on the ventilator
lying flat on his back, eyes closed,
skin warm and wet, still sweating,
every vessel dilated,
the green line on the monitor
cruising jaggedly along,
a fast regular rhythm.
I stand there and cry
thinking breathe, breathe, breathe
and pulse, pulse, pulse
and almost believe that if I stop
saying the words his heart
will stop pumping.

    I mean this, I mean
    to keep you alive.
    I don't want to be
    an only child after all.
    If you leave now,
    I'll hate you forever.
    You fucking bastard,
    don't you dare die.
    I've only just told you

I love you.
I know I never chose you
and surely told you
to drop dead
and go to hell
a million times.
I take it back.
I'll share this family
with you after all.
It's you I want,
the only one on earth
who shares this history.
I need your one year older eyes
to tell what happened—
the things we saw
and never said.
I, the thorn in your side
little sister, whining
take me with you,
I say stay.
I say breathe.

I stand and watch him lie unconscious.
Mom comes in, I look at her and cry
and she hugs me hard for the first time
in twenty years or so and she says
"he'll be ok, I know it, I promise you."
I know another lie when I hear one.
The nurses tell us to go home and sleep.
We go, she to the Chateau Laurier,
I to his daughter's room to lie awake
and listen to the night noises
in his solid house I've never visited.
I think how little it takes to turn
the world on edge. I remember the smiling
people in the hospital elevator and wish—
your brother not mine. Then I go back to this
personal form of magic, imagining maps
of arteries and veins and concentrating
to keep everything open and I think—
if he dies what a large blank space
there will be in the universe.

In the morning I am up by five
and have to wait for all of them.
The children get up,
have cereal and go to school.
In the hall, my six year old niece stops
going out the door and says
"it's good you're here."
I ask why.
"Because you're a doctor,
you can make him better."

When the nurse finally opens the windowless door
I examine her face for signs. I count machines
to see what equipment has been added or subtracted.
There are tubes everywhere:
one for his lungs, blowing the air in,
one for his urine to a clear plastic bag,
one to a vein in his arm for fluids and meds,
one to an artery in his other wrist,
one to a vein in his neck where a yellow tube
with black stripes curls through his heart,
past tricuspid and pulmonic valves then
into his lungs to measure the venous pressures.
Other lines are all around, one for the suction bottle,
pale green ones for the cooling blanket,
ekg leads from the plastic patches on his chest.
Even the bed is plugged in.
At work we would joke about the seven-tube sign.
With it, most everyone dies.
They call them lines like on a boat.
My brother is moored to the walls.

He is still alive. He opens his eyes, tries to talk
but can't. He mouths words which none of us can understand.
His wife tries to read his lips. I watch. I haven't seen
this body in years, shirtless, arm muscles overdeveloped,
scant-haired chest. The grey at the sides of his head and
eyebrows surprises me. We wait for the doctors to arrive
on rounds. The attending decides to talk to me and have me
tell everyone else. They watch, as if we are speaking
another language, smile to see me speaking it. It amounts
to everything being the same. Stably critical condition.
The whole family goes out to lunch, eats salad and omelets
in the market, with one of the cafe windows open on the first

day of spring thaw. They ask if I want dessert and I start
to cry, thinking how his head fell back on the pillow with
a sound from his lungs that made me wonder if he'd ever breathe
on his own again. They react as if a small unruly child
just peed on the rug. They order coffee, not dessert.

Don't leave because
I'm not done with you,
we're only starting.
I need you in the world with me,
the only creature on this planet
sharing so many double helices.
Your daughters look like me,
the nurses think they are mine,
springing out of the family tree
of which you have all the documents
and the old oil painting that is really
a tree by the water and each twig has a name,
stopping with our father.
You stayed and got the stories
while I wandered off around the country.
You stayed and did the things you should:
the military, marriage, employment
in the family company,
visiting the grandparents,
making the parents grandparents for the first
and second and third times. That's the part
I envy, even while saying I'm not ready
to participate in this spreading
of DNA down through history.
When I look at your oldest daughter
I see your face at twelve,
the freckles around the serious eyes,
the full line of lower lip
that pinches in with worry.
I almost expect her
to call me names like you did
or sidle up to me all friendly
then smash me in the arm and say
got you last and run.

The next day he's sitting up when we arrive. His fever's
down. He tries to talk and again no one understands.
He gets angry. We find a felt-tip pen and paper for him

to write. He asks in gestures, if I've walked around, what
I've seen of the city. I say—Nothing. Slowly, careful
not to hit the IV's, with a weak hand he writes—Go
visit Parliament. And the House of Commons. I say I'll go
today and he falls back asleep.

My sister-in-law makes me look at their wedding book
while we wait for the surgeon to phone.
I always forget their anniversary.
So we sit side by side on the living room couch
both holding the white leather book with gilt trim
and flip plastic coated pages.
Everyone looks impossibly young in 1972.
There are a few long-haired cousins and her brother,
but I notice my hippie boyfriend was edited
out of the book. I look at the pictures of me—
a chubby innocent, hair down past my fingers,
sweating in the high-necked bride's maid's dress
in July, smiling, as the only other one who knew
my sister-in-law was pregnant. In the line-ups
of all the relatives I remember everyone was furious:
mother at me for my fatness in public and bringing
the boyfriend who she didn't want to seat at the family
table; mother at brother for getting married at all,
much less to a blond with loquacious parents;
sister-in-law at mother for wearing a red dress;
father at brother for marrying too young,
at me for not marrying sooner, to someone acceptable;
grandmother at mother for not being invited
to the rehearsal dinner, even though we used her silver;
and me with my smile enraged at them for being
reactionary, overcontrolling, perfectionistic,
insensitive, incompetent, self-involved and disapproving.
We all smile for the camera.

You used to throw my blanket up into a tree.
You would pick a small tree, too skinny to climb.
I'd stand at the bottom and howl at how horribly
unfair it was, until she'd come with a broom handle
and fetch it down. Or we would sit and watch TV.
We'd watch anything, Tarzan movies, Three Stooges,
Pro Golf. This was our contact sport. I'd be
wrapped in my soft and dirty green blanket
sucking one finger, stroking my upper lip.

If one of us crossed the line between the two
plaid pillows—warfare. Hitting, got-you-last
escalated into smashing each other as hard as
we could. When I slammed your hand in the door
of my room which I was running to lock before you
could get me back, I don't know if you cried.
You wouldn't want me to know if I could affect you.
I was the bratty little sister, making your life
miserable. And when I'd really play the perfect
girl you would grab my blanket, run with it,
laugh at my wailing nakedness. This was the sore
you would dig at.

On the first day off the ventilator
with everything still unsure and changing,
with the fevers still high and unexplained,
he got out of bed. He climbed over the bedrails
dangling the plastic tubing and torn gauze
wrist restraints and said to the nurse
who found him standing there naked,
"I'm sorry." Led gently back to bed,
knowing he'd done something wrong
but not sure what, the large and uncertain man
apologized. Confused with surgery
and morphine and a week of almost dying
he must have wondered what planet this was
where women in white and green suits
tuck him in, shave his black moustache raggedly,
bathe him in bed and say no. They say you can't get up
the way they would to a two year old. But this man
is 38 and today is Easter and all his daughters
arrive for their first hospital visit
after church and chocolate eggs.
All in their best dresses they bring cards
they have made and pictures they drew
of the new dog that everyone's forgotten to walk.
Five minutes after they leave, he asks me
when are the children coming. I say they've been
and point to the pictures taped on the wall
and smile at my delirious brother who will live.

In the regular ward, out of the ICU
we visit daily, his family of women:
wife, mother, sister, three daughters.

He looks fine until he moves, and then
we see him cringe. I take the chart
from the nurses station to check
his white count and the results of the bone scan
that I pushed him to in a wheel chair.
Sitting and talking, everyone gets bored.
Each one wants to be with him alone.
He talks about the day they intubated him.
He remembers the fevers, the sensation of cooking
from the inside out. He remembers the helplessness,
feeling himself ebb away. He considered what was
in the bank in US and Canadian and calculated
how far each child could get in school on that amount.
He doesn't remember the next two days. He thinks
the nurses told him he wouldn't make it. So he talks
about wills and funerals and asks what each of us wants.
My mother says where she has bought plots and how many.
She tells how her father's current wife had the first
wife dug up and moved. There is one place left
in my father's side's cemetery. And she has six plots
besides hers. I tell them I would claustrophobically
prefer cremation. He wants to be buried near my mother.
I rethink my choice, imagine the pull—
the picture of my bones slowly decaying
beside my mother's and I compare this to the image
of their bones dissolving together without me.

You're still alive so now you have to tell me.
Tell me if it was as silent as I think,
the soft layer of politeness over everything.
They said we were fine as long as we looked good,
clean, stood up straight and didn't bleed
on the new carpet whenever we needed stitches.
She would take me to the doctor and request repairs—
make her thin, make her feet not turn in so,
make her not be six feet tall, keep her skin clear.
And you, I remember we went and waited in the lobby
of the stutter-doctor's place. I was not supposed
to ask you what you did there and I never did.
Just as you were instructed not to hit me
after a certain age, I suppose when I began
to get breasts. You stopped speaking
to me then. The house bred silence
that each one of us was locked in.

When he's a little better we walk the halls
doing laps on white linoleum. He pushes the IV pole,
which he hates, snarls at me when I encourage
keeping it. He gets exhausted and keeps going.
We unite to corner the resident and ask questions.
I ask for antibiotic peak and trough levels
and the new CT scan results. We circle more
and talk. It's awkward getting going. We aren't
good at this. He is curious about my moving out.
He asks the story, wants to know how bad it was,
what made me leave. And then he asks if I forgive him.
For what? He assumes I know.

You don't understand.
I loved you.
You don't understand
how the hating and hitting
tied us together.
In all of the silence
this was our language.

Bayla Winters

CAT'S CRADLE

I check into Nuclear Medicine
in the basement where the tech runs
her morning mouth:
"Get undressed, leave your shoes on.
Put one robe on open at the back;
put another on open at the front.
Drink half of this. Don't cry!
Come here. Step up. Lie down.
Close your eyes. Have you prayed?
Raise your hands over your head.
Don't move! Hold your breath.
Let it out. You'll feel warm from
the I.V., the machine needs to be
kept cool. Don't bend your arm!
Finish your drink. Don't breathe.
Let it out. Open your eyes. Sit up.
You're finished. Step down. Dress.
See you in six months."
Immobilized in a steel chute,
I have lain in a cat's cradle G.E.
built with my cancer in mind.
Wrapped in a cocoon of coverlets,
I separated sheet from shroud
ready to kill the next cluck that
quacks: *"Did they get it all?"*
Shuffling across Sunset,
I tackle the table for my young,
cherry-sweet doc;
"Let's look at your belly;
where does it hurt? How often do you
go? Much or little? Does it burn?
Sit in a Jacuzzi. Stretch. Try
these pills. It might get better.
I don't know. Take these referrals.
Leave some pee. See you in two months."
I'm in my red Honda going home
thru Griffith Park passing
joggers golfers horse and rider

sweating out their Friday
while my bike gathers a rich patina
of rust in the garage.
(Who's going to nail a large peg
alongside to hang my pain?)
Meanwhile …
I'm thinking of palming off this poem
as a metaphor for the statistic
I've become

See ya!

Libby Bernardin

ON THIS HEALING POWER
for Patsy

I told you when I was a child
I could heal all by crawling
in bed, hiding under covers
to feel my own breathing rhythms:
The heart's celerity whispering
consolation until I felt morning's
power and self could restore self.
That is what we must do now—
attune ourselves.

We have understood fear.
You waited with me while test after test
proved benign only to find
this loathsome thing in your own body.
Your brother said it would be malignant—
that's always the way with good women
he said and he was right:

> Skulking in you is this vine
> with stone-seeking tendrils
> lacking any grace such as
> we might find in the bemused
> and careless Bankshire Rose.

> It rages at your symmetry.

Yet we will attune ourselves,
leave the vine without sustenance,
send bolts of laughter, fragile blossoms
that scatter in the spring wind,
swirl groundward: If we need to we will gather
them in our hands and crush them—
essence penetrating, like morning.

Karen Blomain

THE ROUTE

Seven years later on my way home from lunch,
I'm wandering in old thoughts like tunes I dream to. So
say I'm half noticing a woman in Rea & Derrick parking
lot shoving a shopping bag into the back seat, her face
buckled in on itself. Maybe that trips me up. Or it could
be the one cluster of notes I can't identify for a second,
that turns out to be a song we used to make up to. But something
happens and I've done it—for the first time in all these years
—turned the wrong way, heading down the street my other life
played itself out on. I can't turn back. Unblinking,
I watch the old trees that no time can change and the holly
I planted, three bushes, now trees, one for each clumsy
little helper, all of us pricked at least once
before we patted in the mulch. Or maybe
it's just registering: my friend in the hospital
this morning, explaining the tumor that has grown
in her brain, how she has to turn it into an enemy,
Mafia man, I suggest, joke about the cliché
fedora, the gold tooth. I want her to imagine
a shoot-out, her hand on the trigger. Gun him down,
I say. Later she imitates the hospital p.a.,
a thick sweet voice: Admitting condition, Black.
The code for no more beds. After three weeks,
she knows the jargon. Red top means fire.
It's easier to move everyone quickly along the yellow
lines to exits if no one suspects. More benign
inventions that keep the terror away.
But I'm safely in the car driving by, and nothing
in that house with the stone wall can harm me. I whistle
in relief, like when you're afraid of something
you can't put your finger on, but there's a sting
and you know without looking that you're bleeding,
and somehow it's important to retrace
the route your mind traveled to put you there.

Gary Aspenberg

IN THE BOOK OF TEA

In Okakura's *Book of Tea*
the zen student becomes
a vacuum—open
to all. Today
your best friend
is having her breast
amputated for cancer;
one of my students comes in
to tell me she is going
blind in both eyes;
yesterday afternoon
you longed to make love,
feeling it would be a long time
if we didn't—and now
you're packing to leave town.
I remember you last summer,
depressed, half asleep, you whispered
"Write something nice
about me. . . ."

Walter Peterson

OCTOBER TURNS THE CORNER AND I THINK OF CELLS

In at 8 a.m.
they have completed two small tests:
"Cough, now cough again,"
sent two smiling nurses
and a serious intern by one.
Finally, I stretch out on your bed,
lay my book down on the stand.
You curl up at my hip and fall asleep.
Outside the window, October turns the corner
toward winter and I think of cells.
How cells divide sometimes like an unruly child
growing in unchecked self division within
another's body. I envy my friends
whose wedding we may not dance at tomorrow,
how wedding dresses look best
when wantonly flung
to the far corner of a Holiday Inn room,
how hands look cupped around the areola
of a rose. I have loved breasts
before I have known the difference
between them and me
and you only afterward.
I have kissed them and you,
their memory
and the air where you have lately been
and will do so in the future
if the chance or that need
should arise.

Marion Arenas

LETTER TO AUNT LUCY

I'm mad at you, Aunt Lucy,
I'm mad you didn't tell us
they cut off both your breasts
when you were my age,
you didn't tell us,
the daughters and the nieces,

and now you can't lift up
your arms because they cut out
all the muscles, and when it sneaked
into your backbone and your lungs,
you didn't tell us.
Bald and skinny in a nightgown,

you tell us it's arthritis and pneumonia,
but then your daughter got it
so they took off her right breast and now
she pokes the left one all the time.
I'm mad because we daughters and
we nieces still sit here around your bed

telling lies about arthritis
and then go home to check
each bump and pucker on our chests,
but soon we won't have you to check,
Aunt Lucy, and I'm mad at you for that.
I'm really mad at you for that.

Ingrid Hughes

FEMALE

At the doctor's office where I went about the pebble in my breast,
I looked with jealousy at the lovely clothes of other women,
fear pumping through me. I tried to tell whose breasts were real.
A woman about my age, her eyes riveted to a magazine,
had prominent breasts so bound and anchored
that I thought they weren't alive.

I could see the doctor was a knowledgeable man, and kind.
His fingers working the flesh mine had probed and pressed,
he said, "It's probably nothing, but it should come out."
Can the person announcing you just might die be kind?
"It's the size of an olive," he said.
It's small, I protested. He agreed: a small olive.

At dinner my friend said that when she had her cancer scare
she occupied herself with thoughts of dying nobly.
But I'm damned if I'll let go without a struggle.
Sweet or mean, I'm greedy for this world,
and both my breasts, marked only by my times of nursing.
Darlings, I pray, holding one with each hand,
good globes of sex and life, fight on my side.

Sue Walker

REMEMBER THE PATIENT IS AWAKE
for C.R.

She stares at the O.R. lights
as strong as God's eyes blaring,
hears Country Western music play,
her surgeon say "Take a deep breath;
let it out slow—words she translates
to a mantra: "Breathe in peace, healing;
exhale pain."The anesthetist suggests
a brief sleep—long enough to deaden
the needle piercing her areola,
her chest, but she begs to stay alert,
seeks to address the upper left quadrant
of her breast, divert blood from the site
where the soft snip, snip snip
of scissors cut a mass away.
No one speaks of Love
in the midst of an operation,
so she imagines the word in stitches
the doctor sews—she knows
it is important in the covenant
that exists in this theatre:
surgeon, nurses, patient,
and above all
those eyes.

Marion Arenas

THE SOLARIUM

The spring I got chicken pox Madame put me
in a small room off her bathroom with glass
on three sides, away from the other children
who boarded with her. I was up there
for three weeks, alone but for one angel fish

in a small glass bowl that Mother sent
and the Dionne quintuplet paper dolls:
Marie, Annette, Cecile, Emilie, Yvonne.
My five babies slept in a paper bunting
with five pockets, like a bicycle

built for five, with a name on each slot.
I dressed them in their pink paper dresses
and talked to them about the angel fish.
Their hands and faces turned different ways.
I could tell them apart. I warned them

not to get chicken pox, stood them
on the window sill next to the bed
and chanted their names over and over:
Marie Annette Cecile Emilie Yvonne.
I wasn't allowed to get up except

for the bathroom, but in the late afternoon
I did, looking down at the children, home
from school in the fenced-in back yard.
Madame brought me soup and bread every day.
I ate everything, then fed air soup and air bread

to MarieAnnetteCecileEmilieYvonne.

Ruth Daigon

THE OUTER EDGE

And the blind
whisper to each other
in rinsed voices.
They ask me to describe
darkness. I begin with
the charred edge of the sea,
winds trapped in caves,
a wheel turning away from itself.

I have gone into the hollow place
behind my eyes,
to the outer edge of sight
moving on white lizard feet.

No longer blinded by the visible
the world is nearer in the dark.
Light sinks inward to its core
and the wind on its ghost crutch
brushes the hard limits of a star.

Lisa Schafer

SESTINA

Father gave me a silver key
on a shoelace and told me to mind
Aunt Audry, to stay off the blue
velvet sofa and not to crawl
in the flowerbed or act like a child
when I wasn't. Mother has a disease.

I loved Mother better without her disease
that locks doors and grants a key
and makes me a grownup when I am a child.
She lies on the bed and asks if I'd mind
holding her hand. My fingers crawl
toward hers to embrace bones as pale blue

light sifts through the venetian blinds, making blue
the mirror, water glass, and sheets. Mother and her disease
are close now, she says she can feel it crawling under her skin. She touches the key
swinging from my neck and shining. In her mind
it is a diamond or the sun. She is a child

reaching for magic. I am not a child
because I know better—I know the blue-
ness of this hospital room and I mind
the stream of doctors who find her disease
to be "quite interesting." The key
makes mother smile. I see a spider crawl

through an obstacle course on the nightstand, it crawls
inside a box of kleenex. A child
would think it went in for a reason. The key
to being a grownup is to quietly accept blue
light, bad smells, spiders, and disease.
I watch colors reflected in my mother's eyes. Her mind

holds pretty, unarticulated pictures; my mind
and throat fill with heat and slow tears crawl
down my face. I don't like her disease.
I want to cry fast and loud like a child,
I want to kill blue
and not have to wear this silver key.

But the silver key is imprinted on my mind.
Blue is just a color. Spiders without reason crawl.
And I am not a child because Mother has a disease.
But the silver key is imprinted in my mind.
Blue is just a color. Spiders without reason crawl.
And I am not a child because Mother has a disease.

Glenna Luschei

VISITING HOURS

My aunt tells me she's writing a story
just by turning the leaves of the pad.
Beautiful
not a word on the page.
It's light, pure light.

Against her hospital screen
I sense Nebraska wheat,
touch the wooden wagon Grandpa pulled me in
nights too hot to sleep,
feel ants crawl from the peonies.

Our lives grow bound
through every year
by every wind.
I am reading your story.
My heart turns page after page.

Mary Beth O'Connor

THE EYE DOCTOR

"The little girl has a lazy eye." The doctor squinted at the man in the long camel coat. "We could operate but I don't really see the point." He chuckled to himself at his little opthamalogical joke.

"It's not serious?" the man asked.

"Well, no. Not unless you want to enter her in beauty contests." He laughed heartily at that one, and reached down to give the little girl sitting in his dentist-like chair a squeeze. Her cheeks were still red from the November cold. She watched the conversation between the two men as a spectator watches a tennis match, back and forth.

Back home, the little girl wriggled out of the Sunday clothes she'd had to wear to go see the doctor. She finally could relax and stop worrying about a shot. "It didn't hurt at all," she told her turtle. "They just looked in my eyes and talked." She didn't speak in regular English, but in a special language she used to communicate with her amphibians.

"Oh, oh," she exclaimed, putting her hands on her hips the way she'd seen her mother do. "Where has Jojo gotten to?" She was forever finding that her favorite frog had hopped away into the closet she shared with her older brother, and would be nestled sleeping in one of her shoes. She was always careful to look before putting them on.

By Christmas the little girl's eye wandered so badly that her father took her back to the eye doctor.

"Hmmm," he said importantly, "what have we here? We'll just have to see about this." He refrained from chuckling, since the little girl's problem did appear to be worsening. She sat stiffly in the chair, thinking this time there would be a shot. She didn't even glance around at all the marvelous instruments and machines. Maybe the shot would be *in* her eye! She winced as if she'd been hit.

"Does it hurt you?" the doctor asked.

She shook her head. He frowned. So she squeaked, "a little."

"Why didn't you tell us that it hurt?" her father said gruffly, his concern sounding like anger. The little girl shrunk back in the big black chair and refused to say another word.

The men talked in hushed tones, every now and then glancing at the little girl, who could see perfectly well with her good eye. She heard them say words like "aggravate it" … "operate … " "patch …" … "grow out of it … " … "hurt … ". She began to hum to make herself feel better. She hummed every song she could think of.

The next week at supper the little girl announced that she was going to have to get rid of Albert. Her mother looked surprised.

"He has a lazy eye," the little girl explained. "He won't be able to fit in any beauty contest." She shook her head. "I don't think he'll grow out of it."

258

"Ohh," said the little girl's mother. She was having a hard time looking at her daughter's wandering eye. "Where's your patch?" she asked. Her daughter shrugged. "Why don't you go find it—you look so much like a pirate with it on." So the little girl ran to her room. The patch worn over her good eye seemed to bring the other one into line.

Later they all stood solemnly in the bathroom, as the little girl flushed Albert down the toilet. The mother was relieved because that was one less goldfish and there were already way too many. But the little girl began to cry and wouldn't stop. She went to her room and took off the patch. She stared in the mirror and tried and tried to make her eye look the right way. "Over," she said, but it wouldn't work. She looked for a long time at her goldfish, at how their eyes got huge and funny as they swam past a bubble in the glass. She went to find Jojo in the closet and sat with him among the shoes, hiding until the time they would come to take her away.

Susan Policoff

WORLD WITHOUT END

A storm rattles the windows, and I jerk up in bed, mistaking its force for the outward sign of an old need—to transform my anger, my sense of betrayal into forgiveness. I must've been dreaming of my father, again.

Outside my apartment, the storm whips branches, bends the limbs of a fir. Pale forms wheel around and around the fir with the monotonous rhythm of recurring thoughts. Gulls, by their shape. Harder to pin down numbers because of the wind and the rain, and because I am going blind.

***

My father was thirty-three, seven years younger than I am, when he lost the sight in his left eye. The right lasted another seventeen years. On my thirty-seventh birthday, possessed of two good eyes, I risked hope, but life has to have its little jokes—both of mine are going at once.

"You've inherited the wrong kind of retinal degeneration for the lasers, Cal, not much we can do," my doctor said.

"Not much I can do to change your feelings," my father wrote me, a few weeks before he died. "For your sake, I'm sorry you still feel bad about me."

I shredded the letter, never answered it. Sympathy wasn't what I had needed or asked for.

***

Blindness is a kind of treason of the body—the eyes, the 'windows of the soul'—against the spirit. I can feel my spirit withdrawing. "Going blind's a kind of shrinking," I tell my buddy, Jake.

He drives a cab. Till recently, I did, too. He and I hung out at the race track, angling for fares, watching the races, betting, in between passengers.

"Shrinking?" he asks.

"If I'm invisible to myself, I'll fade out of other people's sight, too."

He squirms, a good friend, but uncomfortable with such talk. "It's not a death sentence," he reminds me.

"Plenty worse things," I agree.

"Right. Famine, war, mental illness, incurable cancer...."

I nod at each item in his litany of lousy fates I don't have to endure, but I hate being grateful someone else is suffering them. I've seen on the street, on television, in the papers, the faces of people who do suffer things more terrible than blindness. Once I can't see them, will they lose reality for me? I'm afraid of this narrowing of the world.

***

Four days have passed, and the world has dissolved into the dreamlike rain. It floods basements, sewers, streets. Helicopters whirr north to evacuate the river towns. The radio reports they're submerged to their rooftops.

The rain pelts down with a sound of hard laughter. The newscaster announces the deluge of water won't alter the region's usual drought next summer. The earth can't absorb it, neither rivers nor reservoirs can contain it. Torrents of it rush away, wasted.

I'm losing my sight in a manner equally dreamlike, amid an overabundance of visual hallucinations. Everything skitters, wavers, dances, as if charged with electric current, shot through with a beam of glorious, unbearable light.

***

My father's sight failed completely in his fifty-first year. He lived on for ten years more, blind, but there was a moment during that year I have always counted as his true death.

He was a big-boned man, but that year, his cheeks acquired a sunken look. I'd get steamed when I noticed a shirt hanging on him, his pants sliding. Before then, he had been so solid. My first memories are of trying to climb his legs, of him hoisting me up to his shoulders. Once, in exuberant play, I slammed into him, and was shocked by his gasp, by my ability to hurt him. He caught a lungful of air, and tussled me down. "You'll be the death of me, Cal," he said, laughing.

He taught me to shoot, and we went hunting together, for pigeons, quail, pheasant. Remembering this, I poke out a finger, idly say, "Bang, bang, you're dead," to the gulls. I can't quite make out my finger. It's engulfed in the beam of light, which originates in my eyes, but I aim at the vibrating shadows surrounding the fir. Bang, bang, you're dead....

As a child, I refused to admit to missed shots. "I hit that bird," I insisted. "It just doesn't know enough to know it's dead."

"Maybe it thinks you don't know enough to know you missed," my father said. "I don't get every bird I aim at."

Pride soothed, I grinned up at him ... But that was long before that moment of betrayal.

***

We lived on a farm converted to a horse-boarding stable. My father managed the stable and the land—acres to ride and hunt in, fields of timothy grown for hay. My mother had died when I was a baby. The nearest town, where I went to school, where my school friends lived, was seven miles away.

We owned a horse, a brown gelding named Lightning. When we rode together, I used a horse we stabled, whose owner wanted it exercised. Not a bad horse, but it lacked Lightning's proud gallop and sleek beauty.

I fed, watered, and groomed Lightning as part of my daily chores. I told the horse my secrets, and found as much pleasure in the nudge of his muzzle, the rasp of his tongue on my skin as I ever found in a woman's touch.

In the fall of my father's fifty-first year, while gentians in the fields glowed like blue flames, he avoided riding and hunting, due to his deteriorating sight, which he never mentioned. I wasn't sorry he stayed away, since I got to ride Lightning. I was eleven. What my father faced in silence had less substance for me than my life of horses, school, and chores. We both considered him a strong, self-sufficient man. He didn't ask for help. I didn't ask if he needed it.

One day, he came into the barn with his rifle. I remember he trailed his free hand along the barn's plank wall, his gait cautious, measured, and that I was careful to ignore this.

"I'm going after a pheasant," he said. "Saddle Lightning."

"He's skittish," I said, tightening the girth. "I didn't get to ride him yesterday."

"Think I can't handle a horse?"

"I'm just saying, he's jumpy." I handed the reins to my father, and began saddling a horse for me.

"I'm going alone," he said.

His harsh tone prevented me from fetching my own .22, but I didn't unsaddle the horse. The day was meant for riding. The intense blue of the sky roused me to an exhilaration all the keener because the wind had an edge, because I knew winter was creeping in, dusk arriving earlier each afternoon.

We both knew a particular section where you could always flush a pheasant. A circular trail enclosed it, opening out into a stand of maples. I decided to watch my father hunt from a distance. I waited till he and Lightning trotted off, and headed down the other fork of the trail.

I veered off into towering wheat grass, which camouflaged thickets of blackberries, elm stumps, bits of rusted machinery. Despite its concealed treacheries, this stretch was the surest place to shoot a pheasant. I could already hear them: Cookcook, cookcook, and a drumming of wings on the ground.

I spotted my father near a dead elm. The ghostly-silver trunk rose above a blue blaze of gentians. My father threw a stone. A pheasant squawked and surfaced, wings thrashing. It honked again. My father fired, missed, cursed, and urged Lightning forward.

After two steps, the horse whistled, and shied. Another pheasant flapped above the weeds. Again, my father's shot went astray. Snarling, he prodded his heels into Lightning's sides. The horse pranced a step, balked. He rolled his eyes, tossed his head, legs stiff and planted.

My own horse snorted, and I allowed him to retreat a few paces. From my new position, I spied what had spooked Lightning, a piece of barbed wire that coiled from the elm to a tangled end among blackberry canes. Most of its twisted length was rusty, but a single strand flashed in the autumn sun.

"Dad, watch the wire," I called, but my father's roars, Lightning's furious whinnies, drowned me out. Panting, red-faced and shouting, my father rammed his boots into the horse's sleek, dark flesh. Lightning danced aside, and bucked, heaving my father into the gentians.

"Stupid horse, I ought to...." My father brushed himself off, still yelling. My horse snuffled, and sidled further back. My father kept bellowing. Frenzied, Lightning flattened his ears, and reared, teeth bared, hooves flailing. With a shrill neigh, he thudded his hooves down so close to my father that both man and horse stumbled.

"What are you, blind? You useless ..." My father seized his rifle and sprang to his feet.

***

The image, the memory, freeze, only to unwind in my dreams, sometimes in slow motion, other times at a jerky double speed: Arm and rifle leap up, finger presses trigger, the air thickens with my cries, Lightning's frantic shriek, my father's hoarse shout. Lightning tumbles to the ground.

I dream this over and over, have, for years. The images never move past that moment. The horse lies still, the known world annihilated. And yet, a sense of incompletion hovers, the moment poised to repeat itself without end.

This, too, repeats—how I stand, mute and paralyzed, staring at Lightning, his dark body reduced to a stain on the glaring blue flowers; how, suddenly, I hate the gentians for their vivid life; how the hole in the horse's chest resembles a different flower, one with a black center and red wet petals.

I wake, certain that the light swallowing my vision is the final burst of that long-ago shot.

Even awake, if I shut my eyes, my father appears, swaying above the fallen horse. His breath hisses, my own sobs in my chest. The odors of spent shell, horse, sweat, and the earth's moist moldiness assail me like fists.

***

An aunt came to collect me two days later. My father had kept to his room those two days. The first I knew of my aunt's coming was her knock on the door.

Numb and confused, I stood in the driveway, my suitcase beside me in the gravel. I waited for my father to speak, but he said only, "Mind your aunt."

For several years, I rejected any contact with him, though once, I asked my aunt, "How could he, how could he?"

"He was upset over his eyes, Cal," she said. "He thought you'd be better off here. But you best ask him."

I refused. To me, his faltering sight wasn't reason enough for so monumental a treason. I mixed up Lightning's death and being sent to live with my aunt into one indigestible lump. I couldn't ask him about it. What if he had no better answer than my aunt? Yet, at last, need overwhelmed me. I had to give him a chance to explain. He had to try, he owed it to me.

He had moved into a cheap residential hotel, in a city north of the farm. Most of its residents lived on pensions. I recall a man of huge bulk, who had to be hauled up from the chair in the lobby where he spent his days, and a withered woman who talked to herself in a low, angry mumble. To see my father among them made me want to smash something, to smash him.

His room reeked of cheap wine. Remote as an indifferent god behind dark glasses, he settled into an armchair that leaked stuffing, and told me to sit. Instead, I paced. We bandied around awkward small talk. Curious, despite a growing misery at his reticence, I asked how he passed the time.

"I go out to the racetrack," he said. "I listen to the horses, smell 'em. I miss horses. You know I love them."

"Like you loved Lightning?"

He must have expected the question, yet, he jerked back as if I had smacked him, and gripped the arms of his saggy chair. Slowly as a man feeling his way along a path he can't see, he said, "Sometimes, Cal, things just happen, and you have to find a way to live with them. But there's things a man has to fight against, any way he can, before he accepts them."

He bowed his head, chin resting on his stained shirt, and I realized he had given me all he meant to. It wasn't enough.

I blundered out of the hotel, out of his life. I never saw him again. I never went riding again, either. But, like him, I missed horses. I resisted their lure for years, but finally, fell into the habit of frequenting race tracks. I guess I, too, will keep on going, to hear the horses, to smell them.

***

The dream, again. After Lightning tumbles to the ground, I moan, toss, drift back to sleep, and confront my father. He huddles in an armchair that trails stuffing, in his hotel room, except it's also my apartment. I start toward him. Something heavy drags me back. I'm holding his rifle, and I lift it ...

***

I keep thinking of him, of his cramped, sour room, of the long hours when the horses weren't running.

I wish I could ask him, when the beam of light that's consuming my vision like a bird of prey is done feasting, and has left me with two black holes, will I be trapped inside them? Were you? Is that why you didn't try harder to tell me?

Bang, bang, I whisper to the unseen gulls. As though I'm really armed, a jolt like a gun's recoil shoots up my spine: How hard did I try? I should have given him as many chances as it took, should have demanded he rouse himself, persisted, until together, we wrestled from the darkness between us, a scrap of grace.

Bang, bang.... Maybe all the chances in the world wouldn't have done it. Maybe only my own blindness can, for my hands are clenched as if they're wrestling, now. I can see the shape of my clawed fingers, but I can't see the gulls. One cries out, a note of piercing sorrow like a lost child, so I know they are there. I guess once the world slips away from me, that's what I'll cling to—the belief that it's there.

264

I unclench my hands, and light from my eyes spills over them. In its shimmer, I picture my father as he appeared in that last dream, slumped in his chair. I see myself, throwing off a thirty-year old weight to cross the room to him. It's too late to matter to him that I can picture this, but it matters to me, and to some balance the earth needs in its swing between the light and the dark.

I envision myself walking toward him, saying, I hope you had something to cling to, those ten years. I'm saying, Dad, I'm sorry it couldn't have been me.

Brian Cronwall

MID-WINTER FLU

It is like forces have invaded the country of my body. Not
just potshots across the border, not just a small foray into
the northwestern corridor, not even just a quick dart for a
regional center—no, it is a full-fledged attack on all
fronts: a coup d'etat in the capital city; troops overrunning
towns, mountain outposts, strategic passes; the navy controlling
several major straits and waterways; troops marching through,
pillaging villages …

But they don't control it all. In a small hideaway in the
dense woods, plans are being made, tactics and strategies
devised to fight a guerilla war against the occupiers:
opening up a vitamin front, sneaking declomycin into the
enemy's maps at night, dropping cough syrup on unsuspecting
guards, ambushing with lemon-and-comfrey tea, generally lying
back, biding time, conserving resources, secretly building a
determination to throw the bastards out …

Jeanne Foster

THE FOOT

When I saw that man's foot
I thought of George,
petrified arches, tendons
like stripped gears. Each year
the leathermaker fitted him for sandals,
the kind that strap to the dumb big
toe, over the purple instep, and around the pounding heel.
George could be a healer.
I saw him lay his hands on a writer's strained back
and ease the pain. I saw him pull
roasting ears from the pit and feed
a whole flock of us. But the longer I lived
with him, the sicker I got.
Everything of his that was twisted,
everything that was dark, everything
that was mean, shuddered into me
when his whole body knotted like his foot
lay on me.
I cried myself to sleep.
I cried myself to sleep.
I cried myself to sleep.
Then the locusts came into the trees,
their noise unceasing, grating and sawing.
Through the night the full moon gave off heat
equal to the sun.
And I arose knowing I was my own
salvation. After that, I began to give him back
the concavities, the convolutions,
the trunk and the seeds.
I let him shake in his own fear.
I let him stutter through his fate. In this way,
I extracted myself bit by bit.
More and more eagerly, I reached for my life
and left him with his.
By God in Heaven, I let him have
himself to heal.
I had not thought about this for years
until I saw that man's foot.

Sue Walker

LIVE OLD SOLDIER, LIVE

Never mind old Soldier,
This is one battle
I'll see that you win.
I'll write the scene,
Place the characters,
Arrange the lines;
Reality is what I make it.

That stroke. It never happened to you.
The word is wrong; I'll change it
To an active verb
Like LIVE.

Arteriosclerosis. That's a medical term.
Ugly. Too long. It has no meaning.
Doesn't fit the context of this passage;
It isn't you at all.

What does the doctor know about your heart?
It's a pump to him, a mechanical thing—
Lines and squiggles on a graph,
A chart he marks: HEART FAILURE.

I refuse to let you die, Dad,
See you suffer, struggle for breath
Flat on your back in a hospital bed,
Your life an electrocardiogram.

I'll stage it all another way.
The month is April,
Azaleas blaze with color in Mobile.
I wear the wishbone pin you gave me,
And when you drive up,
We'll lunch at Korbet's as we always do;
I'll order shrimp cocktail,
You'll have chicken and dumplings
And turnip greens...

Old Soldier, your heart is forever
In the sanctity of a moment like this.

Karl Shapiro

THE FIGUREHEAD

Watching my paralytic friend
Caught in the giant clam of himself
Fast on the treacherous shoals of his bed,
I look away to the place he had left
Where at a decade's distance he appeared
To pause in his walk and think of a limp.
One day he arrived at the street bearing
The news that he dragged an ancient foot:
The people on their porches seemed to sway.

Though there are many wired together
In this world and the next, my friend
Strains in his clamps. He is all sprung
And locked in the rust of inner change.
The therapist who plucks him like a harp
In a cold torture: the animal bleats
And whimpers on its far seashore
As she leans to her find with a smooth hunger.

Somewhere in a storm my pity went down:
It was a wooden figurehead
With sea-heard breasts and polished mouth.
But women wash my friend with brine
From shallow inlets of their eyes,
And women rock my friend with waves
That pulsate from the female moon.
They gather at his very edge and haul
My driftwood friend toward their fires.

Speaking of dancing, joking of sex,
I watch my paralytic friend
And seek my pity in those wastes where he
Becomes my bobbing figurehead.
Then as I take my leave I wade
Loudly into the shallows of his pain,
I splash like a vacationer,
I scare his legs and stir the time of day
With rosy clouds of sediment.

Karl Shapiro

THE LEG

Among the iodoform, in twilight-sleep
What have I lost? he first inquires,
Peers in the middle distance where a pain,
Ghost of a nurse, hazily moves, and day,
Her blinding presence pressing in his eyes
And now his ears. They are handling him
With rubber hands. He wants to get up.

One day beside some flowers near his nose
He will be thinking, *When will I look at it?*
And pain, still in the middle distance, will reply,
At what? and he will know it's gone,
O where! and begin to tremble and cry.
He will begin to cry as a child cries
Whose puppy is mangled under a screaming wheel.

Later, as if deliberately, his fingers
Begin to explore the stump. He learns a shape
That is comfortable and tucked in like a sock.
This has a sense of humor, this can despise
The finest surgical limb, the dignity of limping,
The nonsense of wheel-chairs. Now he smiles to the wall:
The amputation becomes an acquisition.

For the leg is wondering where he is (all is not lost)
And surely he has a duty to the leg;
He is its injury, the leg is his orphan,
He must cultivate the mind of the leg,
Pray for the part that is missing, pray for peace
In the image of man, pray, pray for its safety,
And after a little it will die quietly.

The body, what is it, Father, but a sign
To love the force that grows us, to give back
What in Thy palm is senselessness and mud?
Knead, knead the substance of our understanding
Which must be beautiful in flesh to walk,
That if Thou take me angrily in hand
And hurl me to the shark, I shall not die!

Tom Crawford

THE HEART

The heart, we tell ourselves, is a pump
like any other.
Some things are just true: the fist
we are asked to tighten
brings up the large vein.
How much grief is enough?
Old Mrs. Vorhees
standing on swollen legs
on the front porch
waving at us, believe it or not,
with a red handkerchief. Now she's dead.
I don't know why we won't listen.
If someone holds up a sign which says,
"You're next," we all look around
for the unlucky one.
Aren't we numbered among the chosen,
what's measurable? The walk to the gate
before boarding. The solitary ride home.

Connie Hutchison

PREPARING FOR THE LIVER BIOPSY
for Francine

She draws the world a curve in Prussian
Blue, slashes the page to threshing blades,
calls the series Tilt of Axis. Flame
and more incisions over pastel hues,
the tulips, mint and yellow,
trodden, smoked.
Paper boils
with her liver's essence they will tap.
The nurse compares it to a bee sting
then the pow of impact with a truck.

In rebound, she will order, cleans the house,
begins by opening the bottom drawer,
touching piece by piece the bureau's horde;
clusters of memories, dried lavender,
the skin she hesitates to scrape, all
mingle their perfumes.

I ask her where she sees herself,
what color? Does she hover in the air
above the shining house,
lie tethered to an ochre field?
She answers blue
and I see water, streams.

I remember when she painted liberation:
after viewing Rothko's closed rectangle, canvas tomb,
(one woman fled his airless shout, hand to her throat),
Francine painted her escape:
      wide swathes of orange wash,
      a pendulous drop with transverse orange arms,
      the passages a gentle V, Fallopian.

I see her red, a speck
and growing brilliant.
She gathers calmness
in the orange flume.
Streaming the narrow pseudopod,
             she glides out, protean.

Lynne H. deCourcy

HER SUITCASE PACKED

Her suitcase is packed
to carry into death,
                              but the nurses are plain sick
of her whining about it; she's got maybe six months left,
after all, of this slow closing of her lungs, these trips
in and out of the hospital. They don't understand:
she knows her gasping is worse from the heaviness,
dragging it around on bad days, but it keeps her
alive, too, its weight pinning her
to the earth.
                    Sometimes she opens it to check:
yes, there's Jr., that son of a bitch
who drank himself into an early stroke
after he drank up all she worked for, stuffed
into a small side pocket, finally
out of the way. In other pockets, packed
with more care, her sons. When she looks
at them, sometimes she strokes their soft
baby hands reaching for her
and sometimes she sees them grown, folded into their jobs
and wives, and then she pokes at them angrily, stirring
and jabbing; they don't come often to see her.
There's Reba and Marie, too, her lying sisters
who pretend the Dr. hasn't said
what he has about her lungs
to tell her to buck up, fakely cheerful
and irritated as the nurses
                              when she cries
into the dank, suffocating center of the suitcase,
filled with the raw, wild fear she breathes. It trembles
out through her fingers as she feels the length of clear tube
pumping oxygen into her nose,
                                        when she thinks she hears
the hiss of life escaping through minute leaks.
They fuss at her for the great bruises that stain
the soft insides of her arms like spilled
burgundy, from yanking out
the tubes that feed her
                              when she has gone mad

273

and tried to yank free, drop the suitcase
and dance,

as though she had lived a different life,

out the door of her room
into another whole morning, to open
unweighted arms and embrace
the good air,
                believing it would embrace her back,
like a kind lover; the good air, good air
would embrace her and she could open
her mouth and it would come inside
to fill her, fill her.

Jack Coulehan

THE MAN WITH STARS INSIDE HIM

Deep in this old man's chest,
a shadow of pneumonia grows.
I watch Antonio shake
with a cough that traveled here
from the beginning of life.
As he pulls my hand to his lips
and kisses my hand,
Antonio tells me
for a man whose death
is gnawing at his spine,
pneumonia is a welcome friend,
a friend who reaches
deep between his ribs without a sound
and puff! a cloud begins to squeeze
so delicately
the great white image of his heart.

The shadow on his X-ray grows
each time Antonio moves,
each time a nurse
smoothes lotion on his back
or puts a fleece between his limbs.
Each time he takes a sip of ice
and his moist cheek shakes with cough,
the shadow grows.

In that delicate shadow
is a cloud of gas
at the galaxy's center,
a cloud of cold stunned nuclei
beginning to spin,
spinning and shooting
a hundred thousand embryos of stars.
I listen to Antonio's chest
where stars crackle from the past,
and hear the boom
of blue giants, newly caught,
and the snap of white dwarfs
coughing, spinning.

Jack Coulehan

The second time
Antonio kisses my hand
I feel his dusky lips
reach out from everywhere in space.
I look at the place
his body was,
and see inside, the stars.

Dannie Abse

TUBERCULOSIS

Not wishing to pronounce the taboo word
I used to write, "Acid-fast organisms."
Earlier physicians noted with a quill,
"The animalcules generate their own kind
and kill." Some lied. Or murmured, "Phthisis,
King's Evil, Consumption, Koch's Disease."
But friend of student days, John Roberts, clowned,
"TB I've got. You know what TB signifies?
Totally buggered." He laughed. His sister cried.
The music of sound is the sound of music.

And what of that other medical student,
that other John, coughing up redness on
a white sheet? "Bring me the candle, Brown.
That is arterial blood. I cannot be deceived
in that color. It is my death warrant."
The cruelty of Diseases! This one, too.
For three centuries, in London, the slow, sad bell.
Helplessly, wide-eyed, one in five died of it.
Doctors prescribed, "Horse-riding, sir, ride and ride."
Or diets, rest, mountain air, sea-voyages.

Today, an x-ray on this oblong light
clear that was not clear. No pneumothorax,
no deforming thoracoplasty. No flaw.
The patient nods, accepts it as his right
and is right. Later, alone, I questing for
old case-histories, open the tight desk-drawer
to smell again Schiller's rotten apples.

Clark Powell

POEM FOR THE DEPRESSED

Beneath your chair
gravity reverses itself
at the center of the earth!
Think about this. Think
how ceilings are shaped,
like floors. Think of words
like *mango*.

Remember golf balls, and how
as a child when you cut them
they ran across the rug
unwrinkling their little cores
in a frenzy of rubber bands?

Listen: right now out there
somewhere a recess bell
is about to ring!
And right now
a diver waits deep
in some sea for his body
to change its pressure, to rise,
as a just-born kangaroo rises
through miles of fur
toward a pouch—its mother cannot help,
if it falls it's lost.
But one kangaroo will not fall, will make it
out there, right now, while you read this poem.

This poem is for you.
Stop reading

and go outside.
In winter trees are plans in the sky.

Joanne Seltzer

JENILU

The psychotherapist
who eavesdrops upon
my innermost world
doesn't expect me
to notice hers
because listening
is what she does with her life.

Propelled by the spoken word
my fifty minute hour
moves aimlessly
as in a dream
while the grandmother clock
in the waiting room
ticks away the dollars.

Considering the expense
of a vocalized pause
talk is cheap:
cheaper than cluttering
both hemispheres of the brain
with unsolicited
catalogues of troubles.

Kathleen Newroe

PSORIASIS

For a long time I really didn't think I itched. People would ask me, doesn't it itch; but I'd say no, not really.

I don't mean I itch all the time, but if I stop in whatever I'm doing and see what else it is I'm doing just then, it's itching. I'd have to say that at any idle moment, at any time in my life, I would be likely to find my hand in my hair or at my ankle or behind my elbow, itching.

For a long time I really didn't notice that that was what I was doing. Later in life, when I was a teenager, those commercials came out—well, two of them, really. One was about how a guy would see a girl and think she looked great and then she'd itch her head and he'd be turned off.

It didn't surprise me; this was what my mother had been telling me anyway, along with how I should start wearing lipstick and a girdle.

But then there was that other one, about the "heartbreak of psoriasis."

And that one did get to me because everyone laughed.

It became a big joke, you know. You'd hear it everywhere. "Oh, no! It's the heartbreak of psoriasis!" It was the sarcasm of the times.

It offended me, though I wouldn't have known how to say so then. I mean, I had lived with psoriasis since I was eight and I wasn't walking around all day, everyday, with tears in my eyes. If I was the one who had it, and I could overlook it, I sure thought everyone else could, too.

I guess I got a kind of chip on my shoulder after those commercials. The second time I was in the hospital (I'll tell you about the first time in a minute) they had me wrapped up in Saran Wrap. It was a teaching hospital and all these doctors and interns would come in and look me over like I was some kind of larva ready to pupate. I wore my hair in a towel like a turban. They let me walk downtown like that one afternoon. I pretended I didn't speak English. The rest of the time I stayed in my hospital room. I remember I didn't have much of an appetite. Mostly I dumped the food out the window into this big pine-tree after the nurse left. It was a good contest to see how much of the food hit the tree and how much of it fell the two stories to the ground. The rest of the time I watched the birds and the squirrels come pick at my food.

When I went to college I developed a pretty good answer for people who just couldn't resist asking me what had happened to my legs, or my arms, or my forehead. One day, waiting for the elevator to our dorm rooms, a girl who lived on my floor gasped and asked me.

"What happened to your legs?" she squealed in a particularly offensive manner.

"I was caught in a radioactive cloud," I said.

"Really?" she said. I could see she was impressed.

"Really," I lied.

I don't lie anymore. Recently I remembered the first time I was in the hospital. I was ten years old and four hundred miles away from home, at one of the Mayo Clinics's hospitals.

My mother and father had had to leave me there for ten days. I was so covered with psoriasis, the doctors couldn't get a needle into my arm. They had covered me with tar. It was the only way they knew how to get rid of the old outer layer of skin and let the new skin get through. The nurses were sweet to me. The doctors had put me in the geriatrics ward because usually people are pretty old when they have severe cases of psoriasis.

It was the night my parents had to go home and leave me. I suppose they couldn't afford to stay, and besides it was time for school, and they had to get my brother back in time. I wasn't going to start class the same day as the other fifth graders. The nurses had given me a glass of orange juice from their own refrigerator down the hall and I had been covered, for the third time that day, with the black, ooky-gooky, coal tar.

I was snuggling down in my bed, as well as you can snuggle when your pajamas stick to you everywhere and you smell like a newly-surfaced county road. I had ahold of a clown doll my father had brought me. It was red and white silk and had a wind-up stick of a nose that played a lullaby. It was getting all tar-covered, of course, and I felt badly about that but I held onto it anyway.

I rolled to the side of the starchy white bed and looked out the window. Way across I could see another building, or maybe it was another wing of the hospital I was in. I could see four or five stories of it, standing solid and square and black in the night.

And then I saw a light come on in one window, just one window. It was on for just a short time, and then it went out and the light in the next window came on. Then that one went out and the next light came on and the next, on and off, you see, all the way down the hall.

I suppose it was a janitor moving from one office to the next that night, emptying garbage cans or picking up newspapers. I don't know. What it seemed to me was how like those little lights going on and off we are, separate from one another, and alone; just lined up, one after the other, with some random or ritualized duty or habit holding us together.

I wasn't mad at anybody then. I knew it would be up to me. I knew there would be people who would try to help and I knew there would be people who wouldn't understand or whose curiosity would get the better of them.

I do itch. Sometimes I try not to because I don't want to make other people uncomfortable. and sometimes I go ahead and scratch where it itches because I have to.

David Hood

RHEUMATIC FEVER

Elizabeth is sick,
The doctors say
it might be
rheumatic fever.

Her joints are swollen
and ache when she moves.
Elizabeth's mother
touches her legs
and feels small suns
burning in the bones.

A kitten rubs my ankle.
I pick it up
and put it on the bed.

Tomorrow at the clinic
the thermometers
blood tests
stethoscopes
and probes
will announce
an antiseptic answer.

But what murmur
of the heart
can purr loud
as the kitten
she holds
in her arms?

Jan Epton Seale

THE DAY I WENT TO VISIT MY INNARDS

I never intended to make an appointment with my innards. You might have to make a date with your girl or the dentist but not with your innards.

But then again, I never intended to have some of them out. About a year before, I woke up one morning north of Albuquerque and passed a bunch of blood. When I saw it, I said flat out loud, "You've got cancer. You've gone and taken up with cancer."

Well, I just pulled on my pants, went out to my rig, made my delivery, then let the throttle out all the way back to Texas.

I don't know what I thought crossing the state line would do for me. My mind was batting around like one of those bingo number-picking things that blows a bunch of ping-pong balls around in a little cage. I guess I was hoping my lucky number would land in the little cup and that blood back there could be a secret between me and New Mexico.

Still, when I got back to Borger, I told Sue about it and she threw a fit so I told myself I'd see about it to satisfy her.

Dr. Winkel's been our doctor since before the beginning of the age. His office is at the corner of Main and Juniper. I've often wondered what a family does when their doctor gets old and dies. Funny, but it seems kind of disloyal of the doctor. I mean, he goes and does the very thing he's been fightin' against all these years. Well, but why am I talking like that? Of course, Dr. Winkel wasn't dead when I went to see him.

I wouldn't say he and I were good friends but we had a kind of tie and that was hunting in the fall with the same group of men on the same deer lease. Some years that's the only time I'd see him. Other years, I'd see him quite a bit, because he doctored Donald Joe and Jeanie Sue when they were little. For that matter I knew Dr. Winkel's nurse Mari about as well as I knew Dr. Winkel—though it goes without saying that I'd never gone hunting with *her*. But Mari is a real sweet woman. She was just as nice as could be when Sue had the kids and then she was nice to them when we'd take them in over the years with runny noses and for their school shots and so forth.

The night before I went in to see the doctor, my stomach hurt like crazy. I kept getting up all night to go to the bathroom until finally the cockroaches didn't even seem to mind me turning on the bathroom light. They went on about their business right there around my feet. Whatever their business is. I'd never seen one doing anything productive. At least ants carry crumbs and mosquitoes bite you.

Finally there wasn't any use making the run back to bed so I sat there and counted the tiles on the floor and wondered who Sue would marry after I died in about a year, and whether Donald Joe and Jeanie Sue would get to college if they wanted to.

Even though I knew better, I dreaded that appointment like I dreaded a haul to Houston. Once I got lost in Houston and it was 24 hours before I found the warehouse. At least I was going to a familiar place. But when I got there, I saw Dr. Winkel had bought new flowered furniture for his waiting room, taken in a new man, added another nurse, and put up a little glass cubicle with a woman inside at a computer. You can't believe how it unnerved me.

Sure enough, the new nurse, a little slip of a thing, came to get me. Kathi—I got that from her name tag—said, "Right this way," and then is when I realized Dr. Winkel had remodelled throughout—with a low ceiling, more exam rooms, lots of indirect blue lights, and a carpet. I wanted to bolt. If I hadn't felt so bad I would have bobtailed it out of there.

Kathi weighed me and took my temperature and asked me why I was there.

I didn't want to hurt her feelings but I wasn't about to tell her anything. So I said, "I'm just here for a check-up. Kinda tired lately. When you get to be 45 years old, you'll understand."

She smiled and rested her pen on the chart. "It says here 'rectal bleeding.' You must have talked to Dr. Winkel over the phone."

My stomach hadn't been feeling too good and it'd been well over an hour since I left the house, so when she caught me in that lie, it *really* knotted up and I thought I was going to have to excuse myself.

Instead, I crossed my legs fast as a jack-knife and laughed—kind of a careful laugh though. "Oh yeah. I did mention that to him."

Kathi got ready to write again. "Okay. When was your last bowel movement?"

I was beginning to understand the lay of the land. I knew perfectly well it had been about an hour but I studied how to say it. Seems like to say, "One hour and fifteen minutes ago" was showing you were paying too much attention to that sort of thing. So I said, "This morning." Kathi made a notation.

"What was the consistency?"

I felt like I was on a quiz show going for broke. I hadn't ever described to another person what I did in the bathroom, much less to a nineteen-year-old girl named Kathi. Now that I think about it, her not having a "e" on the end of her name kind of unnerved me.

I searched around for a word. "Loose." I know I colored.

Kathi wrote. "Did it have blood in it?"

"Yep."

"Was it a black tarry substance or bright red?"

"Pretty red," I said.

She stopped writing and looked straight at me. "Was it a little or a lot?"

I felt something inside my head crack open. I think I even heard it. It was the sound of a turtle or armadillo shell when it's hit out on the road. "You mean the blood or the whole thing?"

"I'm sorry," Kathi said, "the blood."

I was hurting real bad by that time. "Beats me. Hell, I don't know what's a little and what's a lot."

She looked sort of disappointed. "Maybe like a teaspoon, or like a half a cup?"

I had to admire that little gal. She was bound and determined to do her job. I sighed and shifted around on the stool. "All told, it must have been a half a cup."

"What do you mean by 'all told'?"

The armadillo was just lying there on the road, guts strung out, the echo of that crunch going on and on like in a shooting gallery.

I looked straight at her. "I mean I was on the toilet the better part of the night and I guess I lost that much all told."

"I see," Kathi said, and wrote some more on the chart.

When Dr. Winkel came in, I noticed he had grayed more in the months since I'd seen him. We talked a little about the deer lease and whether the season was going to be any good or not. Then I told him all in one breath about the blood in Albuquerque and hightailing it home. I hadn't really spelled it out over the phone. I even beat him to the draw and told him I knew it couldn't be much else but cancer and how long did I have.

He said, "Not so fast, Bill. We're going to take this thing slow. I'll order some tests, we'll look at the results, and if it's the big C, we'll get you the best help we can find."

He wrote a little more and handed me some papers. "Bill," he looked at me in that I'm-telling-you-the-gospel-truth way, "the next few days you'll feel like you was on the business end of Roto-rooter."

He slapped the chart shut and started for the door, then said over his shoulder, "We'll talk some more later about huntin' this year, okay?"

I've already told you more about my guts than I first intended to so I'll skip over the next few weeks by just saying that I got so used to taking enemas and dropping my drawers and having people run tubes and lights in me that after a while, it seemed like these things had been happening to me all my life. And that there was a big industry of this sort of thing, generally hidden and secret from the public, but at least as big as IBM or Ford when you got into it and found yourself a customer or stockholder or whatever.

Then you started meeting the same people over and over again. First in the drugstore the evening before the tests, buying their Fleets and that awful yellow liquid dynamite that would blow you out of bed at 4 a.m.

And lo and behold, when Dr. Winkel sent me over to Big D, there they were up in Dallas again at the Medical Complex. We looked like a bunch of pervert choir members standing around in the doorways of the x-ray station in our short white gowns. I never got one of those little cup-towely things that had a decent tie or snap on it and it looked like neither did anyone else so we spent the whole time clutching at our behinds to keep from exposing ourselves. We made up our own little games to keep ourselves from dying of shame on the spot. The object was to tell how your body had let you down worse than all the rest.

"Fell unconscious in the bathroom and lay that way four hours until my son happened by ..."

"A wonder you hadn't died, but listen, I lost a quart of blood inside of an hour ..."

"But at least you're here to tell about it. I know I had this friend ..."

And then's when we started on the second generation stories.

The long and the short of it, and believe me, there was more long than short by the time I got through, was that I didn't have cancer but I did have something else I'd never heard of—CUC—and wished to God I never had. Seems I'd had it for a long time. Some people were sick for years and some, like me, just showed up with it after it had done its dirty work and ruined their colons.

The trouble with CUC, besides having to quit your job, losing weight, sitting on the throne day and night, having constant fever and pain—the trouble was two things: you couldn't get any sympathy from people because you couldn't spell out the details, and eventually, you had to have an operation and have it all taken out or you'd get cancer.

That's how I wound up at the Medical Complex making an appointment to visit my colon.

"Will Friday at 4 p.m. be all right with you?" the lady beside my bed asked. At these big hospitals they have people that are like USO directors. They go from room to room asking sick people if they think they can possibly squeeze in time for physical therapy on Thursday morning or a sugar diabetes study first thing next Monday, or in my case, a trip to the pathology lab.

"I had planned to go dancing that afternoon but I guess I could call it off," I said.

She grinned. "An aide will take you down in a wheelchair; I'll set it up." She patted my arm and was gone.

When I started all this, I liked to never got the hang of staying alive in a hospital. The things they do to you in a hospital—well, you think at the time you'd just rather go ahead and die than endure them. You have to give up, give up completely, just pull her over alongside the road and take the keys out of the ignition and say, "I quit." Many's the time I felt so bad, all that saved me was knowing my pants and boots were in the closet. The real me was waiting in there in the dark, my belt buckled up, a bill of lading in my hand.

Now I don't want you to get the idea I'm some kind of prig. Truckers' stop johns are not for the faint of heart. And I've told and listened to my share of doctor and nurse jokes. But let me tell you, you hit that hard white bed and they start coming at you with all those rotten things they do, well, it's not funny like those dirty jokes and sex gizmos.

After a while, giving up felt good. Maybe I went a little overboard asking to see my colon. But after all people took their gallstones home in a little bottle. My sister's appendix sat pickled on the shelf over her bed for five years.

I readjusted the tubes out of me and took a peek at the 13-inch scar going down my middle. It took a little detour around my navel so that the whole thing wound up looking like a giant question mark. The bag with the "efflux" (they have a nice clean name for everything nasty) lay on my right side like a forgotten water balloon.

Sue had gone back to Borger to be with the kids and it was just as well. She was a pretty unflappable girl but I didn't know if she'd think I had cracked up for wanting to see my colon.

I hadn't told anyone else after I told my friend Tom. It's something I have to do. I want to make sure it was bad," I explained. "I wake up nights wondering. Just sit up and sweat about it. At the time, I was hurting so much I didn't care. Now I think if I could have held out a little longer ... some people get over this thing. Maybe I traded my birthright for a mess of pottage, you know."

I saw Tom's hand go to his throat and then he pretended to scratch a mosquito bite. "Yeah." He looked across my bed and out the window. "Do you think the Cowboys are ever gonna' get it together again?"

Friday afternoon dragged by. I got up a couple of times to watch the Med-vac helicopter taking off from its pad. It made me want to get back behind the wheel of my rig and see that flashing center stripe again. I wondered if I'd ever have the balls to haul cross country again. I stood straight and the new scar pitched a fit.

"Mr. Watkins, you ready?" Joe stood in the doorway. "I understand you've got a 'pointment' with pathology." There was a little tease in his voice.

Joe was huge and he and I had been through a lot together. I know it didn't mean a thing to him but I was beginning to feel he and I had been lifelong buddies.

We got the damned ostomy bag emptied and cleaned and then he helped me in the chair and started on the tubes. He changed the IV over so that the little bags were swinging on a pole attached to the chair. He emptied the catheter bag—thank God—and hung it on a hook on the side of the chair. He put little temporary doo-dad stoppers on the two drain tubes coming out of my sides and pinned them to my gown. Then he put a temporary clamp on the tube coming out of my nose.

He laughed softly. "Don't you look fine, Mr. Watkins!" Right at that time, Joe was the only person on earth that could get away with saying that to me. Oh, my friends had said other things when they called or came to visit. Some said they sure were glad everything had come out all right, or that I'd got this behind me. I'd think about those expressions and laugh my head off when they were gone. One of my trucking buddies came over here and told me I sure had a lot of guts, going under the knife. He colored real deep after he said it. The one I like the best was when somebody asked me what by gut-level reaction was to something. I couldn't help it. I said. Hell, I don't have one of those anymore."

We started out. Once, going down a long hall, I thought of telling Joe I'd changed my mind. Take me back. I felt like Aunt Bertie who lived across the street from the funeral parlor and made herself unpopular by regularly visiting the lying-in-state room so she could tell the family of strangers how "natural" their loved one looked. But it was too late to back out. Besides, I'd never know whether I'd made the right decision or not. For that matter, I might look at it and still not know.

We stopped at a door that said "Pathology Consulting." Joe wheeled me through. It was a small room with a low counter. Joe went around to a phone, punched a button, and said, "Mr. Watkins, four o'clock, is here to see his specimen."

In a minute a door bumped open and man in surgical greens, complete to the mask, came out carrying what looked like a turkey roaster pan covered with a napkin.

Now this took me completely by surprise. I had been prepared for a snake-looking thing sloshing around in a big pickle jar but not a piece of meat in a turkey roaster.

The man behind the mask set the pan on the counter in front of me. He told me his name—it was a foreign one—and that he was chief of pathology. Then he took the napkin off.

I didn't know whether to say hello or spit on it. It was gray, about three feet long, and one big mess—but then what did I know? It wasn't like link sausage, like the encyclopedia pictures. It wasn't all gleaming pink and red either. I tell you what it looked like, and excuse me if this is—was—your favorite barbecue cut, but it looked like the world's biggest fajita.

"Vee cut it laterally for zee examination," Dr. Gorba-somebody said, moving it around with some ice tongs. "And it has shrunk considerably."

"Show me the bad part and then show me a good place." I wanted to make the comparison with my own eyes and know for all time that it'd been necessary.

Dr. G looked at it for a moment, then said, "Oh, zat von't be possible. It simply von't be possible."

So. They didn't know after all. They just guessed. I was madder than hops. "Why not?"

"Because zere are no good places to show you. It was totally diseased—one of zee verst ve've ever received." He bent over the pan and pointed. "See all zeeze little ripples? That is zee disease."

I strained to see what he saw. The little ripples looked like the tenderizer had gone berserk on the fajita.

I sighed and stared at the poor lame thing. It had caught some kind of fever or been trapped in a germ war and that's about all we knew. It took sick and died inside me and would have taken me with it if it could have. It was just as tormented and sad as could be. I'd miss it, but I wasn't going to act like a man with no guts (ha ha).

Dr. Gorba-something showed me which end was which. He showed me the appendix, dangling there like a little baby. He showed me a piece of the small intestine they'd snipped off for good measure. "In-tes-stein," he said every time.

"Anything else you vant to know?" He had obliged me about as much as I could stand.

"Thanks," I said. "You can throw it away now."

"Oh no," he said, "vee keep zem practically forever. You can come back years from now and see it again. Zey are studied over and over."

So it was to be like an old truck tire. A tire could lie around for a lifetime unless someone poured gasoline on it and burned it. Then it would make one last hoot and holler with black smoke seen all around the countryside.

"Well, whatever." I turned to go. Joe took command of the wheelchair. I knew one thing. I wouldn't be back and I wouldn't be crying over spilt milk.

We were almost out the door when Dr. Gorba-whatever stopped us. "Oh, Mr. Vatkins, one more zing." He stood pointing down at the pan. "You have just seen a perfect example of a cancer host. If zis vere five years later, I vould be showing you your cancerous colon."

That did it. "Joe," I said, once we'd bumped out into the hall, "floorboard this thing. I gotta' get the lead out."

He did, and we didn't hit a single armadillo or turtle on that haul back to the room.

Lila Zeiger

EGRESS

"I'm terribly sorry but I seem to have lost all control of my bladder." It was difficult to sound dignified when there she was, peeing all over the goddamn floor. She was mortified to be laid out under such a bright light with so many men in the little room—especially since someone had taken her glasses away so she couldn't see what they were doing down there between her thighs. As they scurried about in their white coats with what looked like large blotches over them, she suddenly realized that it was not urine that was gushing out of her, but blood.

The gynecologist, who had been hastily summoned that evening, was the biggest man in the field—but he was so tiny, actually, that she hoped that his grasp would exceed his reach. And she was really infuriated to be here with all these men, and none of them paying any attention to her as a *person*. Big G was actually teaching the others right inside her crotch, one could say. She thought of her father's sad admonition to novices: "You are learning to cut hair on *my* beard!"

"Now here's where we have to be careful of sepsis," the gynecologist was saying with certainty. "Just at this point we must provide egress."

"Egress!" she yelled. "That's an odd way of putting it. It's like Barnum's sign, isn't it? TO THE EGRESS!" When she laughed aloud at her own remark, he said quickly to the others, "She's becoming hysterical. Too bad we can't sedate her."

And that was when she could no longer make believe that all this was happening to someone else. She stamped her feet (as best she could in the stirrups) and wept. "How can I be hysterical, when my womb was taken out just last week? And don't be so smug about the egress—you can read it in a book. Barnum put up a sign to keep people moving. They thought they were going to see a marvelous beast, but it was really the exit."

No one was listening. They seemed to be snipping away at something down below. The pain was so awful that she couldn't locate it exactly. So she decided to hell with them all. She'd just keep shouting to the ceiling about Barnum's egress until they let her out of there.

Safe in a hospital bed that night, she made solemn preparations for her funeral. Important questions presented themselves, like who would take care of the baby, and would it be more appropriate to play the "Bach Oboe Concerto" or "Greensleeves."

By morning, however, the nurses were finally taking her pressure in as much as half-hour intervals, and it looked as if the blood had decided to stay inside her for now. Indeed, it was never to come out of *that* place anymore. And sure enough, in about two months, there she was back home again holding the baby. And it was really amazing how quickly and easily she caught on to fucking again.

In time, as such things do, the whole thing became quite a funny story—something like this one. But what stayed with her was the certainty that she would never let herself be ushered to the egress before she was quite ready to go. In fact, she decided, they would probably have to remove her bodily.

Michael Chitwood

WHAT WE DO NOT KNOW

He called it "Taking the steam," and it began the winter after his return. We would find his suit pants neatly draped across the seat of one of the dining-room chairs, which he had placed outside the bathroom door. His starched white shirt and coat were hung on the chair's back and his shoes, each with its sock, stood formally in front of the chair. Inside you could hear the water pouring.

This was also when he began to use his power, which he said he always possessed but had never felt possessed by. That is, never until he saw the large woman in the white, billowing sweater and white knit pants tucked into tight black boots. She looked like a cloud on stilts, picking her way through the mud puddles of the feed store parking lot.

It came up as a humming in him, as though, he would later describe, he had suddenly been inhabited by a swarm of bees.

He stopped her as she reached the steps to the loading dock and took her hand, which had a large wart, just back of the first knuckle. He lifted her astonished hand to his mouth as if he were going to kiss it and began to speak in a low voice. Neither she nor I could hear him distinctly enough to tell what he said or even whether what he said was in a tongue recognizable to us.

He finished what he had to say and placed her hand back at her side as if he were putting a cherished object in its resting place.

"That blemish will trouble you no more," he announced and turned toward our car, leaving me with the bale of peat moss and bag of seed packets.

I questioned him on the way home but he just watched the landscape feed into where we had been. After telling the family over cocktails and everyone saying Papa this and Papa that, we very nearly forgot about the incident until the woman knocked at our door with members of the Firefighters' Ladies Auxiliary in tow.

When I opened the door she presented her hand to me and at first I thought she had decided that taking a woman's hand and speaking to it was a custom with the men of our family, a custom which she enjoyed and was here to honor. However, I quickly saw that she was displaying the hand he had held and that the wart was completely gone without any mark remaining.

The other women then began to show me hands, knee caps, big toes, forearms and one brazenly lifted her blouse to reveal, and this on our street-side porch, a very large wart and the edge of an extra large, lacy bra cup.

I explained that I shared their enthusiasm for what had happened, but that they would have to speak, or show themselves, as the case might be, to Papa.

Since then the wart-afflicted make regular calls. The old gentleman has his ritual—he emerges from the steam in a long, red bathrobe and announces whether he will see any callers that day. He does not always see them and if he "isn't square" that day, those who have appeared must return another time. If he is giving an audience, he conducts the whole process clad only in the bathrobe. He moves in close to the wart no matter its bodily location and speaks to it. He has yet to fail.

For our part, we have made no protest. My wife did suggest, early on, that he conduct the business in some other attire, but he shushed her with "Do not speak of what you do not know."

Since then, we have not spoken of it, even to each other, for it is true that we do not know what language the flesh obeys.

Christopher Moylan

RECOVERY

Here, in your east of unfinished
novels and talk, you boast
of dangers overcome, long exile—
way-ward surge of blood on bone,
billowing skin, downward drift
of wit your own, not your own,
to its sink of corrosive metals
and cold fire. You've no gift
to still your own wasted gifts,
their incessant singing in shadows.
You fear you'll end your days
dry and stale, watching
detritus of family, career
vanish in riots of dead time
that cry from waves of the tv.
Who will know or care, years hence,
you kept your eyes open,
your ears unstopped with wax
when facing siren song of career
and hard cash? That life is gone …
Yet each line is a charmed circle,
a still spot in cracked bell
of a chest cough, in clash
of cymbals and tiny hands
on alarm clocks winding back.
There, the day is young. Islands,
flora and fauna, relieve blue—
white symmetry of cloud and sky,
and pleasure beams its milk—
white nimbus deep in knotted
belly of approaching storms.
Each word you write springs
chameleons and spotted birds
greening, yellowing, fading
to diamond black and white,
till these reduce to one beam
of light, one simple unspoken
line suspended, like the cord
on bedside lamplight
between darkness and desire.

Marilyn Kallet

LANDSCAPE WITH BLUEBIRDS

Winter colorless after a long illness,
at last I see Paul Klee's "Landscape with Bluebirds,"
a score of red, green, and seablue trees,
a small blue mosque, canvas alive with color.

At last I see colors, Paul Klee's landscape alive
like the wrap of a woman washing clothes in the sun,
and a small blue mosque, a religion of color.
The text of his journal alongside: "Color possesses me."

Warm like the wrap of a Tunisian woman.
"I don't have to pursue it … That is the meaning
of this happy hour." "Color possesses me."
"Color and I are one. I am a painter."

Red, green, seablue trees, bluebirds on clay roofs,
Healing colors after a winter's long illness.

David Ignatow

FOR MY MOTHER ILL

I'll join you in your sleep,
into the same darkness dive,
where dead fish float together.
But we shall be communing,
blindly and without feeling;
but by knowing now,
as I lie back upon a pillow,
as you close your eyes,
the comfort of it.

Barbara Crooker

ON LOSING MY ANTERIOR CRUCIATE LIGAMENT
for Jean Pearson

One way to speed the body's healing,
according to the Christian Scientists,
is to imagine that love is radiating
out from the injured part.
And so I think of this creaky hinge,
my wounded knee, filled with blood & pus,
bits of torn cartilage,
the last scraps of the ligament
that held it together;
I think of it opening
like a sunflower,
the noon sun's double;
I see sprays of forsythia
crown the patella;
hear daffodils sing a cappella
on its knobby tor.

Rochelle Natt

EULOGY FOR MY MOTHER

This is a eulogy written before death. It is for my mother who is locked in purgatory. The clinical name for this state is Alzheimer's disease, which is a progressive loss of memory until ultimately, the mind forgets to tell the rest of the organs how to keep the body alive. The cause is a matter of speculation and the cure, or at least, control, is unavailable at this time. Perhaps prayer will soon release her to embark on the celestial journey. I don't visit her anymore, but I write about her or to her everyday, and thus, the relationship continues although she has long ago forgotten who I am. My last physical visit was when she was still in a private nursing home. She had to be transferred to a state institution because she screamed continuously and it was too disruptive to the other patients.

I passed the entertainment room. A row of elderly people in wheelchairs were being serenaded by two guitarists. I can still hear them singing: "Through all kinds of weather, what if the sky should fall? Just as long as we're together, it really doesn't matter at all."

An eerie howl drowned all sound. I couldn't tell whether it was coming from me or my mother as I looked into her reclining wheelchair. The stalk-like limbs crossed themselves. I picked up the gnarled bird-like hand and called, "Ma," across the barrier of gibberish. "It's me, Rochelle." Her magnificent blue eyes opened for a moment. She began to cry. I heard her say, *"Hob rachmones oft mir"* I couldn't be certain that I hadn't rearranged her invented language to extract the Yiddish plea, "Have pity on me." Or was it my own heart making that request? Her eyes sealed again. She couldn't look with me at the framed photographs of all our family that my sister had so lovingly brought. Had they given her a moment of comfort? I looked out on the faces of my sister, brother, nieces and children and thanked them for being there with me.

I cannot connect this being to my mother who could never stop moving. She used to come home from a full day's work at my father's grocery store and hang wallpaper or antique the living room furniture for recreation. She filled every moment. I can still recall the clacking of knitting needles coming from behind the closed bathroom door. Productivity! My mother had her fourth child, her only son, when she was forty-two. Both my parents often referred to him as their "Kaddish," the one who would say the prayers of remembrance after they were gone.

How I wish that her closing years had reflected the boundless play and joy she contained! When she was in her fifties, my mother would take a running slide over a snowy sidewalk shouting, "Whee." At all the weddings and bar mitzvahs, my mother whirled solo across the dance floor, singing loudly. I shrivelled with embarrassment as any teenager would. I resented her not being sedate like the heroine of the old television show, *"I Remember Mama."* However, I continued having those feelings through adulthood. When her behavior became bizarre, I reacted as I used to as a girl.

I was so involved with my own feelings that I couldn't discern that the new experience were outgrowths of a physical condition.

Two years before she was hospitalized, I took my children to visit her. She ran across the boardwalk singing, "Stay young with youth." I winced. This had been a theme of my childhood. Mother wanted to be as young as her three daughters. My children, as usual, were wiser than I. They loved it. They already had a sensible grandma who read them stories and wiped their noses. Here was one that could dash about like a small child.

Incidents began dangerously escalating. My mother wasn't eating and grew seriously malnourished. Several times, she was picked up by the police for vagrancy. Once, when my sister brought her a chicken, she put it directly on the flame without benefit of a pan. The fire department began making regular house calls. Neighbors continuously phoned us, but we couldn't understand. Whatever measures we took were like putting bandaids on a swollen dam. We couldn't see the obvious. This woman, who single handedly nursed all of us through pneumonia in staggered succession without ever coming down with it herself, was totally incompetent. We hired a full time companion, but mother's situation was far beyond the ability of one person to handle. She was like a large toddler, constantly pulling everything down, running with sharp objects and toying with the gas. There was no time to get her into a nursing home. I had to bring her straight to a mental hospital to await placement. Along the way, she kept shouting, "I want my son, my son, the only one." I felt the knot of jealousy tighten my stomach. I still couldn't stop my role in a tired old drama.

After admission, when she was settled in, I watched her lie back on her bed. Her last coherent words to me were, "I'm not as young as I thought." I wanted to scream, "Run, Mama, run. Stay young!" It was too late.

If I could waken her from this nightmare, I would say, "Ma, I hurt so much to see you like this. I know now that any pain I experienced in connection with you at any other time of my life was inflicted as innocently as it is now. Thank you for my birth."

Elspeth Cameron Ritchie

HOSPITAL SKETCHBOOK
Life on the ward through an intern's eyes.

ON THE WARD

I carry three AIDS patients, about the same as any other intern on the medicine service at my hospital. One is a young black male, one a young white female, the third a middle-aged black male. The young man received a lethal blood transfusion three years ago. The black man, married with children, has told us of his homosexual activity. The white female has known no risk factors, but we suspect IV drug use. She may simply have slept with an infected man.

A scant two years ago, in a hospital that has a high proportion of AIDS patients, an intern would average only one AIDS patient. I was a third-year medical student then. I cared for, and became close to, my intern's AIDS patient.

His name was Dave. He was attractive, very thin, and gay. He ran fevers and we could not find the cause. So we drew culture every night, seeking the bug that shot his temperature up to 104 degrees. He would ask me late at night, while I was setting up the tubes and bottles, why I was planning to hurt him. I never had an answer I believed in. The blood cultures were always negative. We finally treated for pneumocystis pneumonia. Then he spiked fevers in reaction to the antibiotic.

At first I gowned and gloved whenever I entered his room; I hated to draw his blood, fearing needle sticks and contamination. I grew more relaxed; sometimes I almost forgot to put on gloves when I drew blood cultures.

He hated being in the hospital. He could not eat the food and seemed thinner every day. I tried once bringing him his favorite flavor of ice cream, butter pecan, from the cafeteria. He thanked me for it but I think he just let it melt.

I rotated off service. I remember his fantasies of leaving, going home to Florida, and floating downstream in a leaky canoe. I'm sure he is long since dead.

Now, with so many patients to care for, both tragedy and precautions are routine. Any patient is risky. I recently stuck myself with a needle for the first time in my life. Fortunately, the married lady had no risk factors. I sent off hepatitis screen and HTLV-3 (now called HIV) tests anyway. They are due back in two weeks. Should I sleep with my husband until then?

All of my HIV patients are sick, hurting, up here on the medicine ward. Asymptomatic ones wait for disposition on the self-care ward. They also wait for the first signs of real illness: the white thrush over the throat, the purple spots of Kaposi's, and shortness of breath of pneumocystis.

My middle-aged black man will die soon. He has cryptococcal meningitis and pneumocystis pneumonia. The titer of cryptococcus is the highest that this hospital has ever seen. Recently he has become even more short of breath and his tremor has gotten worse. He also has painful rectal herpes. Today his bronchoscopy specimens show an acid-fast bacilli, probably a special form of tuberculosis that immunosuppressed patients get. He is already on four toxic antibiotics. What do we do now?

He finally allowed me to tell his family that he is very sick. They do not know of his AIDS diagnosis. His numerous and respectable family arrived last week. They questioned me as to whether he has cancer. I hedge and talk of his pneumonia. They ask me whether he will come home soon. Not yet, he's very sick, I answer. They suspect the truth, I think, but do not ask. His wife has not called.

Interns see a lot of sickness and death. We build up protective mechanisms: she was old, he drank too much. If somebody our age is dying, our mental dams sway. It could be my best friend (who is gay), it could be my college-age brother. There, but for the grace of God, go I.

My young black male received a blood transfusion after he had a minor accident two years ago. He developed a painful throat ulcer and fevers. He was diagnosed six months ago. He did not tell his family for three more months. He is from a remote town in Kentucky and he did not know how his family would respond. They are angry that he did not tell them sooner. He is about to go home for a convalescent leave. What will his neighbors say? Will they believe the blood transfusion or suspect his morals? Will anybody enter his house?

He is still attractive and personable, if thin. This morning he told me how nice I looked. I replaced his feeding tube; his throat hurts too much to swallow. We are doctor and patient. Two years ago I would have hoped that he would ask me out.

I tell myself severely that it is no good crying for him. He has five sisters who will weep. I have other patients to care for.

The third patient, the young white female, is hostile, remote. She has end-stage renal disease and is on dialysis. You have to coax her into drawing her blood. I don't want to do it either, but the consultants recommend an antibiotic level. Of course, they are not the ones who stick her. I am her intern.

I have other patients, patients with heart, lung, liver, and kidney disease, but they come and go quickly. They die or leave. Except, of course, the elderly waiting for nursing home placement. I hope to send one to a home soon. He has been in the hospital for ninety days.

I also care for healthy HIV-3 positive patients. They are still working and active and only come to the hospital for staging. While here, they have their blood drawn for T-cell count and their skin pricked to see if they react to allergens. Then they return home. One to their jobs and families. One recent twenty-nine-year-old admission was diagnosed eight months ago. His wife was initially negative; a month ago she converted. They have two children, six and eight, who have not yet been tested.

In a year or three, they will probably be lying in a hospital bed with pneumocystis and cryptococcus raging through their brains and bodies.

Fortunately I am HIV negative. I feel lucky. My husband cooks me supper when I surface after call. My older brother and his wife just had a healthy baby. I know infected two-year-olds.

I warn my younger unmarried brother. My friends all question me. I have only moralistic-sounding statements to make. Don't sleep around!—or even occasionally. I am glad that I am married and tested negative twice. If I were single, would I insist on a blood test before sleeping with a man? I hate to sound so pessimistic when friends grill me at a cocktail party—but I don't want my friends to die that kind of death.

I wish the families of AIDS patients would come more often. You won't catch it by persuading them to eat! They need their mothers, wives, sons here. They are hurt, sick, dying. They need family. I substitute where I can. It is too little for them and too painful for me.

THE INTENSIVE CARE UNIT
DECEMBER 25, 1986

The lady lies
surrounded by a court
of alarmed of machines.
They record life:
blood pressure, pulse
and respirations.
The lady does not talk
so we read her numbers:
the language of
her failing heart.

Her daughter questions
incessantly,
her husband is mute.
Grandchildren in the waiting room
watch Roadrunner.
Over the thicket of IV poles
nurses snatch glimpses
of M*A*S*H and St. Elsewhere.
Electronic Christmas carols
spew over her bed.

Once she ate, excused herself
to her powder room, breathed on her own.
Now, her body is helpless
and her mind.
Perhaps her soul
wonders at her ruined holiday.
She did not mail her Christmas cards.

I draw the bloods,
apologize for sticking her again.
She does not twitch.
Only the ventilator answers.
The Redskins' field goal
should excite her to wake.
Instead her heart throws a
crazy beat.
Then another—
time for another EKG.

I sigh; no sleep again
tonight, Christmas night.
I nibble microwave popcorn and
stale fruitcake, swig Diet Coke.
A tube bears Osmolyte for her.

The clouded moon through the window
over her busy bed, reminds me of
when I believed in Angels.
Every Christmas, when I was a child,
I searched the orange city skies
for their shining.

I seek again tonight.
No answer.
Winged men triumphantly
should bear her soul to Heaven,
bring me a festival stocking.

Yet, I hope she does not die today
(though my tasks would be fewer).
Her grandchildren should not remember
Christ's birthday and new toys
by her death.

Her blood pressure is dropping.

I will try to keep her
breathing until tomorrow.

LANGUAGE BARRIER

It gets hard to communicate in the old language.

When I started medical school, our courses were basically word lists. The lists were anatomy and microbiology. We memorized the eleven muscles of the thumb, chambers of the heart, classification of diseases of the colon. It was like studying French. All those nouns to memorize!

We all studied how the organs work, of course: the lungs exchange gases, the heart spins blood around, the kidney filters the waste. We peered at purple-painted bacteria, watched antibiotics scour those bugs from the petri dishes. But it was the names that we were tested on, the vocabulary that would isolate us as physicians.

In medical school we were taught never to refer to patients as a disease. To say, "the gall bladder down the hall," was demeaning. We resolved always to give our patients due respect.

Back in those pre-war days, they also warned us to continue to communicate with our families, friends, and children. "Spend an hour with your child every day." "Take time out to go running." "It's important to keep up with politics."

Then came third year, the clinical years. The dicta were moot. Even if we had a free half hour it was more important, it seemed, to polish up the history and physical for presentation to our preceptors, to volunteer to hold retractors for another choles-tectomy, to scour the library for articles on esoteric aspects of lupus.

Shakespeare, botany, evolution were lost fantasies. Once, I learned how many petals adorned roses. Now, flower petals are submerged beneath liver enzymes.

The gap widened. How could our husbands know the frustrations of missing a blood draw three times, then have the intern draw pints with ease? When eating with in-laws we could not talk at dinner of the smell of melena (old blood leaking out of the rectum), nor of the skin lesions on our AIDS patients.

As time rolled by, life outside the hospital dwindles. Now I am an intern.

"How was your day, dear?" I politely inquire at home at eight p.m. after a night on call.

"Terrible. The computer went down on a very important project. I was at work from eight this morning to seven tonight. Then the bus broke down. I need a drink. Oh, yes, how was yours?"

I am silent for a minute. "Well, I was lucky last night on call. I slept from one a.m. to four a.m.. Then I got a drunk hit from the nursing home with chest pain. But I slept again from six-thirty to seven-thirty. So, almost four hours." Of course that is in a cell-like call room in the bottom of a creaky bunk bed. Meal carts creaking and nurses gossiping loudly outside. Another thirty-seven-hour shift. But I got close to four hours. These days that's cause for celebration. Almost.

So, my sympathies for others' trials are slight. Unfairly, I become impatient with their tribulations. Sometimes I explode.

"Don't tell me about your difficulties with your computer. My favorite patient is dying. And one of my AIDS patients developed pneumocystis pneumonia. And you're whining because you partied too late with friends when I was on call and only got six hours of sleep."

Non-medical friends sympathize. "Oh, you poor dear." They try to help and are puzzled when I am nasty and irritable.

In cocktail conversations acquaintances say: "That's a terrible system. It should not be allowed. I wouldn't want to be cared for by somebody who had been up all night." Noses tilt. Their anger descends on me. I'm a doctor.

Thanks. I don't want to care for them either after I've been up all night. But I can't afford the energy to waste on rage at the system.

After all, it's a privilege to be a doctor.

My fellows on the battlefront become my in-arms comrades at least until we rotate to a new service. We joke about the drunk hit. We share doughnuts and popcorn. On rounds we talk about the gall bladder down the hall and the valve in Room 4116.

We develop sexual fantasies about those in the trenches with us. At two a.m. your resident is your staff. When a patient is spurting blood out of his tracheostomy and you together insert a central line (an IV in the neck), transfer him to the unit, and save his life (at least for now), then you are brothers. Afterwards you raise Diet Cokes in companionship.

How can your husband compare to him, the man who just helped you save a life?

Marriages are made in medical school and dissolve in internship.

But the deans who pontificated in medical school about the values of outside interests were right. We—the battered products of medical school—know that to be true. It just gets harder. The gap widens.

"She didn't make it. We coded her and shocked her and put a pacemaker into her. It didn't work. Why, I'm not sure. We asked for an autopsy. What should we have for dinner?"

HOSPITAL SPACES

Life is defined by bounds:
here, sickness and health are also sequestered.
We have the isolated rooms of infection,
and social wards of men whose
efforts are limited by chest pain.
They play spades with vigor.

Metal rails surround the beds with
air bubbling up through fluid plastic beads.
confining and relieving the comatose.

The staff have large hectic rooms
with multiple desks and phones ringing.
We report local recoveries and deaths,
call the public health department,
and field calls about AIDS and angina.

Chairs are constantly swiped from one desk
to another, as an intern dashes in to
scribble a note, feet hurting,

or to try to turf a patient to a nursing home.
This one has been in for ninety-seven days.

The hallways link the separate worlds.
Like salt sea barnacles
groups of doctors cling on the walls,
discussing their patients' potassium
(barely out of earshot),
drinking instant coffee, grateful
if a stretcher appears to perch on.
Two hours sleep last night.
A long day's journey ahead.

The pantry is guarded by fierce ladies
microwaving the trays of hospital food.
Medical students sneak in to steal
leftover chocolate pudding.

Elevators frustrate. Waiting,
pondering my clipboard,
I can hear them ping at every floor.
Rumbling food racks are loaded.
To the lab, to x-ray, then to surgery clinic.
to drop off another consult.
I wave to friends on contralateral trips.
How many romances start, and stop,
with the opening and shutting of doors?

Sometimes a patient crashes on the
seventh floor.
With cardiac monitor beeping,
and code drugs on the stretcher,
in case his heart stops,
we transport a patient vomiting blood
to the ICU on the fourth floor,
squeezing past the linen carts
in the narrow hallways,
hoping that we will make it,
before he stops breathing.

So far, so good.

More lines intersect.
The snack bar, the chapel, and barber shop,

the clinics and the morgue.
The library offers a soft chair for sleep.

My beeper is a leash,
jerking me back
to headaches and chest pain.

When I finally break out into the
winter evening,
after 38 hours of the hospital,
it is amazing that
I can remember where the car is,
and that
yellow crocuses are blooming.

Nathan Slack

THE FAMOUS CATCH
For Ryne Sandburg

Me and my friend Bryant
was playing pitch
and if you miss
the ball
you have to get the ball.
I standed up very straight
and thought about Ryne Sandburg
catching a ball
and Gary Matthews—
they are some of my favorites,
and I thought for awhile
I saw the ball.
I was nervous.
The ball went straight down
very close to the ground
and I kneeled down
and leaned over,
put my glove on the grass
and my feet in the air,
hanging there
doing three flips
and kept the ball in my glove,
so happy that I caught it
it was just like a
major league
catch.
I don't even play baseball
because I am a hemophiliac.
If I *could* play baseball,
I would be very glad
because some nights
I cry because I can't.

* Nathan wrote this poem in 1985 at the age of 7.

relationships

*...I thought you knew
you were beautiful and fair
your bright eyes and hair
but now I see that no one knows that
about himself, but must be told
and retold until it takes hold...*

Peter Meinke - "untitled"

John J. Brugaletta

DISAPPOINTED FATHER

Some men there are who look upon their sons
And wonder if the world will last a year
Or if, like cities razed by drooling Huns,
Their right response should be disgust and fear.
Such men regard their wives and wonder how
An honest woman hid such thieving genes
Or if his field had known a neighbor plow,
So spotted and so wrinkled are his beans.
I know a man who wonders so and frets,
But I can only pity his poor taste
In publishing details of his regrets
And thinking his unswerving wife unchaste.
     Had he the plain, unwrinkled sons I grow,
     His soul would blaze so angry, Mars should glow.

Sharon White

MARRIAGE POEM

You
left me
slowly
your mind a map
of detours

even though
we walked
familiar roads
as the aspens
turned
their brittle
golds

My nephew
born
not long after
our
wedding
uses his finger
to trace what
he wants
in the air

you used
your hands
to draw
words
you couldn't
remember
except the few words
to tell me you loved
me you lost almost
everything
but that

B. B. Adams

MARRIAGE

You came from another state
crossing the border
when the guard was asleep.
You left rocks thick as death
and hard as frozen dreams.

I spoke your language,
an ancient code
meant to ward off danger.
Even I—your translator—
could not decipher some words, however,
the *hapax legomena* of your tribe.

You've abandoned the customs
of your country,
eating the meats, drinking the wine
of mine,
your hand at home on my breast
which you know better than your own.

The climate here is softer,
if somewhat damp,
but you miss the game
though you always missed the deer.
In bed beside you,
I feel your dream, the pristine stream
leaping with wild trout.

Sometimes I wonder
if we know only the half
that faces each other—like the moon,
one half forever turned away
peering into the unknown.

Laurel Speer

48 YEARS MARRIED
AND NOT A HAPPY ONE AMONG EM

Here's the old man determined to hold
his mountain of junk against the state
buyout. He's the crusty geezer; the rusted
out part; the principle on which this great
country is built sitting up there with his
long rifle shooting the eyes out of squirrels.

Those're my squirrels, mister. I can do
with em whatever I want.

Now his woman Edna Mae is expected
to go along, shut her mouth
and do the wash.

When two people agree to spend their lives
together, you gotta know she'll scrub
the inside of the pickle jar when it's empty,
if you'll unscrew the lid when it's full.

But Edna Mae has burned down the house
with a grease fire in the kitchen
wearing an apron and high-heeled shoes.

Lost all our chickens when it spread to the coop.
Smashed 16 mason jars full of pickles
and handed me the lids.
There was some sweet ones in there, too.

Judy Goldman

CALLING OFF THE WEDDING

It was buying the bed that did it.
Suddenly I knew I'd never
polish the pieces of sterling
people were sending like messages,
never set a table
with the salt and pepper shakers
showing up in pairs. Coiled words
no bigger than good luck coins
were sliding into the margins
of ivory invitations mailed weeks before,
all those stamps coming unglued.
Bridesmaids' dresses danced like paper dolls,
flapping their sashes into fuchsia tongues,
spitting satin-covered buttons
all over the floor. Impossible
to take a step.

And there we were in the right department,
a bright young couple making a choice
between French Provincial and Early American.
Bedside tables, chests and chairs were stacked,
waiting to topple. Why didn't I say it
when he gave me the ring? When I bought the veil?
When the gifts began to arrive
like exquisitely-wrapped warnings?
Why did I wait until everything turned white
and voices were begging, loud as organ music,
don't do it, don't do it, don't do it.

Dorothy Sutton

FED UP WITH LEFTOVERS

You were surprised
at my initial fear, but I'm only human,
dear, and haven't humans always
been afraid of falling and of fire?
That heat had me leaping pretty high.

So I get burned again.
I *wish* you could have loved me,
or if you did, I wish
you could have known how to show it
in ways I could have understood.

I'm fed up with leftovers,
you recycling your trash on me. Slipping
all them extra sinkers on my line,
me struggling already not to drown.

In high school I learned pain
is good, your switchboard flashing disaster,
warning you to do something quick,
to needle out that embedded thorn
or jerk away from the flame.

I know it sounds strange,
my health teacher said, but pain's not the worst
thing in the world: not being able to feel
pain is.

You want me back. Too bad, honey—
trouble is, I done turned that burner off.
That supper's done got cold.

Janice Townley Moore

THE TAXIDERMIST'S WIFE

Don't all obsessions start innocently?
In early marriage she watched him mount
behind glass a pebble from every river he fished,
and each fly that caught the fish—
unlike other newlyweds counting pebbles into a jar
the first three years.

Now the frame exhibits neat rows of
stones and lures next to names:
Tusquittee Creek, Hiawassee River.

Daily in the dim cellar
on her way to the washer-dryer
she passes the baby raccoon climbing a stump,
bass and trout in their last grins.
As some kind of vengeance he placed at her eye-level
the heads of three angry bears.

It is the boar she hates. How its head had glowered
at her from the refrigerator that day, the tusks wedged
between the mayonnaise and the milk.

This morning frying his bacon, poaching his eggs,
she recalls last night's dream; the palmist examined
her hand, closed it quickly, and said
*Look, my dear lady, you have already lived
longer than anyone expected.*

Daniel McDonald

THE SUMMING UP

It's the right metaphor.

When the Shah was overthrown and his
    prisoners freed, the torturers waited
    outside the Teheran prison and assured them:

        "It was nothing personal."

Isn't that the line we need

    —when our kids leave home?

    —outside the divorce court?

    —after the party celebrating a twenty-fifth anniversary?

Oh, we'll remember the chains, the
    electrodes, the tricks with the
    bayonet. We carry deep scars.

We were a family.

Maybe it will help afterwards if we
    can say

    "Sorry about that."

    "We're all good people."

    "It was nothing personal."

Pamela Gross

IDENTIFICATION AND FITTING OF PIECES

For My Mother

When the plate's crazed pieces are pressed
together just so, the crack almost
heals, and this miracle
of edges—that hands' satisfaction
in the fusion they have worked—flows
like a current to the body's
core, where its benediction is felt
as if the hands themselves had sealed
in prayer: prayer which is not
words or thoughts, but the perfect
union of all surfaces whose meeting
is both supplication and answer.

This is not to deny
that for such a holy
piecing together to take place,
something must be broken.

Isabella Halsted

THE MGANGA

"I am looking at you with one eye," Nzamba said. We were talking about the last faculty meeting, having a drink in his apartment, and waiting for the chicken to cook.

"What does that mean?" I settled back, and prepared for fun.

"If I looked at you with both, I would go blind with love."

I flushed with pleasure; then I laughed. African sayings are like that; you think you know exactly what they mean, then you get tangled in their many shades; there's no one answer. It's a little like being in love with the wrong person: at a certain point, you give yourself up to confusion, rather than make up your mind.

The first time we went out together, he said, "You shouldn't look into my eyes when you talk to me!" I was startled, then worried—had I offended him? But then I saw he was smiling. "At home, when someone looks directly into your eyes, you know he's not telling the truth."

He said this, I pointed out, while looking straight at me with his. They were the most beautiful eyes I had ever seen. They tilted slightly at the corners, were set deep and thickly lashed. In certain lights I saw a tantalizing fleck of gold in the bottomless brown.

My own eyes are pale blue. "Eyes of the Devil," said Nzamba. I'd heard of that before. I'd seen an old sailor in southern Spain who had looked straight at the sun for so long, his eyes had turned blue, and then milky white. "I'm sure he was blind," I said, "but people kept him apart, as they do in small villages, said he was possessed."

"Blue eyes, Devil's eyes," Nzamba repeated. "Goes with red skin. Did you know we called the British 'Redskins'? They looked so funny to us with their sunburns. British skin is very white, you know; in the sun it never gets brown. We used to make fun of the red *mzungu*, and if they caught us, they'd beat our hands with their sticks and make us squat in the dirt and say 'I'm sorry, Bwana, I'm sorry!'" He laughed and took a long draw on his beer. "The first day of school, this tall skinny *mzungu* with a red horsey face looked down his nose at us and said: 'Natives! Stand up, boys! You there, come here! What's your name, boy?'"

I laughed aloud. Nothing was funnier than to hear the clipped dry British accent coming from this comfortable black man in his brightly striped dashiki.

"I told him my name was Nzamba. 'No, No!' he said. 'Nevah, *nevah* use that evil, pagan, African name again!' and he rapped his ruler on the desk. 'Your name shall be, let me see, ummmm, Richard Jonathan. Mr. Richard Jonathan.' 'Yes, Bwana,' I said. 'Call me *Sir*, Richard.' 'Yes, Bwana Sir.'"

Nzamba loved to tell these stories, partly because he was a natural teacher and excellent imitator, but also because remembering his childhood, he said, kept him sane—even the worst parts. Sometimes his face seemed to go behind a mask—his mouth smiling, but his eyes somewhere else. He drank a lot—not to wash the hated away, which would be impossible, but to keep it at a distance so it wouldn't consume him, so he wouldn't explode.

Nzamba always said, and I believed him, that I was the most African *mzungu* he'd ever known in the States. He also said he loved me because I was white—one of those contradictions I gave up trying to understand. For that matter, wasn't I always drawn to darkness and to worlds other than mine? When it came to Nzamba, I felt sure that destiny was part of it. The time I visited his village in Africa, his wiry old father Tata, a traditional doctor and shaman, declared that I had lived among them before. He blessed my return by pouring homemade honey-beer into the dusty ground for all the ancestors, theirs and mine. As the gourd of sweet and heady *pombe* was passed around, I called out the names of the people I loved, living and dead, and felt truly at home for the first time in my life.

My mother said it was rebellion. After my father disappeared, she had let me have my own way too much. Far too much, she often said—with all that freedom, I'd gone wild, always playing with fire. She'd say this as if it were all her fault that I had turned out so badly: here I was over thirty, still unmarried, without children, and living with an African.

"An African, darling!" she said. "How fascinating!" which meant, of course, "how unthinkable." In those days, an African was still exotic; Nzamba had been among the very first students brought over to the States on scholarship. I reminded my mother she had brought me up to be a citizen of the world, and a nonconformist, too. Hadn't she herself stepped out of line when she married my handsome, dark-haired father? "Penniless upstart from the Midwest," the family had called him, and then he'd left when I was only four. True, she said, but at least she'd married him, at least she'd had me. Nzamba and I had been together for over five years. How long would we go on like this?

"We should get married one day, Bwana!" I said to him. I thought I meant it. Only a few things bothered me when I pictured life in Africa—for we would surely live there one day: I hoped I would never have to see the slaughter of a goat or a cow, ritual or otherwise. Polygamy was hard to understand. Most of all, I hated the circumcision of young children, especially of girls—so much so that I wouldn't even think about it. But I thought I might even accept these things in principle. You had to take the bad with the good, I said.

"You would be miserable, married to me," Nzamba replied firmly. "Mixed marriages don't work at home. The women hate it. Besides, I am going to marry a village girl, one who can bear me many children, and bring me soup and *pombe* whenever I want it."

"You could never give me up," I said. "Who would you have to talk to? Besides, I'm always bringing you soup and *pombe*."

"You'll always be First Wife," he said. "But Tata had six; I'm entitled at least to two!" The gold speck in his eye was dancing.

I refused to believe him about the village girl, but I thought about her. I thought she would look something like the Masai dancer in the poster by the window at the end of his bed. The first time I stayed there, I woke up in the morning to her friendly face and felt we were sisters in our happiness. The brightness of her wide, humorous eyes. Her broad smile and perfect, white teeth ("That's from all the milk and blood she drinks," said Nzamba. "Raw?" "Raw.") From the base of her neck to her chin, she wore a rope of many colored beads, wound round and round, that matched the triangle hanging on her forehead from a leather thong, its tip resting exactly between her eyes. More beads, braided on wires, fell across her chest in widening loops, and from her ears, there were multiple coils. Though she was so different from me, we had a lot in common: her nomadic ways, her softness, her gaiety, her love of jewelry and bright colors. But one morning, she looked strangled.

"Look at her eyes!" I said.

"What now?" said Nzamba. He was buried in *The Chronicle*.

"She's terrified! Don't you see? Those beads are choking her."

"It was just a passing glimpse. For that brief moment, all the happiness I saw in her face had suddenly vanished. Her eyes looked so fearful, they were almost empty of self. Suddenly she seemed a very young girl, caught in a smile that stretched far beyond laughter. Almost a grimace, really, for a white tourist with a camera.

"Don't be silly," said Nzamba, and went on reading.

The summer we went to Africa together, Nzamba took me to meet his sister Syungo, a traditional doctor, or *"mganga,"* who was living in the city. I was excited and happy. He'd told me so much about her and about African medicine, which fascinated me. "She is not a witchdoctor, by the way," he said emphatically. "Witchdoctor is one of those *mzungu* words, like 'medicine man' or 'native'." Syungo was also 'family'—and I was always looking for family. Nzamba was my lover, I was First Wife, so we were all connected. She could be my sister.

"Syungo is me," Nzamba said—but what I often thought was cryptic he assured me in Africa was literal. "Who you are about to meet is myself."

The self he might have been, that is. As he told it, Nzamba had been torn away from his beloved father and deprived of his heritage by their mother, a fanatic Christian convert. She had pushed him into a colonial missionary school, which eventually led to many years away in America. So it was Syungo, as next in line, not Nzamba, who inherited their father's medical knowledge, as soon as she was old enough to toddle after him in his wanderings. She had learned all the secrets: the different herbs and trees and where to find them, the recipes and songs, and how to recognize and treat disease, physical or mental—if the two can be distinguished. She practiced her medicine in the course of having seven children, four of whom had lived, and was now pregnant with her eighth. Though she could neither read nor write, Syungo had become so wise at forty-two, Nzamba told me, she would be chief elder in Kibera, if she hadn't been born a woman.

"I hate her," he said, laughing. "She knows too much."

We turned in from the highway and bumped along the rocky dirt road that was the main street of the oldest African quarter in the city. Most of the houses were like village huts—made of clay with twig rooves, instead of the collapsing corrugated iron shacks you saw in other parts. Things looked clean and people seemed well fed, busy and happy. The sun was bright. I felt joyful. We parked the car at the end of a road, at the top of a rather steep bank, and walked down a winding path to the cluster of houses below. Nzamba went ahead, and little children followed us, waving and laughing and pointing, the bravest coming up close to me, almost daring to pull at my skirt, calling "*mzungu! mzungu!* munnie! munnie!" Except for the children, people seemed not surprised to see a black man with a mzungu woman—they hardly looked at us. I didn't feel white, anyway—in fact during those days in Africa I saw myself in a mirror only once, by chance, and was shocked when I saw the pale face and blue eyes. Nzamba was the one they thought was strange, not me. He was the Prince who had flown across the big lake in the silver bird and returned—so they said when he first came back, the village women dancing in a row to celebrate. Unlike most educated men, he wore the dashiki and called himself by his African name instead of Charles or John or James—names he was quick to tell anyone who carried them were the names of slaves.

The mganga's wooden house was a luxury made possible by money Nzamba sent home from America. Syungo lived there with her husband, one unmarried daughter, another married daughter, son-in-law and baby, and four younger children, two of them hers, two her grandchildren—all eight in a single, modest room. But it was cool and comfortable. Cots lined the walls, and we sat on these and on low chairs. Light came in where the walls met the slanted roof, and from the door that was left open during the day. A brazier was in one corner, and on it, a simmering pot of beans, I was glad to see. Mealtimes in Africa, I'd already learned, were always uncertain. I was often anxiously wondering when we would eat, and so far that day, we'd had nothing.

We opened the beer we had brought and passed out gifts—printed fabric, jewelry, clothes for the adults, pencils and pens for the children. Then we settled down to talk. As she was far along in her pregnancy, Syungo lay back on her cot, her head propped up on one elbow, an arm slung along the broad mountain of her hip. She was smiling and warm, her eyes bright as obsidian. She looked like a queen, or a bountiful odalisque, relaxed and familiar. Nzamba translated for us, back and forth, listening, then speaking, then taking a pull from his beer, his face expressionless, his voice soft and rapid. It was as if he were not there and that Syungo and I were speaking the same language.

"How many children do you have?" was the first question she asked. Any African woman would. It was as natural to her as "how's the weather today?" or "what do you do?" would be to a Westerner.

"I have no children," I said, feeling my face grow warm with embarrassment. The world never stopped reminding me that I was childless and never more so than in Africa.

"No children?" As I expected, Syungo looked surprised.

I've had some difficulty...." I hesitated, ashamed and confused. A lame excuse. Syungo would never understand. Who will replace the children that regularly die? Not to have children, Nzamba had explained, was a curse brought on by evil spirits.

"Ahh," said Syungo. She gazed at me for a long moment. Then she leaned forward and touched Nzamba's arm, speaking rapidly to him.

"She says you must come back and spend the day with her. She will help you. Then you can have as many children as she does."

As he spoke, Syungo nodded and smiled from her cot. Yes? Yes? She laughed, and I laughed back. A wonderful joke had been told, I thought. Yet I knew that what she said was true—not that I could have seven children, but that if I came back, whatever it was that stood in the way would vanish. It was time to have a child, whether or not we ever married. My heart quickened with happiness ... or fear. Would Nzamba bring me back? Could I find my way by myself?

I wanted to ask many questions, but Nzamba had turned to chat with Mbiti, and without him there could be no more talk. Syungo seemed to have dropped the subject and now was gesturing to one daughter to serve the beans; were they ready? Come Kidogo, more beer—go, take this (she reached into her blouse, pulling out a bill) take this and get more beer for Bwana! Kidogo snatched the bill and ran out the door. Soon we were all eating, balancing tin bowls on our laps. The beans were just cooked through, crunchy and a little sour—coming through a mix of hot spices. I found them delicious, washing each bit down with the sweet warm beer and finding out how hungry I was. We ate with occasional noises of satisfaction coming from this or that corner of the room, with smilings, belches, a few words passed here and there.

Suddenly a dog barked raucously outside the door; a rooster and hens started up with a shriek and a flutter of feathers. Then there were voices, first far off, then coming closer in an undistinguishable mix of spiraling murmurs, muffled cries, shouts. Angry, or afraid—I couldn't know, except by how the atmosphere in the room seemed to change, go tense. I moved to the edge of my chair as the voices grew closer, clearly the voices of men, excited, talking over each other. Brother Mbiti stopped eating, set his bowl down on the floor, and leaned forward slightly as if to get up, hands on knees, eyes fixed on the door. Nzamba continued silently drinking, his eyes half closed; he glanced at me, in an expression I couldn't read. Kyathe held the baby tightly to her chest, her eyes perfect rounds. The little boy ran over to his mother's knee and leaned against it, whimpering a little, and the older one jumped up and down in excitement. Only Syungo, still half lying on her cot, gazed peacefully at the door with a look of expectation, as if she had known about this all along.

Footsteps were now on the wooden porch outside, loud and purposeful. The door pushed open wide, swinging against the wall with a sudden blare of sunlight, as Mbiti jumped up. The man standing there said something to him, low and insistent, while outside the voices had gone to a murmur. Slowly, Syungo pulled her blanket around her shoulders, swung her legs to the floor, and pushed herself up from the cot. With a hand on Kyathe's shoulder, she went to the door.

I glanced anxiously at Nzamba: "What's going on?"

"They've come for the mganga," he said, getting up. "Come and see. You'll be interested."

Outside, a large crowd lined the top of the bank, while three men came down the path, half pushing, half carrying a struggling figure. When they got to the bottom, they approached Syungo, who was now seated on a chair, facing them. The crowd at the top of the hill fell silent.

It was a young girl they held, perhaps twelve or thirteen, tall and leggy and thin. She wore the short blue pleated skirt and white blouse of a schoolgirl, but it was smeared with mud, her hair was dusty, its braids undone, as if she had been rolling in dirt, and she wore no shoes. The men had tied her arms firmly behind her back, and her body writhed, her head rolling from side to side. Her mouth was open, saliva at the corners, and her throat worked painfully up and down the length of her long neck, though she made no sound. From where we stood to one side, we could see her eyes—thrown into the back of her head so that only the whites showed. I clutched Nzamba's arm.

"What's wrong?" I whispered. "What has she done?" But he didn't answer, only drew me slightly away from the scene.

Syungo waited quietly, hands resting on her knees, her back perfectly straight. As soon as the men untied the girl's arms, they stepped away hurriedly, pushing her forward. She fell to her knees, bumping her forehead on the ground in what looked like prayer, but in seconds her head was up, as if jerked from behind, her arms flailing, her body rocking. Syungo reached into one pocket, drawing out a small bag which she put on her lap. Then she placed a hand on the girl's shoulder.

"What's she doing?" I whispered to Nzamba.

"She's going to exorcise the Devil," he whispered back.

"The Devil!" I felt slapped in the face with anger. "The Devil? Why—she's just a young girl!"

"Shh!"

Everyone leaned forward as Syungo, one hand on the girl's shoulder, took her chin in her other hand, while the girl's head snapped back and forth. She then held it firmly and looked intently into the girl's face. Soon the shaking body began to still, and as she gazed back at the mganga, the girl's eyes seemed to clear.

"Let's go," said Nzamba, turning away from the scene. "She won't do anything now."

"Who won't, Syungo won't?" I said, anxiously, my heart racing, my eyes fixed on the child. "When will she then? What is she going to do?" The girl was so alone—the men standing arms crossed between her and the path leading up the bank; Syungo sitting, so rigid, so silent, before her. I wanted to protect her, to free her from the trap she was in. She was innocent, a pure spirit, and I was her ally, I who had spent my own life refusing narrow boundaries. Alone and vulnerable, this girl was being choked by tradition, by superstition, by ignorance. She was like the Masai dancer in the poster, with coils of tightly woven beads twisting around her neck, the heavy beaded loops pulling at her ears, the band of embroidered wire tied around her matted hair. And Syungo, who I'd thought knew everything, was only a witchdoctor, after all.

Taking my arm firmly, Nzamba started towards the path. I pulled away, and went quickly over to the girl. Syungo looked at me, unsmiling, but without sending me away, so I knelt down between the two, facing the child, and held out my hand to touch her. "Hello," I said, as calmly as I could, in English. I was sure she would recognize me. I had to tell her I understood—no matter what it was they were doing to her. "Hello," I repeated, softly. "Are you all right?" She turned her head towards me, her dull, blank eyes, still tear-filled, widening, and suddenly there appeared in them an expression I had seen before on the face of the Masai girl. Slowly, her mouth began to stretch into a smile, almost a grimace, as she looked at the mzungu. All that was left in her eyes was the fear. I lowered mine and withdrew my hand.

"Goodbye," I whispered. I got up slowly and turned for a moment to Syungo, who nodded at me. Then I followed Nzamba up the hill.

Nzamba inched the car along the bumpy road, watching for potholes and for people in the way. I peered into the oncoming darkness, wanting to give in to my exhaustion, but once again alert and anxious: we were in the poorest African quarter of the city at the end of the day, in a car ready at any moment to break down. Here and there, people had already begun to light their fires—bright yellow torches beaming out of the developing velvety black, beacons without hands or bodies. The car slowly moved past a bonfire on the side of the road where three small children were playing. I was suddenly enraged by the sight. Why couldn't these people take care of their children! They could set themselves on fire!

"What's the matter now?" Nzamba's voice was cold, flat. Uncanny how he could always sense how I was feeling.

"I hate the way your people treat children."

"*My* people. Yesterday you were saying there were yours, too."

"Look at those kids," I went on, ignoring his remark. "What if they burn themselves to death? Who'd care?"

My bitterness came not from this sight but from the opposite, how the men had bound the girl so roughly by the arms, the wild whites of her eyes.

"The girl just now—you just let it all happen! What they were doing to her!"

"They weren't doing anything to her. She was hysterical. That's all. Children her age get hysterical, you know that, anywhere. If anybody was doing anything to her, it was you."

I stared at him.

"But ... what was Syungo going to do?"

"Probably give her something. A placebo."

"But what about the Devil ... you were just making that up?"

"Of course not. Both are true."

I gazed out the window again, my stomach in knots. What he said did nothing to erase my fear. Syungo knew too much, that's what I felt. Especially about me, far more than I knew myself.

The right wheel of the car sank into a bad pothole, and I saw now that night had completely fallen, in the sudden total way it did every day. There was light and then there was darkness. It was cooler—but that wasn't what made me shiver. I felt totally alone. Scared. White.

Nzamba returned to Africa for good. One day he sent me a picture of his village wife. She is a young, pretty woman, dressed in the country manner with a loose white blouse and a piece of bright kanga cloth wrapped around her waist, a yellow scarf on her head to keep off the sun. She is lifting the baby high up in the air with her strong bare arms, face turned towards the camera, her eyes caught in the middle of her laughter. Syungo knew I never meant to have a child with Nzamba, nor he with me. We never meant to marry. Nzamba never pretended otherwise.

Melissa Kwasny

THE MASSAGE

These feet are large
as those in Kollwitz's drawings,
the thick, arthritic ankles,
peasant ankles crossed one
over the other as a sister
lovingly holds another's arm
while talking. Two plain sisters,
opaque as soapstone. They
are long as two carved fish.

Old roots,
they are crippled,
cave in on themselves
like the hunched men
in folk-tales, grimaced,
who live in German forests.

These are my grandmother's feet
and I am cupping them
like a prayer between my hands.

In the kitchen, Duty
is steeping herbs: slippery elm,
cohosh, skullcap and rue.
She avoids cooking yang foods,
coffee, sugar, meat, washes
the down of the old woman's hair.

Answer it! Sacrifice
is knocking, a sister delivered
to the back door, hands tied.
Another arrives later
with open arms, humming polkas
and old tunes, "Irene Goodnight."

And the hidden one,
who cries at odd hours
and in company, her hands
orange and slick from the oil
of corn. She is getting old here.

The younger, betrayed,
an intricacy of worlds and words
between them, saying:
No, Grandma, it is not a Lord
who works through me.

The grandmother saying:
But who will heal, who
will stay with me the winter?

Mario René Padilla

THE NAGUAL

the beast upon which the weal and
woe of a man's fate depend ...
The Golden Bough

... and like the cats who animate the night
who turn the garbage
and walk along the fence in defiance
who stalk and cry till
routine sounds of milktruck sunrise
scurry them off to benevolent strangers
to beg a morning feast
I never sleep
but move through the dark like a Mayan beast
to watch and prowl these alleys of the night

and when I return
you are there
standing by the stove in early light
making love with Bach, eggs and butter
and you turn your face reaching for a kiss
that sometimes comes in sympathy
for all those days I strayed
and you were alone with my ritual letters
sent from a jungle in Mexico
where I go in the time of the Nagual

I have come to know the self as other
I have learned all his secrets
like the dream mortals dream of immortality
the trace of ashes the soul also makes
so I turn the garbage
and watch how the night sleeps
how trees *are* in the absence of light
how black shadows reach and sway
how senses react when cornered
by the dark and unknown leaf
until I break and slip quietly into your bed
where you stroke that part on my back
and I curl into your breasts
so that I might sleep

but something to do with being an other
my eyes open into a non-being creature

330

when I hear mysterious sounds
that others only dream
when I hear the rustle of leaves
dropping stem by stem
and feel in the dark such unconfessable things
these words cannot express
I stalk the slow and coming end
that creeps   *creeps*
like rats
through endless
alley nights

Sandra Love

PSYCHOLOGY IS THE ANSWER

The sign was yellow with moveable red letters and protruded from a low-slung storefront of colorless concrete block. The sign, bright against the tedious blocks, said: JESUS IS THE ANSWER. Nell always thought: What is the question?

Inside was a carpet store.

Nell could picture the owner, a stout, red-faced man with a large nose who had the courage of his convictions, but she could never imagine what he might ask of Jesus. Better business? A new building?

What would I ask? she mocked herself, thinking she'd waste her request asking for mornings to be calm, her older son more light-hearted and her younger son less. She'd want her mother able to keep all her teeth instead of needing an upper plate and her husband Ken to get his promotion soon. When what she'd want most would be—

To be more like Joan?

The thought startled her, as truth sometimes does. After she parked, trudged over the crisp morning frost and hurried upstairs, greedy for the first cup of coffee and the precious minutes before her first client, she told herself she'd talk it out with Roger at lunch today.

"Perfect, isn't it? Jesus obviously answers for the carpet store. Lovely cushion," Roger said at noon. He was a Gestalt therapist and everything was a pattern. The two of them shared office space, traded therapy sessions. "How's Lena?"

"Oh … Lena. Do you know that she spent more than $12,000? All the money she made from selling her house. She doesn't have anything to show for it, nothing—well, a TV and a stereo, I think. Otherwise she blew it."

"You're smiling," Roger was frowning at her.

"Well, of course I am. Who wouldn't? The thing that worries me about Lena is that she doesn't enjoy it. Any of it. Saving it or blowing it."

"I still think she plugs into a problem of yours," Roger said, and insisted on picking up the check.

Nell let him, but then worried so much about when she would repay him that midway through the afternoon, she realized what she was doing to herself and chuckled.

During her ten-minute break before Lena was due, the phone rang. Joan's ever-calm drawl came through, as clearly as if she were in the next office, not an hour and half away in Louisville: "What're you up to next Wednesday?"

"It's the worst day of the week," Nell snapped. "I have an appointment with the school super in Loveland about a year-long contract—read lucrative—and then clients all afternoon. Not good to cancel clients."

"But it can be done?" The drawl went on. Nell could hear her draw in the smoke that made her voice thick. She was the only person Nell knew who had not given up smoking.

"Yes, of course it can be done—if Mom needs it." Nell knew that Wednesday was when her mother was scheduled to have the oral surgery for her upper plate. "Why?"

"You know I don't usually ask, but Frederick's been having pain ... we changed medication last week and he's supposed to check back with the cardiologist that morning."

"Oh, God," Nell said. "That's terrible, Joan." She felt worse about Joan's husband because she didn't like him. "Look, I can't talk, but it's do-able. Barely. I'll reschedule, and I'll be there at eight-thirty to take Mother in. I'll phone back if there's a problem."

"You're a miracle worker," Joan's throaty voice was soothingly honied. "Thanks. See you then."

Lena came in and started talking while she dropped her coat on a chair. Thrown by the phone call, Nell stared at Lena's familiar mass of freckles and pudgy folds. "Wait. Hold everything. What's the question we're dealing with?" Nell's mind worked in jerks like her car engine had in the cold of the morning.

"I don't want to live with my parents." Lena's violet eyes, hidden in her puffy face, scrinched into a pout. She looks awful, Nell thought, her natural sympathy stronger because Lena had been a friend before she'd been a client.

"But what is your main objective?" Nell repeated, tapping her pencil.

Most of Lena's conflicts had nothing to do with money. She dwelled on events, combing through details over and over, and in the end misreading everything, perceiving the world upside down. Nell was amazed by this talent, only partly because it rendered her usually effective tactics powerless. "What difference does it make? I'm stuck living with Mom and Dad."

The strains of every day survival in the same house with her parents and a 17-year-old son showed around Lena's eyes and chin, and she'd begun to have circulation problems in her legs.

"Try to choose what you want." Despite Lena's convoluted view of the world, it was Nell who felt frustrated: she could not move Lena one inch from where she'd been when they started.

"To get a job, a good job, that's my purpose." Lena spoke promptly and obediently this time—maybe too obediently?—and blinked three times. Lena had had a goal since childhood that she managed, neatly, to miss: she wanted to be a housewife.

"You're an excellent secretary. There's no reason you can't get yourself a good job if you want to." Nell had felt Lena's solid support and used her skills when they both worked at Proctor and Gamble. Lena had the same inborn aptitude for being a secretary that Nell had for therapy. "What keeps you from getting a job?"

"*You* know," Lena reproved Nell, honestly puzzled that Nell would ask. "You know me better than anyone—even better than my sisters. *Much* better than my sisters," she amended. "Why do you ask when you already know the answer?"

"I'm not the person who has to hear the answer," Nell said. "Am I?"

Lena looked away. "True," she admitted.

"Life isn't perfect," Nell said. "But you can do better than no job, no money, a son who drains you and a father who cuts you off from your friends." Deal with your problems, leave them behind you, let life give you what you want, Nell urged Lena with every technique she knew.

Nell glanced down at her notes from Joan's phone call. They stood out on the white pad, big black letters from her Flair pen. She recognized the angry frustration she felt with Lena, suddenly—the same emotion she felt when she dealt with Joan. Lena outmaneuvered her the way Joan did, never doing anything Nell thought she should, but coming out on top more often than not. Lena looked up with tears in her eyes. "Dan never had a real father," she half-whispered. "Except for Terry, when he was real little, and Terry was too irresponsible to count." Poor Lena, Nell thought. Lena was not on top of anything. "I—I want Dan to have a real family, like yours. Mine sucks," Lena said. Her voice was barely a whisper. Then the dam broke, and tears came.

Nell brought Kleenex and let Lena cry, her touch offering sympathy and readiness to go on whenever Lena could. She glanced at her notes. "Something major escapes me," she'd written after one of the first sessions. She remembered worrying out loud to Roger about having been Lena's lunch buddy, thinking their slight friendship kept her from seeing her correctly. Nonsense, Roger said. Keep looking.

When Lena stopped crying, she looked accusingly at Nell. "You did that on purpose."

Nell sighed. Lena freely admitted that the only reason she was trying "this psychology stuff," was that Nell had helped her at P&G. Nell had been the Employee Assistance Program counselor there before starting her own practice.

"Yes, I did it on purpose. Sometimes if you get pushed you can knock down a barrier and get to the truth."

Lena nodded. But Nell knew she'd already used her standard defense: divert the thought, stay blind, don't see what you don't want to see. "Why do you say your family sucks?" Nell asked, trying once more.

"Of course they don't, not really. I only feel that way sometimes," Lena was smooth, all right. Her eyes were still ringed with red, the too-white flesh swollen where she dabbed them with a fat finger wrapped in one of Nell's tissues, but her voice didn't quaver.

Push, Nell told herself. She's never been this close before. "You had a reason." Nell kept as calm as she could, held her breath. The silence lengthened, deepened.

"I—I—uh ..." Lena trailed off.

Nell felt her feet wobble onto dangerous, and therefore possibly fruitful, ground. She spoke slowly into the second pause once she felt it die: "You once told me you went into a church and knelt and cried for an hour."

Lena nodded. "I get pushed and pushed and then I fall down," she said thickly. "I—get—pushed and poked and he pushes and pokes and—" she was looking into space, beyond Nell—" and I break. I crumble into tiny pieces like one of the cakes I make and then God comes along and puts glue on the pieces and sticks me back together on the plate."

Her eyes were clear, innocent, looking back into Nell, drawing strength through a straw.

"It isn't that I hate my father," Lena said. Her eyes wandered to the wall. "He's—who he is, that's all. Strict. He thinks he's right. Maybe he is. He doesn't care that it makes him hell to live with. Anyway, they have plenty of space. They don't mind."

"You pay for it," Nell cautioned.

"It's my house, too," Lena said.

"Is it?" Nell waited. Lena merely looked expectant. "What about your mother? How does she cope with your father?"

Lena shrugged. "She's mental."

Nell sat up. "Mental?"

"She wigs out," Lena said. "Acts like she doesn't know what she does. Little things ... she carries his beer down into the basement refrigerator and he thinks he's out. She acts like she doesn't remember doing it. Once the downstairs refridge ended up completely full of Budweiser. Daddy was furious."

Nell laughed. Startled by the sound, Lena almost smiled, hesitated, then let herself. "It *is* funny, " she finally said. "Most of the time mother's okay, though." Nell's heart sank as Lena added, "It's time."

Nell pressed: "Wait. Your mother. Did you see her when she took the beer? "Why?" Lena dropped her head to the side like a cocker spaniel.

"Do you know why she's doing it?" Nell said, but she rose, defeated, knowing it was lost, the hour gone.

After Lena left, Nell hurried to write down what she'd seen, thinking she should not have laughed: Try mother again, to get to father.

Nell got up, paced, sat down again, chewed the end of her pen, switching her thoughts back to Joan, to the change in plans for next week, her own mother. Her mother had always given in to what Nell's father wanted, and when he'd died five years ago, she and Joan worried. But their mother had survived. Eventually, she branched out into new friendships, came more often to see Nell and Ken and the boys. Nell realized long ago that it was Joan, not her, who took after their mother in that; Joan gave in easily to men, had never been really happily married.

But she pushes my buttons with cool precision, she thought. Nell jumped, scaring herself, checking to see her pen still in hand. She felt giddy with insight.

She'd never thought of Joan and Lena being alike before, but today it seemed obvious.

Damn Joan! I end up feeling guilty when it's my schedule she rearranges ... and because she has a husband with heart problems everyone feels sorry for her. *You're the one who moved away,* she could hear the familiar tape inside her head, playing her tune. But it was Joan's voice, not her mother's. How was it possible she'd never noticed that before?

She called Rob in, her last client of the day. She was glad when he was done and she could start making the phone calls she needed to make in order to free next Wednesday, part of Thursday, for her mother. It was blowing outside, the sky a dull steel, spreading clouds that made the November outdoors look as unappealing as a leftover baked potato.

When she went out to the waiting room, Rob was gone, but Lena was returning, coat tight around her, sweeping cold air back into the small anteroom that served as a lobby.

"Well?" Nell asked.

"My car won't start," Lena said. She gave a full body shiver. "Whew—ee! I thought it was time for Dad to show up so I went out, but it's too cold. I'll watch from here."

Nell checked the time. "Let me call home and I'll wait with you."

While she was talking to Ken, Lena's father arrived. Nell clicked off and hurried to catch up, dropping dirty coffee cups in the sink, snapping lights. She pulled her coat on against the dark as she went down the steps.

Lena's father was a short, dark haired man, as meager as Lena was plump, an older version of Lena's son Dan except that Dan had red hair. The father was balding, but looked fit and taut, muscled like a weight-lifter. He stuck his head under the hood as Nell approached. Lena stood to the side, elbows on the fender, butt out, a teenage posture. Lena saw Nell first. "Oh, Nell, I'd like to introduce you to my father, Sergeant Vito."

"Nell Thomas," Nell put out her hand. "I didn't catch your first name?"

"Don," Lena supplied.

Don Vito looked at Nell, but his hands held a dip stick—he turned over his palms to indicate the grease and did not smile. "Pleased to meet you," he said, but he stared so unblinkingly it was hard to believe him. She should be able to see, he seemed to say, that he had more important things to do than to stop and shake hands or even talk to her.

Lena seemed oblivious to *his* body language, filled the silence with her chatter: "It could be the battery, but if it isn't, can we leave the car here until tomorrow?"

"Sure. That's no problem. No one will bother your car in this lot." Nell looked straight at Don Vito, but he ignored her a second time, concentrating on dipping the stick, drawing it out, measuring. It was necessary to check things like oil when something was wrong with an engine, but his obsession with it was unusual. Don looked through Nell and said to Lena, "Bring me the rag in the back of my car."

At that, Nell turned sharply to leave. What was going on here?

And then, as Lena called out, "See you next Thursday!" her cheer overriding her father's bleak rudeness, it came to her. Lena's earlier speech about being pushed and poked, her uncanny ability to turn everything inside out, not to see things, her inability to form close relationships. A classic case of sexual abuse.

"A breakthrough," Nell told Ken later that night. On the drive home, her thoughts danced wildly, and she felt like a dog trying to nab its fleas. Ken had a fire going and dinner ready to reheat in the microwave. Nell felt as if her wishes from the morning had been granted: Ken was looking after her, Roger bought lunch and she'd be able to help Lena now. Finally.

She ate in the living room, the ugliness of her insight about Lena stayed by the warm arms around her, her two boys's sloppy goodnight kisses, sweetly brief. Fourteen and twelve were not her favorite ages, but at least they were self-sufficient about homework, bedtime. She told Ken about Joan's call, her plans for driving to her mother's and circled back to Lena, wincing. "Poor Lena."

"What can you do now that you know?" Ken asked.

"I'll have to be cautious, not to frighten her. There are steps to healing." Nell stuck her toes toward the fire and felt the warmth start. She stretched. It was good to be home, to let go of the day's work, the pushing into the unknowable. Lena needed so much—was it more than Nell had to give? Not until Ken came to rub her shoulders could she let go and allow the warmth to creep the rest of the way up her body.

When Nell arrived in Louisville the next Wednesday, her mother was dressed as if for a party in a tasteful skirt and sweater that matched, low heels. She made a face at Nell: "This is not going to be fun," she said. "But it will be easier with both of you.... Joan wants you to call." Nell kissed her mother, went straight to the phone.

"You made it," Joan signed with relief.

"You didn't think I would?" Nell asked.

"Well—no, that isn't what I meant." Joan backtracked as smoothly as Lena. Nell smiled. "How's Mom?"

"Fine," Nell told her sister. "Go take Frederick to the doctor. Come on over after lunch." She was the one who said goodbye and hung up, leaving Joan a little doubtful.

"You didn't argue?" her mother asked, shaking her head the way she always had when sensing disagreements.

"We're not going to because I'm not going to," Nell grumbled good-naturedly, thinking Joan didn't have to choose a second husband ten years older than she was, one with heart problems.

Nell couldn't concentrate on the story she tried to read in the dentist's office as she waited for him to yank her mother's teeth. It wasn't going to take half an hour. That shocked her. In less than half an hour, you could lose all your upper teeth, replace them with acrylic.

When Nell was finally invited into the inner office, her mother was upright in the chair. She smiled and, though part of her face would not respond, she could talk. "It's done," she said. The new teeth were in place, and the dentist reviewed with Nell the procedures her mother needed to follow until he saw her again the next day. "She'll rest, go to bed early," the dentist said. "I recommend it, in fact."

Nell exchanged a look with her mother, who winked.

Aunt Sarah called, Clara, Dorothy and Aunt Corrine. Uncle John called later. Nell reassured everyone. She stirred the soup, coaxed her mother into eating.

After lunch, her mother napped. Nell brought out her paperwork, the proposal for the superintendent's office. When she finished reading, she was glad she hadn't gone today. She could do a better job. As she started to rewrite, the doorbell rang.

Joan let herself in, flopped on the chair across from Nell. Her hair was blonde and swept back from her face, the latest style. "How's Frederick?" Nell asked.

"Better," Joan said. Joan lit a cigarette, even the gesture part of her role: older-sister-in-charge-of-everything.

Nell pushed at her own short hair, flecked with gray. Dowdy, she thought. Joan was the pretty one. If I am the smart one, then why do I feel so damn stupid?

"You should've brought Frederick," Nell said, then could have bitten her tongue. Joan knew perfectly well how she felt about Frederick. But if he had come, Nell wouldn't have had to face Joan alone.

Joan said, "Ha!" and added, "What will we do when Mother gets really old?"

"She's healthy and she's only seventy-four."

"Just remember you're her daughter too," Joan snipped, but she looked vulnerable for a minute, as if she knew that the club of guilt she had always used on Nell wasn't working the way it should. But they stopped talking, because their mother appeared, wrapped in a housedress. Shaking her head at both of them, the familiar scolding, she said she'd heard them arguing.

A few minutes later they were all in the kitchen, freshening up the soup for dinner, clattering easily, noisily. Nell couldn't dictate Joan's happiness any more than Lena's, and, anyway, how did she know how happy Joan was?

By the time Nell left for home the next day, in time to catch her afternoon appointment, she felt refreshed. She had enjoyed cooking for her mother, their long talk over dinner and breakfast. Even her mother's fussing and Joan's stubbornness seemed to underline how fine everything was, how strongly their lives marched forward, how easily they lived. Joan would stay in that warmth forever, and part of her was jealous, would always be jealous.

What made children leave home? Having Lena as her client underlined the problem. Too much closeness brought disaster, she knew. She wouldn't want her boys to stay home forever—would she? Joan thrived on staying in their hometown, instead of feeling stifled, as Nell would. Who was right? Who was wrong? Both of them? Neither?

That afternoon, Lena was five minutes late, then ten. Finally, Nell's phone rang. "I'm sorry," Lena said. "I can't make it. Mom's gone into the hospital—gall bladder. I'll get back to you when I can." She sounded shaken.

Lena hung up. A bowl of silence descended over Nell with awful suddenness. She took a deep breath, put her head down on her desk; some sixth sense was saying Lena would not be back.

To keep from crying, Nell wrote notes furiously, completing all her reports. But she couldn't shake her vulnerable, lost feeling of failure.

Days, seven of them went by. Nell called Lena. The first time she reached the father and she was sure Lena never got her message. The second time, Lena's son Dan answered, and Nell wan't sure he was any more reliable. The following week, though, Lena sent her a card explaining that her mother was recuperating from gall bladder surgery, she couldn't leave her, and that she had to discontinue therapy because of the time and the expense. "Nell, you have been wonderful to me," she wrote. "And I am better because of you. You're the world's best therapist!" Lena had drawn squiggles and hearts all over the bottom of the paper.

Nell felt sick. She put the note in the file with Lena's session notes and closed the drawer. Even the slender edge of understanding, of hope that Lena would heal, was lost. The drummer Lena followed was inaudible to her.

It was days before she could even try to tell herself that there were compensations: Lena had given her a newfound ability to deal with Joan. She'd remember her for that.

Months later, when Nell could almost believe in the compensations, she ran into Lena at the mall. Oddly, Joan was the one she told. They were on the phone, discussing what to do for their mother's 75th birthday. "I saw Lena today," Nell said.

"Lena?"

"The woman I told you about ... who never could leave her family."

"The one that reminded you of me?"

"That one."

"I remember. How is she? Did you find out you cured her after all?"

"Why not?"

"Not exactly. She's working now, parttime. Not that she needs the money."

"Her father died, as it turned out; stroke. She's living quite comfortably with her mother. It agrees with her—she's even lost weight and she's not so puffy. Can you imagine?"

"That's what my children would do if I let them. So she still lives at home?" Joan's sigh sounded like wistful admiration.

"And the grandmother's going to pay Dan's way through college—he's doing fine. Loves being doted on by two women, I'm sure. At least he seemed to." The brief meeting at the mall had brought Lena clearly into focus—as confused as ever, but coping somehow. She thought about the yellow and red sign, and wondered if Jesus had done better with the carpet store.

Joan laughed.

"What's so funny?" Nell asked, irritated. No reason for Joan to sound superior.

"Well, she's a housewife now. You said that's what she wanted. Never said she wanted to get married, did she?"

"No, I guess not," admitted Nell. She hesitated, then told Joan what she was thinking: "Look next time you take the brains and I'll get the looks and we'll see how it comes out, okay?"

Peter Meinke

(untitled)

This is a poem to my son Peter
whom I have hurt a thousand times
whose large and vulnerable eyes
have glazed in pain at my ragings
thin wrists and fingers hung
boneless in despair, pale freckled back
bent in defeat, pillow soaked
by my failure to understand.
I have scarred through weakness
and impatience your frail confidence forever
because when I needed to strike
you were there to be hurt and because
I thought you knew
you were beautiful and fair
your bright eyes and hair
but now I see that no one knows that
about himself, but must be told
and retold until it takes hold
because I think anything can be killed
after a while, especially beauty
so I write this for life, for love, for
you, my oldest son Peter, age 10,
going on 11.

Deborah Partington

IN SIMPLE WORDS

We were lovers; but when you said, on that snapping-cold night back in December, I got in your way, I knew it was time to cross the ocean. Christabel and I had been saving our money to do this ever since graduation. Over the last few months I've learned how much I love being here and how much I still miss you, but I don't tell Christabel that. You can't talk about certain things to people; they don't want to hear. I'm telling you all this stuff that you know already because I want to get the setting right; I want you to know where I am. I'm telling you the truth in this letter.

Each morning I awake and heat some water for a wash. It's not like it is at home. Here, you have to switch on a heater each time you want hot water. In about thirty minutes there is enough for both of us to wash face and arms. Only on weekends do we take baths. After I wash and have coffee, I go for a walk if I don't have to work. I waitress; so does Christabel. My favorite walk is along the Thames.

To get there, I walk past the homeless camped out near Charing Cross Station. The sound of the trains slurring into the station at night is their lullaby. Their morning alarm is the trains hustling commuters to work. I hurry past those patched coats and dirty trousers, that seem more alive than the bodies shaping them. Some mornings I kick discarded newspapers scuttling along the ground in my path.

The boats on the Thames remind me of Cape Cod. Unweighted by people and cargo, they bob up and down. Sometimes I think they are old men see-sawing on rocking chairs. In windy weather the water reminds me of you, your body rising over me, like a swelling wave, then you come breaking on the river bank or against the flank of boat.

It was on these morning walks that I met Stafford, the guy I mentioned in my last letter. We tended to walk the same path in the mornings. This letter isn't about Stafford though; it's about you, so I won't bother telling you about last night and how he and I had supper at a pub near the University of London.

Remember your birthday last November? We had a beer at Barnacle Bill's and sat at the table cornered between the fireplace and the wall. The fire gave a lambent glow to your face. The lobster trap, retired from duty, that supported the glass table top still carried the sea smell. Its wood was encrusted with sand and little shells. Over our heads was an old fisherman's net. You said you had a steak in your refrigerator and a bottle of Chianti. Hand in hand we walked to the two rooms you called your apartment. The walk chilled me. I remember thinking that afternoon, deep into fall, we will make love, not for the first time, but it would be special this time because this day is special. As we walked to your apartment, the sun setting behind us, you put your arm around me. Every time you moved an arm or a leg, your muscles shifted. You were the wind, and I was a November leaf being blown along. I feared you were laughing at me shivering beneath my heavy woolen cape. But you stopped dead in your tracks and kissed me and then grabbed my hand yelling, "Come on, I'm getting cold." We raced to your apartment, but I was always a half pace behind. That afternoon I fell in love with you. Oh, I thought I loved before that, but it wasn't really love.

The wine was cooling on the window sill while we made love on the mattress in your living room, under the quilt your mother had made out of little scraps of cloth. She'd seen one like it in *Women's Day* and figured it was something she could do between chauffeuring growing boys to basketball games in the winter, to beaches in the summer, and cooking meals seven nights a week. Didn't you tell me she used to sit on Nausset Beach stitching cotton squares together while you and your brother kicked up the sand with your running feet?

For the first time in my life that November afternoon, I had someone I never wanted to lose, and I was someone that I always wanted to be. That was how I knew I loved you, you and the crisp air promising Thanksgiving, and the leaves jumping under our feet as we walked. Cold always makes our senses much keener, don't you think?

Today when I received your letter I slipped my brown woolen cape from the wooden peg on the closet door, wrapped it around my shoulders and fastened its clasp and hopped on a red double-decker bus for Oxford Street. To read your letter I had to be as anonymous as possible. Above all, I couldn't let Christabel see me read it since she always speaks your name with spite. Time spent talking about you was time wasted. She does not like wasting time, and I am amazed at the facility with which she glides in and out of lover's arms and beds. Where she is fluid, I am solid. I have to feel every nuance of love pass through me before I am free to accept a new lover.

Christabel and I usually arrive at the same point; we just take different routes to get there. Once she convinced me to call you a bastard. Does that surprise you? Does it hurt you? At the time I laughed sarcastically and hoped that it would. We were drinking bitters in a pub, The Royal Rose, in Oxford.

"Why do your think about him all the time?"

"What makes you think I do?"

"Because you walk like a person weighed down."

"Really?"

"So do you?"

"Yes."

"The man's a bastard," she said with conviction.

"I don't think that is true."

"Come on! What's your definition of a bastard?"

"Mine?"

Christabel looked at me unflinchingly. I had to answer. "I guess a bastard is someone who is selfish enough to think only of putting himself first and uses people for his own good and ..."

"And ..."

"And doesn't understand how much hurt he causes others."

"And?"

"And doesn't care either."

"Did Don think of you when he started sleeping with Ann?"

"No, I suppose not."

"Was he thinking of you when he didn't return your phone calls?"

"No. Probably not." I sighed deeply.

"Does he care that he hurt you?"

"No."

"So, does he fit your definition of a bastard?"

"Yes. He does."

"Then Don is a bastard."

"Yes," I consented, "Don is a bastard." At the time I really wanted to admit the truth behind those words, though it sounded weird to hear myself saying them.

Because I am still hacking away at the foliage of emotions that gets in the way of seeing you clearly, I had to read your letter in some utterly public, utterly conspicuous place like a cheap coffee shop or a Golden Egg—as far away as possible from some cozy corner. I wanted to be where no one would care if I burst into tears; where I would just be another stranger having morning coffee in the presence of another perfect stranger.

The bus let me off into a queue of people waiting to board it. The British custom of queuing still amazes me. It's so solid, so rooted in tradition, so un-American. Christabel is going to know just by looking at me that I have heard from you. I headed for the Golden Egg; the American equivalent is the old red and white McDonald's, the kind that were around in the sixties.

Two days I stood at the edge of the Thames and watched my shadow playfully flicker in the water. I picked up a handful of reddish brown pebbles and threw them at my shadow. I wanted to kill it. As it lay there on the water sparkling and wavering, I thought it was laughing at me and saying I was a fool to be expecting a letter from you. I didn't see Stafford that morning on my walk. If I were standing there today, I would just laugh right back at that watery shadow. Your letter said what I wanted it to say.

After reading it, I imagined myself withdrawing money from the Barclays down at the corner, going to Cook's Travel to purchase a plane ticket to Boston, and then going to the room Christabel and I shared. She would be out, and I would write her a note telling her that you wanted me to come back. Then I would leave her some money for the rent. I even saw myself carefully placing the note on her pillow so she wouldn't miss it. Then I'd throw my things into the pack and lift my heavy cape from the closet peg and wrap it around myself and head for Heathrow. Maybe I'd leave it for Christabel and just wear a sweater. She loves it and wants one like it, but I don't know where to get her one. Mine came from that second-hand store in Hyannis. Remember the evening we wrapped it around our bodies as we sat on the dunes outside of Provincetown? It was only September, but chilly, and you were wearing a thin sweater. We both wanted to watch the sunset and finish our wine. I don't want Christabel to think I harbor any hard feelings toward her. I've really enjoyed being here with her these past few months.

She's shown me how to enjoy experiences I never could have by myself. Just last week we visited Kenilworth Castle, you know the one that Sir Walter Scott wrote about in his romances. After climbing around the ruins, we got hungry. As we were sitting on the sunny patio of a pub (I don't even remember its name) devouring a ploughman's lunch between us, a guy deep in a wooly sweater sitting at the other end of the table starts talking to us—well, actually to Christabel. Had I been alone, I would have ignored him—or told him I wanted to read my book and eat my lunch undisturbed. Not Christabel. She invites him to share our lunch. Turns out he's a student at Oxford, Keeble College, offers to take us pub crawling through Oxford. So that's what we did last Sunday. I liked The Bear the best. It's right near the center of the city. The walls and ceilings are covered with ends of neckties that the publican snipped from the wearers. It's a small pub, intimate. Of course, the Turf Tavern is nice too, tucked away in its own little corner. Luke Islington, that's the guy's name, and two of his friends, we all went out together. Christabel opens up all these new experiences for me, so if I left, I wouldn't want her to think I'm leaving because of any hard feelings.

She wants us to go to Paris next, then maybe to Brussels. She has always wanted to see both of those cities. By fall, we should be in Greece. And you want me to come back to Cape Cod. If I told her I was going back to you, she'd remind me of the nights I called her, in tears. The night, two weeks after your birthday, I went to meet you at Barnacle Bill's; the night I tried phoning you and you weren't home even though you said you would be; and the third, which I don't need to remind you of since you spoke of it so eloquently in your letter. But what about that night right after Thanksgiving at Barnacle Bill's? I knew you slipped money to the bartender every time you went to the men's room. Funny, how you had to go to the men's room so often that night. You were flirting with that woman near the bar. You were buying her drinks. You were trying to be cool. When I got up in anger and disgust, you just sat there. That evening wasn't written away in your letter. If I told Christabel I was going home, she'd just fix me with her stare and say something like, "You're just going to forget about Stafford for that creep?" I need to feel every nuance of love before I can really move on.

But you did ask me to come home. You told me what I wanted to hear. Your letter spoke of jealousy and how much you really wanted me around. You said you wanted to make it all up to me. My coming to England proved how much I respected your need for freedom. With those words, the love I feel for you, the love that is being sheltered by hurt, wants to bloom again. But this is a letter, and I'm taking a long time to get to the point, am I not? Then again, we're not in any rush, are we? Except that I can hear you saying "Why doesn't she get on with it and tell me when she's coming? I'll go to Logan to meet her, or pick her up at the Hyannis bus depot. If she's not coming, why doesn't she just say so?"

You responded right away to my letter, so I should trust your sincerity. Or perhaps, you wrote when some spur-of-the-moment fondness overtook you. Maybe now you're regretting that you responded so hastily, that you don't really want to see me again. Maybe I'll go back to my room and find out that you phoned and spoke to Christabel or left a message with the proprietress. It would be tacked on the board at the foot of the stairs for anyone to see. *Tell Ellie to stay in London. Sounds like she's happy there. I made a mistake. Don.*

Of course I'd prefer to believe that you really want to see me again. And I want to see you. Though Christabel would tell me I'm a fool. Haven't I told you there are more pigs in the sty, is how she would put it. On the spot, I would agree with her. I know she's right. But her rightness doesn't answer the questions asked by my hurt. Her rightness is not *my* solution. That's the problem. That's what I am struggling with. Can you understand that?

We're telling the truth, right? Part of the truth is that I wound each word you ever said to me tightly around my heart. Waiting for the bus at Oxford Street that would return me to our rented room, I unfolded, for the fifth time, the light-blue paper and reread your words; they were almost memorized. But words, Christabel would say, can strangle you if you take them too much to heart. I can still hear you saying "I love you" that first time. The English teacher, Miss Owensburg, you know her, the one who always wears charcoal-grey suits and has grey hairs flying loose from the bun at the nape of her neck, once said those were the three most powerful words in the English language—and they're all one-syllable. Our deepest sentiments, she said, are always spoken in simple words. We should never lose the ability to use them. You signed your letter with the words *all my love*. What is all your love? How do you know it is with all your love that you want me back? Christabel says there's no such thing as pure love. There's passion, she says, and there's affection. Sometimes you feel them both for the same person, but most of the time you feel one or the other. Now I'm sure you'd be telling me not to listen to Christabel so much. What does she know of what you and I shared? And you never much cared for her. Perhaps you were afraid of how she might see right through you.

Before I went back to the room Christabel and I share, I visited the Thames one last time. As I stood on the banks of the river, the airmail paper containing your letter fluttered in the breeze as I reread your words. The last paragraph is the one that moved me the most. *It's too bad you fall for strangers so easily* you wrote. *Our love was different. We were friends before we were lovers. I felt a special attraction to you that fall I started teaching American History. I was fresh out of UConn, with my MA. You were a delightful presence in class, always smiling and eager to learn. Being around you was infectious. I want to be around you again.* These words carved a desire in me to go home. That was the effect you wanted, isn't it? If I had stayed on Cape Cod, I would be encroaching upon your freedom, but now that I'm in Europe, I'm something exotic, something desirable again, like I was last June. Then I was all tanned from lifeguarding at Nausett Beach—and free. I was still in my bathing suit and had sand clinging to my feet that afternoon we chatted at The Lobster Trap as we stood in line waiting to give our separate orders to the kid behind the counter. Shortly after that you called me.

You wanted the words in your letter to chisel, to sculpt, a truth that isn't possible. I'm not a statue; statues can't feel, and all I am is feelings. That I learned without Christabel's help. She helps me to interpret the truth.

The Stafford I wrote of in that letter to you a couple weeks ago was a creation of words. There is no Stafford who lives in London, who studies history at the University of London. There is no Stafford whom I meet on my morning walks, and who became enamored of me through casual conversation, then took me to Amsterdam for a weekend to see the Van Gogh Museum and take boat rides through the canals. Christabel watched me write that letter on that drizzly cold day that kept us inside. We both decided it's the little things that Stafford should appreciate in me, like how I laugh, how I hold my head when I walk along the Thames, and my shyness. That's how we made him, the perfect lover. But why, I ask myself, must I make you jealous to get you to want me back? In simple words, am I, just me, Ellie, not enough?

Christabel is running water in the tub for her bath. I'm sitting on my bed with a book propped on my knees as a makeshift desk, writing, and wishing it didn't matter what you will think of my letter, and glad that I will not see Cape Cod for many more months. Next week we're heading for Paris, and then, I'm not sure where.

Liz Rosenberg

THE GENIUS TEST

A few years ago something sad happened to my sister after trying a long time to become pregnant; she had a fourth-month miscarriage. We were on the phone when it happened. I'm her younger brother by seven years, and both our parents have been dead a long time. I don't call her as often as I should. Her husband was away at the time, visiting family on Barbados. My sister had begun bleeding the day before, so she called me, just to talk, she said.

I'm not used to this. For one thing, she's never alone. I've learned not to call and say, "Yo, it's me," because I never know who's going to answer her phone. For another, she's no conversationalist. Trying to get a full sentence out of her is like trying to pry the can straight off the sardines. First she told me about the bleeding, then about the decor of the baby's nursery, then back to the bleeding again. When I'd start to hang up, she'd change the subject somewhere else. I finally realized she just wanted company, so I rambled on about this, that, and the other thing, carrying on. In fact, I was in the middle of telling her about some of the black brothers in my department at the university when it happened. I heard her gasp into the phone and then she said, "I've lost it!"

I knew right away what had happened, but I pretended not to. I said, "Maybe not, it could be—"

"Shut up!" she said. "You don't know what you're talking about!" Then the fetus, whatever it was, slid out onto the living room rug, and she started screaming. I tried calming her down, but I was sweating so hard the phone slipped out of my hand. I live 160 miles upstate, and my Volkswagen is unreliable.

I made her promise to call an ambulance, and then I said I'd get in my car and be right over, which was a lie, but she wasn't listening anyway. After we hung up I sat on a chair by the phone without moving, thinking I could keep her alive the same way you can keep a plane up in the air just by concentrating.

I called her back a few minutes later, and then every minute for the next twenty minutes, but the line was busy. I figured she had knocked the phone off the hook and was lying on her living room rug in New Jersey, bleeding to death. I was about to call the Fort Lee police when the phone rang.

"I'm all right now," she said in a calmer, subdued voice. "My friend C.J.'s here. She's going to drive me to the hospital."

"Which one?"

She gave me the name and I scribbled it down. "Where is this place?" I asked. "What's the address?"

"Stop yelling." She told me what street. "It's in the middle of Newark," she said. Anyone can direct you there."

"I'm leaving now," I said.

There was a split-second's pause. "You don't *have* to come," she said, which was the closest she'd ever come to asking me for anything.

"You know, Tee, I used to read about this in biology," I said, "It's Nature's way—"

"I know," she interrupted, "I guess it is, but I don't want to talk about it right now, okay?"

"Oh," I said. I had made her cry again. "Okay."

After she hung up I stood next to the phone, staring at it, willing it to ring so I'd have the chance to say something comforting and profound. After it didn't, I picked up the phone and dialed her.

"Yes." It was the way my mother had answered when she was angry or tired or sick. It was enough to make your heart stop pumping, that small, cool "Yes."

"It's me, Jammal."

"*What.*" She was relentless.

"Was there anything you wanted me to bring?"

"Oh." She might have been thinking about it. Her voice sounded thin and far away. "No, nothing. Thank you, honey."

"You sure?"

"Yes. You going to be okay, driving in the dark?"

Ever since I was a child I've been night-blind. You can keep this hidden from the Motor Vehicle Department, but not from your family.

"It's not a problem," I told her.

I was afraid if I arrived at the hospital too late the night nurse would say, "I'm sorry, but she just passed on ten minutes ago," which is what they said about my mother. But I saw a supermarket with all its lights on, so I decided to stop and buy Latitia something; some flowers or a box of candy.

All the fresh flowers were locked up in the cooler and the selection of houseplants was not great. Maybe it wouldn't have been any better the next morning, but all the leaves looked grayish and limp. I'd once read that most people died between eleven p.m. and five a.m. and maybe it's true of plant life as well. Then I looked at my watch and it was after eleven. I started feeling panicky again, the way I'd feel driving to visit my mother in the hospital. I picked out the liveliest-looking African violet, which was none too perky, and bought the most expensive box of mints in the candy aisle. Then I rested the paper bag on the seat next to me in the car, and drove through all the red lights till I got to Newark.

The hospital looked like a big condominium, lit up with street lamps, a small, separate city. I parked in the Emergency lot, but when I tried to get in, the hospital door was locked. That was a new one to me. There was a nurse sitting inside, and when she heard me pounding on the door she slid the glass open sideways, like a woman selling movie tickets. She stuck her face out a little way, and pulled it back as soon as she saw me. "May I help you?"

"I'm looking for Latitia Bridge," I said loudly. I'm a tall, dark-skinned black. People look at me all the time like I'm about to steal their car. I was holding the African violet plant in one hand, and gesticulating with the other. I was ready to get angry, to be belligerent, to demand that I be allowed in to see my sister. Then I remembered her name wasn't Bridge anymore, though mine was. I gave her married name. The woman nodded immediately. That meant she was dead; when you die, everyone knows about it. "Oh, yes," she said. "She arrived a few hours ago. You are—"

"Her brother," I said.

She looked disappointed.

"Her husband is in Barbados," I said. That sounded frivolous of him so I added, "That's where he comes from. It's where his family lives. He's visiting his family."

"Well, I'll call her ward," she said. "But I'm afraid it may be too late." She slid the window shut.

"Too late?" My breath had steamed up the sliding glass window. The steam evaporated in silver swirls, like clouds emptying out to a clear sky, and through the clear patches I could see the woman's mouth moving against the phone.

She hung up and opened the window. "I'm sorry," she called.

"Why?" I said. I came to the window—but not too close, as if bad news is catching—still cradling the African violet in one arm.

"She dropped off to sleep half an hour ago."

"Sleep?" I felt as if I were trying to solve a difficult puzzle. "Dropped off" sounded like a euphemism for something much worse.

"The doctor gave her a shot," the nurse said patiently. "She just fell asleep a little while ago. Can't you come back tomorrow? We open at nine."

"You *open* at nine? What kind of a hospital is this, anyway? I want to see my sister!" Instead of sounding aggressive and self-assured, as I had intended, it came out pleading. The same thing happened whenever I tried to respond to some ugly remark, or argue at a committee meeting.

"I'll give it a try," the nurse said, turning back to the phone.

I stuck the plant back inside my car, so it wouldn't freeze. I turned the engine and heater on to keep it warm.

"I'm sorry," the nurse said again as I approached the window. "The head nurse was adamant. She really needs her rest."

"My sister does or the head nurse?" I said, but I was too tired to fight dirty, and we both knew it. They always hide the real dragon behind some exhausted-looking woman wearing pink nail polish. "What time can I come back?"

"Nine o'clock."

"I made one last stab. "Can I at least leave the plant here? So she'll see it if she wakes during the night?"

"She won't wake up," the nurse said cheerily. "Not with a shot. Come back at nine."

I drove away through the snow and a long tunnel of Route 4 darkness sparked by gasoline stations and all night diners to my sister's house in Fort Lee. The African violet sat propped between the paper bag and the seat back like a pet cat.

I let myself in through the window of my sister's ranch house. Inside, the rooms seemed to sprawl out around and from me in a figure eight. I turned on a few lamps in the living room. My sister had been sleeping on the living room sofa while her husband was away. There were crumpled up bedsheets on the sofa, and a pillow, and an old not very good photograph of her husband James holding up a string of fish on the coffee table opposite, beside a cluster of used tissues wilting like flowers in the ashtray. All signs of her forlorn existence those past few days were frozen in place, as if they had been preserved in Pompei! Her pocketbook was looped over the kitchen doorknob. Inside I found a tuna coupon, a Shoprite photo ID card, two or three lipsticks, and a twenty dollar bill. It came to me like a physical thing, my sister's existence, separate from me, as it had been the seven years before I was born, as it always would be, in a way, and I remembered something from my childhood I had nearly forgotten: the Genius box.

It looked like an ordinary shoebox, sitting on the black lacquer table in the front hall where the mail was kept. Nothing of importance ever came for me by mail in those days, or nothing my mother didn't open first. My sister came out of the kitchen—she had gotten home before me. "I have a test for you," she said. She came toward me smiling and genial, her brown eyes already shining. She rested one hand on the shoebox, as if she were about to take an oath. "My science teacher made this," she said. "It's a genius test. If you pass it you're a genius—and you will!"

"Okay," I said, already nervous. I was a black kid and black kids weren't geniuses, especially not the boys.

"You notice anything funny about the box?" she asked.

It was a Stride-Rite, because I and my sister both had wide feet and my mother bought all our shoes there. I didn't see anything funny in that. "Not yet," I said cautiously.

"Look real close," she instructed me. "You see how it's almost falling off the table? You see how there's just this tiny little part resting *on* the table?"

I looked. The box was indeed suspended miraculously in the air, like Wiley Coyote after he's run off the edge of the cliff, the instant before he looks down. "It's going to fall," I said.

"No it's not. Now, what do you suppose is keeping it there?"

"Magic?" I asked, but she waved me off. "Glue? Scotch tape?"

"Quit." she said. "This isn't a guessing game, it's a thinking game. Now study the box and don't you dare open it." Then she ambled off down the hall into the bathroom—I heard the door click close—and she left me standing there in front of the shoebox. A magnet, maybe? Chewing gum?

Then another thought occurred to me. What if I wasn't a genius? My sister always behaved as if I was one, but she was the only one who did. Even my mother called me thick-headed. I heard the toilet flush, and knew I didn't have much time, so I opened the box. At one end of the box, anchoring it down, was a clock. I stuck the lid back on as soon as I heard the bathroom doorknob turn. When my sister came to rejoin me I had both hands behind my back, and I was looking at the box gravely, like a medieval scholar, Abelard, maybe.

She was already smiling, proud of me in advance. "Well?"

"I think there's something inside the box," I said.

"Like what?"

"A heavy thing."

"What kind of heavy thing?" she asked, excited, but wanting to be exact.

I knew I was not supposed to name the actual object inside; that would give me away. "A radio?" I said. "Something like that?"

And then my face was shoved up against her warm shoulder, brown and light as a bird's bones, already more delicate than mine. "My baby brother!" she sang, her voice motherly and proud. "You're smart!" she cried. "You're brilliant! You're a genius!"

That was before I began to learn my slow, hard, clumsy lessons in life, before I discovered how small the world could shrink down, one good thing after another, till there would be only the two of us left. Meanwhile, my sister raced off on her bicycle, crying up and down the streets our lucky news.

Stephanie Sallaska

FLIGHT

The plane was about to take off from Stapleton Airport on this morning of our wedding night, but Randy reached for a cigarette out of my purse. His breath smelled of bourbon; the red in the whites of his blue eyes dripped like candle wax. It was the most patriotic I'd felt since Kennedy was shot. A magazine in the seat pocket reminded me this month was still April, still 1968. "You can't smoke now," I said. "The plane's about to leave."

He lit the cigarette with a psychedelic match from a book that said, "The Electric Chair." I remembered we both lost our lighters last night at the party, Randy's party, the one where dancing on and vomiting over his balcony were, if not required, certainly electives.

One flight attendant put a yellow cap over her mouth while another stewardess described the procedure. As she stretched the elastic to the side of her head, Randy pulled out the vomit bag in the upholstered seat by his knees and pretended to use it. I smiled and rolled my eyes; humor did not come naturally to me this morning.

Handsome Randy from Ohio, even hung-over, this college senior was almost as good-looking as the photo I had of him in the display case of my billfold. Sometimes I liked his picture better, those times he ran my life like a third parent; but he talked a lot and made all the decisions about our dates.

I was nineteen, just back after my freshman year flunking out of Kansas State which sounded redundant or impossible. Back home in Wichita, my mother begged the board of the commuter college to let me in. She really had begged. I could still see her knees.

"Excuse me—"

The words drew my eyes up the legs of the stewardess. "You'll have to put that out, sir. We're ready to leave."

Randy smiled and sucked the cigarette, then kissed the smoke at her before he stubbed it out. Last drifts wafted up my nose like the end of a battle.

Seated directly over the wing, the revving engines originated in my head. My mouth unquenchably dry, stomach permanently upended, the sense I was doing something my parents would not approve covered me like syrup.

"Tell me again," Randy said, as I felt the earth move, "what you said in your note."

How many times had I repeated it now? Had he no memory? "Dear Mother and Dad," I said, "Randy and I are on our way to Las Vegas. When you see me next, I'll be Mrs. Randall Dial."

"Whoa," he said, as if he were walking a lot of dogs. "I wish I could see their faces when they read that."

I could and did not feel the same amount of glee. My parents had, in fact, twice invited Randy to their house. The first time, he broke one of Mother's Waterford crystal wine goblets; the second, he arrived in time for dessert and argued politics with my simple father whose only dislikes were arguing and politics.

Randy chuckled. "Don't you know they're going crazy?"

I imagined them sitting at the kitchen table staring at each other, which is what they always did those Saturday mornings after I spent Friday nights drunk, this time adding the extra devastation of my marriage so young to someone I'd known only a month, someone they didn't even like. "Did you want them to?" I asked.

"No," he said. "It's just far out, the whole thing."

I looked out the window. We were far out. "Having second thoughts?" I asked.

He paused. "No, are you?"

"I don't know," I said, not wanting to be the first to say anything that might make a difference, anything I would have to take responsibility for.

"We want to go through with it, don't we?" he asked.

Calling for a committee vote sounded like trouble. This *was* more than a drunken ride in the country after all, no road ending to stop me this time, soft earth, or cushion of corn.

"Don't we?" I repeated. The silence made our questions answers.

The No-Smoking sign dinged and faded. Randy and I pulled out simultaneous cigarettes from my pack. He lit a match to his, then mine. Air vents shot smoke back in our faces as stewardesses inclined up the aisles preparing to serve drinks. Randy put his tongue in my ear. "Want a beer?" he asked.

Beer, the word alone summoned the taste of alcohol up my throat. "Pass," I said.

"Pass-Out, you mean."

I remembered that game suddenly, like the bite of a large mosquito. "You play Pass-Out at all your parties?"

"Just the good ones," he said. "Did you see Mitchell attack his blind date after she got doubles, that girl who didn't drink?" He laughed. "I'll bet that's the shortest relationship on record." He dragged on his cigarette. "And Wendy, when she started to take off her blouse?"

"Too bad she passed out."

"Yeah," he smiled until the stewardess came by with the drink cart. Randy bought a beer; I had a club soda, the soda part penance for the headache which geometrically split me. He put his hand on my thigh, but I couldn't feel anything. Numb and sobering, the anesthetic only threatened to wear off as a smoky O coiled into a loose question mark.

What I knew at this moment was I did not want to be 30,000 feet in the air. I wanted my feet firmly on the ground and someone else to answer this question. It seemed so right last night after the party, sneaking into my bedroom, fumbling around my bottom drawer for Christmas money I'd saved, loot which financed this trip. We fell over each other and giggled, slurring words back and forth in some great adventure. Now, I was plummeting back to earth.

"How well do you think you know me?" Randy asked.

"About as well as you know me," I answered, leaving out the part I knew myself about as well. My stomach growled with guilt, the Catholic kind that takes over organs.

"Hungry?" he asked.

"I had that cinnamon roll," I said, remembering the two of us on stools at the Denver snack bar, the feeling I had of sitting next to the stranger I was to spend my life with—marriage arranged by a board game. The pink formica countertop with flecks of gray looked impenetrable, a round and fluted glass bottle with sugar trapped inside the only decoration. And now, the stranger still beside me, it seemed the only way out of this was something dramatic, a hijacking or mid-air crash.

"Kind of a '60's Romeo and Juliet," he said. "Your parents are gonna flip."

"Romeo and Juliet didn't get together just to upset their parents, " I said. "Wasn't there something about love?"

"Love? Love?" he repeated. "Babe, this is the Age of Aquarius. Love is all around."

Suddenly, it seemed I'd worn these clothes since birth. Shirt wrinkled, jeans stiff, my feet glued to each shoe. "What are we doing?" I asked.

"Flying," he said.

"No, I mean after the plane lands."

"I don't know," he said.

I didn't either, and we rifled through travel magazines the rest of the flight.

When we touched down, I touched Randy. "I need to call my parents."

"Why?" he asked. "You left them a note."

"I just do," I said, feeling like a hostage, needing to talk to somebody I knew, somebody who knew me.

"You don't see me calling *my* parents," he said.

"Your parents are in Ohio. As far as they know, you're in Wichita sleeping." Why did it feel like I was the one who had so much on the line, so much to lose, that Randy was just going along for the ride, to upset my parents, a ride I was paying for?

"Sure," he said. "Go ahead. I'd like to hear what they have to say."

I followed him off the plane. At the first pay phone, I deposited two dimes and arranged a collect call.

"Hello," my mother answered, anxiety in two syllables.

"Mother," I said.

"Are you okay?" she asked, without letting me answer, and added, "Are you—" There was a pause.

"No."

"Where are you?"

"Las Vegas."

"And you're not—"

"Not yet."

"This is killing your father," she said.

"I know."

"No, you don't know," she screamed in the phone. "You don't know anything. You don't know how you worried us, how much you've hurt us. Why? Why?"

"I don't know," I said, rolling my eyes at Randy who was jumping up and down as if his team scored a touchdown.

"Your father is crying like a baby," she wailed. "Like a baby! Do you know what you've put us through? Do you have any idea?"

Engines revved again in my head. Picturing my father's rare tears brought my own. I looked at the slot machine in the corner, then at Randy laughing. "I'm sorry, Mother," I said and hung up.

Randy hailed a cab whose driver had longer hair on his face than his head. Take us to the nearest wedding chapel," Randy said.

The driver registered no emotion, acting like this was a destination he drove all day. My fiancé fell back next to me as the taxi pulled away from the curb. "But first," Randy leaned forward again, "Stop at a liquor store."

The driver nodded as if that too were a usual request.

None of us said a word until the taxi stopped in front of Leonard's Liquors. "Be right back," Randy kissed me like a slap on the cheek.

I watched his head travel aisles of bottles, knowing that face would be a pretty one to look at for the rest of my years, knowing too *that* was its main attraction. This time I leaned forward and pulled the driver's seat forward toward me. "Tell him I changed my mind, would you?"

"Sure, lady," he said, stroking a kinky chin hair.

"Tell him—" I opened the door. "Nevermind." There was a casino across the street, cars and taxis nearly shrouding it. I hopped into the closest one. "Airport, please—quick," I said, like a player in a bad movie.

The driver chewed on his unlit cigar and slipped the taxi into drive. "What's the matter, Lady?" he cackled. "Change your mind?"

I laughed as if he were joking but I couldn't know that I would take the return flight without playing one slot, that Randy would return the next day, after playing many. I couldn't know the four of us would meet for steaks at my parents' house and try to do it right which only made it wrong. I couldn't know that Randy would graduate, return to Ohio, marry, have two children, get drunk, manic, then depressed, lose his job, then his teeth in a terrible car wreck and any hope for a normal life. I couldn't know that I would drop acid, careen through six colleges, marry a man twenty years older who fell irrevocably ill a year after our daughter was born, and trap me in bars stiff as prison. I couldn't know what was coming; I just knew it wasn't funny.

Sybil Smith

IN SEARCH OF GREAT AUNT EVA

I often think of the book, straining to recall every detail.

It had a hard, green cover; of that I am sure. The inscription was in lilac, and was to my mother. But was there a year? Was there a "with love, Aunt Eva"? If there was no mention of Eva's name, how do I know (and I do) that the book came from her? Concentrating hard I could almost swear the inscription read, "For Lois, with love, Aunt Eva." But I could be wrong.

It was *The Poetry of Robert Frost.* It was an old book, and may well have been a first edition, since Aunt Eva was a well educated Vermont woman with the money to buy books and the leisure to read them. The book was in our family for as long as I can remember. When my mother died, I made it mine. I carried it with me through college and graduate school, and on my adventures to Mississippi and Alaska. I lost it in 1983.

I don't know how I lost it. I can only say that, like the talisman, I took it everywhere. Why? I am a poet, for one thing. I am a Vermonter, for another. But there is more. I have a memory of my mother taking down the book one afternoon when I was four or five (I wasn't in school yet) and reading the poem "The Pasture"; the one that begins; "I'm going out to clean the pasture spring / I'll only stop to rake the leaves away ..."

I remember the distinct impression the images made on me; the clearing water, the tottering calf, the invitation. Right then I knew that this was something ... Worthy? Precious? Valuable? What words did I have then that I could have applied? Feelings exist before words. Though I mostly find words now; sorting, shoving, herding them around—a bully of words—I didn't have the right ones then. I had a feeling, like warm water or ionized air. What I *felt* was that getting the right words in the right order was a good thing; a worthy pursuit; a power.

Those were the years when Aunt Eva used to come visit. We lived in Massachusetts, so she must have driven from Vermont. Her car was one of those huge, square, grey-upholstered ones. The back seat would be full of clothes, of glasses of jelly with the wax tops leaking, of books, china, stale crackers.

When she left my mother used to laugh. "Good Lord! I'm a charity case I guess. Poor benighted Lois. What on earth does she think I need with embroidered linen napkins? Petticoats? Here chicks, you take them."

The heirlooms of our family are lost, because of her fine disdain. The heirlooms which survived? Chipped, many of them. Ripped, stained, bent.

My mother had been brought up in a family where the silver was polished at appointed times. She was a D.A.R., valedictorian of her class, daughter of a Brandon optometrist. She met my father and was ruined. He was a handsome devil, a rake and a ramblin' man, a jack-of-all-trades. He swept her away, in a gale of passion and radical ideas. She was ambivalent about her ruin, but was in too far to turn back. In five children.

For all her flight from bourgeois convention, I remember polishing silver a few times myself, on too hot or too cold afternoons. My sister, Katie, and I would be set up with pink polish, chamois cloth, and sudsy water. But it was erratic. It was a stab at disorder which had progressed so far there seemed no help for it. For all I know the laundry lay undone while the silver gleamed. Children don't question such things.

I can't remember what Aunt Eva talked about when she visited. I imagine her conversation was laced with references to The Lord. I am fairly sure her intentions were good. She wasn't a malicious busybody, or a bible-thumper, or a flibbertigibbet. She was a well-brought up, well-intentioned, well-educated, God-fearing woman. And no wonder she feared God. He had taken her husband, and both her sons. Her husband died of syphilis at the age of 47. Her son Dennison died of congenital syphilis a few months after he was born. Edward somehow escaped the disease. He died at age 14, of drowning.

He died on June 20, 1930. There was a Sunday school picnic at Lake Dunmore. Back then no one thought a thing of climbing into a boat with three women, dressed in their flouncy best, who didn't swim. I don't know if life jackets were in wide use then, but I doubt it. Life was not as fraught with accident prevention.

Edward, as I have said, was 14. Eva was 49. I confirmed these facts with Dereka, my eldest sister, on the phone this morning.

"Shepard was dead then?" I asked.

"Yes," she said.

"He died of syphilis, right?"

"Yes."

"How do you know?"

"Ma told me."

"And Dennison died young?"

"Three months."

"So Edward was her life then."

"Yes, he was her life."

There was a long pause. We both have children. We didn't need to say what we were thinking. How does one survive such a loss?

And Edward was a beautiful boy, of that there can be no doubt. I have a picture of them on my office wall. They are holding hands, and Eva's cheek is against his temple. They are smiling. Eva is wearing an elaborate dress with shoulder drapes and an embroidered bunch at her waist. The material is shiny, crepe or satin. Her face is large and serene. She is what used to be called, "a handsome woman." Edward has her slightly heavy jaw, but is otherwise even-featured and well-formed. He looks to be about 12, verging on adolescence, but there's not a trace of sullenness or rebelliousness in his face. Horatio Alger material. Bright in school, an excellent swimmer, a treasure.

Another snippet from my sister.

"Ma was five when he died. She idolized him. She would start to cry, thirty years later, when she told about what happened."

Three women in a boat, with Edward rowing. June 20, and it is a sunny day. If it were not, they would not be boating. They have eaten. What? Potato salad, bean salad, and baked ham. Pie, pickles, lemonade. Summer crops are only just in, so people are eating their stored food. Perhaps someone made dandelion greens, for the pleasure of their fresh, bitter taste.

The two girls are sitting on one seat, Edward is in the middle, and Eva is at the other end. She is a bit uneasy, because she can't swim, and the boat seems low in the water.

I blame the girls. They are giggling, showing off for Edward, who is well-liked. One tries to stand and adjust her skirt under her, or one leans to trail her hand in the lake. The side of the boat catches on the water, and it capsizes.

Edward comes to the top, gasping. June 20, the water is still cold in Vermont. He looks for his mother first, and soon sees her, thrashing, her summery dress billowing with trapped air. He grabs her. Mother hold on, I'll carry you in to shore. He hooks his arm around her chin, as he's been taught.

They wouldn't have spoken, on the way to land. They would have needed all their breath. When they felt rocks under their feet, what a relief it would have been.

She shouldn't have let him go back. She should have grabbed a tan, wet arm, and not let go. But she didn't. She didn't know this was the last time they would hold each other, in cold water, in fear, so that later she could not remember, or savor it.

He went back. The boat would have been floating, would it not? Capsized, but providing a raft if one kept ones wits, and held on. Surely that's how the girls survived till he returned. But when he came near, they both let go. They grabbed him. They held him with the grip his mother should have had, back on shore, and all three drowned.

The rest is hard, but easy to imagine.

To recover the bodies, they had to drag the bottom. Possibly she saw him; possibly those in charge thought it best to spare her the sight.

Her three brothers, and their wives would have come. She would have stayed in a darkened room, with the minister holding her hand. The doctor would have given her something; laudanum, I believe, was favored then. Perhaps she shut her eyes, and pictured Edward in God's arms. Limp, dripping. God smoothed the hair off Edward's forehead, and passed his palm over his eyes. They opened. He smiled. He was given a clean, dry robe to put on. He looked down on her, from heaven.

Still, that vision would have paled beside her need for his flesh. Surely she must have questioned God's wisdom.

But she didn't die. Much as we try to deny it, while we're feeling it, grief is rarely fatal. And Eva had something besides God, laudanum, and the family. She had a strength hard to define, a quality refined and handed down over generations of hardship and survival. I know what it is, because it is my inheritance. Tenacity of spirit.

Eva lived into her eighties, and kept a sound mind. She spent her final years in Randolph, in the Eastern Star Nursing Home, having been a matron in the order of Eastern Star, and a Grand Ruth in the Vermont chapter.

But before that, according to the Baker genealogy, she taught music. She had a fine contralto voice, and was much in demand as a soloist. She went to church, went to Eastern Star meetings, visited the poor, climbed into her car and brought us things. And, she wrote poems.

***

The house we grew up in, the house where Aunt Eva used to come visit, was sold recently by my father. It was an old colonial, with 14 rooms, five fireplaces, and a huge, drafty attic. My mother has been dead for 18 years, and my father married again. His new wife brought with her four children.

The rooms, closets, attic, and barn were full of belongings which had to be sorted through. The most recently stored stuff was unearthed first, in the manner of an archaeological dig, and as we dug deeper we went further back in time, till we reached the real treasures. There were about seven boxes in all, full of photographs, tintypes, hanks of blonde hair, hand-tooled baby booties, letters, newspaper clippings, and old Bibles.

My older sister and I split the boxes. Tamar, the middle child, was busy redecorating her home. My younger sister, Katie, wanted nothing to do with them. My brother we didn't even ask.

As to what is in my boxes, I have only scratched the surface. I have read a diary of my mother's, written during the time when she became pregnant (accidentally) with Dereka. I have read two typewritten genealogies, and browsed through another professionally researched and bound, which is far too thick to read, and which traces my family back to Katherine Parr (one of Henry VIII's wives) and Helen of Troy. I have read a letter written in pencil by Harrison Jones, who died in the battle of Chickamauga Creek, during the Civil War. I have studied countless pictures of men in stiff suits and women in long dresses.

My investigation is severely hampered by the fact that I have asthma and am allergic to dust. Dust is composed (partially) of dust mites and human skin flakes. It occurred to me, as I pawed through the memorabilia, that I was surrounded by a cloud of my ancestor's skin. I was breathing it in. What did it mean that this left me gasping, short of breath for hours?

In the end I contented myself with reading the genealogies, with a handkerchief wrapped around my face; (burglaring the past, I liked to think). Before long I knew the names and relationships of ancestors like the back of my hand.

There was Hiram, who gambled away his daughter. (The marriage was soon annulled by Hiram's irate wife.) There was Mercy, who died in an Indian raid. There was Frances Mariah, a photographer who couldn't make tea. There was Elizabeth, who, to prove her daring, whipped up a team and dashed across the tracks in front of a train. There was Ruth, who, after her sons died (one of pneumonia and one when a tree fell on him) wore a deep, deep path between the house and the barn, and refused to speak for months. A prayer meeting was called the day she finally broke down and cried.

Death, it seems, was not the exception. How long has it been?—sixty years at the most—that one expects one's children to live. How long has it been that one expects one's wife to live through childbirth? In the Baker genealogy the marriages of 28 women are charted, my mother among them. Of the 28, three died in childbirth, and six are charted as having no issue.

Fevers, pneumonia, falling trees, wars, drownings, fire, cow kicks; you name it.

It came to me that I was a descendent in more than just genes. The traumas of a family have resonance in future generations. I didn't spring into this world without a history.

A person passes on what they can. My mother had five children. She wrote a diary. She told stories. She saved the boxes. Her father, Clarence, began the Baker genealogy. When he died his brother Horatio carried it on. My grandmother's half-sister composed the Clark genealogy, mostly from memory. And Eva, sister to Clarence and Horatio, what did she do? She brought a book into my life, one that changed it. She wrote poems. She did not let herself be crushed by pain.

You pass on what you can. If it is only children, or china, or the sheer fact that you made it eighty years, so be it. You do what you can in whatever time you have between surviving, grieving, gardening, and wiping babies' chins.

And what you leave behind? Your descendants should grab it, like a baton passed to them. They should make what they can of it. It is wrong to act as if it has no significance or value.

***

It was Katie who lost Aunt Eva's poems. A few months into the house cleaning, when it was almost empty, my stepmother came across a notebook in the back of some closet. She glanced through it, and saw that it was poems. Katie, my younger sister, was the only one around. "Here," my stepmother said, "Give this to Sybil. It looks like something she would treasure." Katie glanced through it. She saw poems, and Eva's name.

"Okay," she said. And lost them.

"I have some poems for you," she told me. "From Aunt Eva. I can't find them in the car. Funny, I thought I chucked them in. I'll look around when I get a chance."

"Poems," I said reverently. "Really? What were they like?"

"Oh, I don't know, they may have been copied out of books, they may have been her own, I didn't *examine* them."

I pressed her a few weeks later, had she found them?

"No."

I called my stepmother. Did she remember them?

(I had to be careful on the phone. Babs takes offense easily at any suggestion that she may have damaged or lost something belonging to our family.)

Yes, a notebook. She gave it to someone. Katie?

Back to Katie, on the phone.

"Babs remembers a notebook. Poems. She's pretty sure she gave them to you. You're sure you don't have them?"

"Positive. I have only one box of personal papers. I threw a lot of junk out. I can't be bothered saving it all."

"Too bad," I said, trying to keep the anger and sorrow out of my voice. I had to be careful if I was going to get anything at all. "Can you remember *something* about them? A line? Were they in pen?"

"Sybil, I really didn't look. I'm not interested in that kind of crap like some people."

Bait. I didn't rise.

"Do you want the oak bed?" she asked, conciliatory.

"Yes, I'd love it. I'll come down, in the truck."

"And the mattress?"

"Why don't you sell it?"

Sharp again. "My time is too valuable to spend trying to find some hippy who wants a mattress for $25 bucks. I'll have my landlord take it to the dump."

My sister, the mathematician. All business and lean flesh.

Then …"Aunt Eva doesn't strike me as a poet."

"Oh yes," I said. "She had leisure, grief, and an education. She liked Robert Frost. She could be a forgotten Dickinson."

There is nothing I can do. I think about the poems, on occasion. I tell myself that they were probably dripping with thous and ohs, and rocks and rills, a mediocre pastiche of Bryant and Longfellow. Still, I would have liked to have seen them.

***

I have one other picture I like, in particular, of Eva. It shows her with Edward on her shoulder. She is looking over her shoulder at him, so her face is in profile. She is wearing a white dress, with an embroidered white yoke. Her heavy hair is piled on her head. Edward looks to be about three or four months old, which means that Eva was 35 when the picture was taken. Edward is wearing an elaborate christening gown.

I keep the picture in my living room. My daughter, playing, knocked it off the shelf one time. She picked it up, worried that she had done something wrong. Then she brought it to me, chirping, "A pitcher of mommy, and me when I was born." I looked at it closely. I do look like her.

I like to believe that her spirit is out there somewhere. Perhaps, since I've been writing this, she's come closer, drawn, as if by a scent. If being dead gives her any power, she will breath some of it into my words. My words will not be perfect then. They won't, as I dreamed in the beginning, get absolutely everything in. There is not room or energy for some things: her face in the wedding picture as she married Shepard, an older man; the look of her gravestone, and Edward's; the smell of the Eastern Star Nursing Home; the years of corsets and flabby arms; arthritis, valentines, sweets, the 23rd Psalm. The words won't be perfect, but they'll have the beat of our combined desire, and will follow each other like water across rocks, never breaking apart, but always moving—changing pitch now and then, braiding around stones, coming together again, always singing.

Amy Jo Schoonover

GRACE BEFORE MEALS

How carefully she used to set the table
for her solitary meal: tablecloth her favorite
blues and greens, English ironstone dishes
just so, and the gold tableware glinting
in an overhead light. Then she sat
down to a supper that would have pleased
any home economist, its balanced flavors
and textures outward signs of a skill
she had not forgotten. Lean meat was done
to a turn, potatoes properly fluffy, and other
vegetables and fruits crisp and colorful
enough for the most finicky palates.
It was her amused or anguished answer
to the doctor who had pronounced
her carelessness in cooking "for one
alone" a disaster to her health.
Not impressed by the old argument,
he had warned her sternly. And now,
grace withdrawn, she lies unmoving
with tubes in her mouth and nose,
perhaps dreaming of food, of dishes
and silver, of a ten-year holding period.
Now intentions count for nothing. Now.

Pamela Uschuk

HEALINGS

Between dusk and the end of shadow
silence keeps this house.
The first autumn leaves dry like tongues
above the uncut lawn.
They say everything in the key of wind,
agree or disagree to each imagining,
each day I've not had
a letter or message from my love
vanished in a foreign land.
Their burnt words love gossip.
I rearrange furniture
as if it were the future
waiting for a friend.
There are no mums brighter
than those I bought, thick constellations
charging the living room with yellow flame.
If I could write him, I'd say
we are made of the same elements as stars
whose constant orbits
we discover each clear night.
But for days, now, it's been overcast,
Cassiopoeia wheeling blind midheaven,
and the mail brings only bills.
Tonight a friend does come to talk
about loss, the fresh deaths
of her father and young friend
she cannot bury in her heart.
There are no biers in the asters
where she'd dance, giving their color
to the hills in this cool season.
We wonder if we can make our marriages last
or learn to let go.
Again. We drink the last of the wine
then hold silence like a lemon's bitter tongue
between us, until only laughter remains.
Fresh chrysanthemums sing from the living room—
and outside,
the Peace Rose I planted blooms
near the front door defying frost.

Ron Weber

THE PROCESSIONAL

All day I walk
the road into sleep
carrying a handful of dust
to drop on my mother's coffin.
Behind me, my brother counts
backwards from a hundred, plotting
coordinates with his engineer's mind.
He knows hard work always provides
a solution—so this must be
it. Behind him
my father wearing dark glasses
taps out his litany of grief,
asking now who will make him
his instant mashed potatoes.
My mother's mother follows
in her wheelchair clutching
a sack of pennies to her breast.
Her eyes sink into
the milk-white distance
as if this was TV and
she was Job taking umbrage
at commercials. After her
come my aunts weeping in black linen,
veils extinguishing their faces.
They carry a baby's casket
filled with fine print
delicate as the wings of gnats. They ask
each other who was
this older sister who insisted
on eating only dead leaves and
dried twigs. They tell each other
she's someone who entered heaven
long ago. Friends, neighbors
are next, whispering
to each other how good
she looks with her eyes painted
blue as the Virgin Mary's,

better than in years. Finally
the priest brings up the rear,
chanting from the *Book of
Sweeping*, "We blame everyone,
it's no one's fault." So
we acquiesce in burying
my mother when she is
still alive, even
my mother. We tell
each other we are planting
a tree.

Kennette H. Wilkes

DEAR MOTHER, I WANT TO WANT TO FORGIVE

I want to forgive the beatings, knotty winter limbs
lashed across my legs, your hard voice, cutting
"Don't scream. I'll whip you 'til you stop."

I could outlast you; my anger could too
after years of turning the other cheek, turning
holy pages written by men speaking of faith.

You taught me to read, said "Bad girl, stand in the corner"
and I saw the rolled newspaper coming fast, the print blurred—
the cheek, the other cheek, blood to the right, blood

to the left. There is a book called *Why Bad Things Happen
To Good People*. I want to teach myself to read, forgive
Daddy for petting the cat when I was in the corner.

For years I have been a hopeful agnostic,
put faith on the shelf beside atheism and the dusty Bible
Daddy gave me, as I waited secretly for a mystical experience.

My best friend has had one, felt God hover like a presence
over her trailerhouse and tested Him—demanded proof
"If You're there tell me how many fabric squares I've cut."

She actually spoke aloud, her needle threaded and the quilt
tight on the frame while God counted the red and blue and
        yellow
in three stacks of squares and got it right every time.

She remembers—there were 37 and 74 and 48. I am almost
48, Mama, and you taught me to read before school, and I read
philosophy and biology and psychology and I want to

forgive and learn to read again. My friend said I should
read Tillich's *Shaking of the Foundations* and I might
because my only phobia after three years of therapy is

earthquakes. The plank floor shook when you came after me,
your eyes flaring, and I stayed scared even after
I came home from college with the degree you always wanted

sat in church and tried not to laugh when the serious choir
sang "Darwin's evolution monkeys ain't no kin to me or mine"
while comparative vertebrate anatomy sang in my head.

Please don't think I've forsaken prayer for a microscope
or drop to my knees in worship of the double helix
although DNA is a fine thing. It's just that believing

doesn't come any easier than forgiving for me, and I can't
help hoping that God is not answerable to me should I inquire
exactly how many words I have taken to say it's ok—almost.

Danielle D'Aunay

Charles B. Rodning

PATIENT-PHYSICIAN INTERACTION:
Healing Power of a Covenant Relationship

The covenant relationship is a valuable concept in the context of healing—independent of the classification of a disease process. This concept implies a reintegration of the individual or self to achieve a state of wholeness. This integration is achieved within a covenant relationship with individuals who explicitly and implicitly communicate caring and hope. This healing relationship is effected at the mental/spiritual level by faith—"the circle of the spirit." Patient-physician relationships are interdependent: physicians function as ministers (servants) perceiving a patient's needs and responding with a demeanor of integrity and candid hopefulness—offering the gift, if not of healing, at least of wholeness. A physician's realistic and goal-directed responses, commensurate with a patient's specific philosophy of life, reduce the angst associated with the clinical situation and facilitate recovery of a patient's self.

> I have come to tell you of the Way
> And the Way is the Circle
> And the Circle is the Source
> And the Source is Life
> And Life is the Light
> Therefore, those of the Circle shall
> Drink of the Source and become as the
> Light that lives and nourishes.
>
> J.W. Anglund, *The Circle of the Spirit*

A pervasive spirit of contemporary society is wholism (Sodel, 1979; Schaffner, 1981; Nouwen, 1971; Glymour and Stalker, 1983). In the context of health-care delivery, it is exemplified by the word "cure," which denotes restoration of an individual's total self. Supplemental terms for cure include salvation, salutary, and even *shalom* ("peace," "unity," "completeness," "being at one with reality," "being at one with the universe"). Each connotes a "well-being of the *total* self" in relation to the community.

The concept of wholeness is derived from Western traditions (Russell, 1977; Bettmann, 1956; Nouwen, 1971; Marty and Vaux, 1982) and from cultural and linguistic patterns developed from several Judeo-Christian concepts. In the orthodox use of these terms, the individual selves were never seen without an awareness of the community of which they were an integral part. All understood that people found completeness, curing, healing, totality, and wholeness within a covenant relationship, and that caring, community, and harmony derived from the covenant. Throughout the societies of antiquity, health, health care, and related ethical concerns were a function of covenants.

When human beings "belong together" (for instance, when they have common blood), they also share a common life, common responsibility, and common will. The personal community of the blood family was only one expression of the common life and wholeness pervading ancient societies. In its antecedent forms, this unity was a result of blood—either of kin or of covenant. As it appeared in ancient Hebrew, "covenant" was something that was "cut," and its ratification involved the shedding of blood. As a consequence of a covenant, individuals became a unity of self, system, and society that possessed one goal: healing, wellness, wholeness—of the total self.

However, later Occidental, Socratic, Platonic, and Cartesian philosophical systems took a reductionistic approach to the self (Russell, 1977; Bettmann, 1956). They divided the self into physical (L. *corpus,* "body"), mental (L. *mens,* "mind"), and spiritual (L. *animus,* "spirit") components. Subsequently, this trichotomy fostered professional divisions, and therapists were educated to intervene at their respective levels of expertise.

Although the trichotomy provides useful definitions, a reintegration of the self provides a more appropriate foundation for human healing. Consequently, the following recommendations apply:

- reacknowledgment of the symbiotic relationship that exists among body, mind, and spirit;

- reintegration of the self, perceiving it as essential in restoring health irrespective of the disease process; and

- "curing of the soul," a valid unifying concept of patient-physician interaction, effected in the setting of kinships or relationships.

There are historical precedents for the resurgence of interest in the concept of wholism. Before modern scientific approaches to the description and treatment of disease, ancient societies used psychosociological diagnostic and therapeutic systems. Within those communities, prophets, priests, shamans, medicine men, philosophers, and wise men assumed the role of healers (Sodel, 1979; Glymour and Stalker, 1983; Bettmann, 1956; Marty and Vaux, 1982). They analyzed and manipulated relationships between individuals and their family and community to achieve healing. These relationships played a central role in "curing the soul."

It must also be acknowledged that despite considerable scientific advancements, knowledge regarding many diseases remains incomplete. Furthermore, because much disease is not amenable to cure, patients must often accept and cope with physical and psychological pain, dysfunction, and disfigurement. As a consequence, because cure is never assured, patients may experience anger, anxiety, denial, fear, frustration, insecurity, isolation, loss of control, helplessness, and hopelessness. Furthermore, if patients are devoid of hope, they withdraw and become passive and non-manipulative; healing may be delayed or negated, and morbidity and mortality may increase.

The healing dynamic implied in the theological precepts of faith and hope has special relevance in the setting of kinships or relationships integrated at the mental and spiritual levels within "the circle of the spirit" (Anglund, 1983). *Animus* (total person or animating spirit) connotes *pneuma* (breath, will); essence of human personality; expression of corporeal life; and temporarily independent possibilities of blessedness and goodness, capable of vast ranges of experience, but also susceptible to anguish, disorder, injury, and pain. In these contexts, the communication of hope is a dynamic educational process. Hope for complete restoration may not be realistic, but hope for the recovery of maximal achievable function must prevail. In this regard, goals are fundamental, because they provide focus, meaning, and purpose to the continuing struggle. Individuals who establish a covenant with a patient and who convey hope function as ministers (L. *minister,* "servants," "service"), because they educate a patient regarding the unknown and unexpected, and thereby promote healing (Nouwen, 1971; Marty and Vaux, 1982; Lasagna, 1983).

Indeed, for the patient, hope may be possible only because of the covenant relationship with agents of healing and the community that results. In this context, the concept of *shalom* is relevant. When and where *shalom* is in effect, partners exchange gifts to strengthen the psychic community that develops. In this setting, a gift is not an expression of sentiment; it is a required consequence of a relationship between those individuals. The gift itself creates and/or strengthens that relationship. Healing (or curing) connotes the transmission of particular gifts—caring, hope, kindness, peace of mind or body. A gift outside a covenant relationship is discretionary; within such a relationship, it is a requirement, a duty, an obligation. Therefore, a fundamental component of "curing the soul" is a covenant relationship between a patient and others (professional and/or non-professional).

In this communicative and educative process, the demeanor of the healer is of profound import. The demeanor of the caregiver is characterized by consistency, equanimity, honesty, humility, perceptiveness, sensitivity, and thoughtfulness. Caregivers engage a patient by eye contact, listening, speech, and touch; they communicate healing by establishing a covenant, acknowledging an individual's integrity, and promising to involve them in all decision-making processes. Only the establishment of a sense of community or covenant will allay a patient's fears of abandonment, extinction, loss of self-esteem, loss of modesty, victimization. The physician or other caregiver thereby embodies someone who cares—an ultimate reality that brings hope, healing, salvation. A caregiver becomes a "curer of souls."

In summary, the "circle of the spirit" emphasizes the continuity of the self and the interrelationship among the three subdivisions. "Curing of the soul," reintegration of self, and restoration of health take place at the mental and spiritual levels when a caring covenant is established between patients and physicians or other caregivers who mirror reality and educate patients regarding options and probable outcomes. The covenant promises the voluntary establishment of an ethical obligation on the basis of and in response to transcendent powers beyond the control of individuals or society. The covenant provides a framework within which healing can occur. Thus it is that caregivers mediate healing.

REFERENCES

Anglund, J.W. (1983). *The circle of the spirit*. New York: Random House.

Bettmann, O.L. (1956). *A pictorial history of medicine*. Springfield, IL: Charles C. Thomas.

Glymour, C., Stalker, D. (1983). Engineers, cranks, physicians, magicians. *New England Journal of Medicine, 308*, 960-64.

Lasagna, L. (1983). The professional-patient dialogue. *Hastings Center Report, 13*, 9-11.

Marty, M.E., & Vaux, K.L. (Eds.) (1982). *Health/medicine and the faith traditions: An inquiry into religion and medicine*. Philadelphia: Fortress.

Nouwen, H.J.M. (1971). *Creative ministry*. Garden City, New York: Image.

Russell, B. (1977). *Wisdom of the west*. New York: Crescent Books.

Schaffner, K.D. (Ed.) (1981). Reductionism and holism in medicine. *Journal of Medical Philosophy, 6*, 93-235.

Sodel, D.S. (Ed.) (1979). *Ways of health: holistic approaches to ancient and contemporary medicine*. New York: Harcourt, Brace, Jovanovich.

Anne George

THE JETTY, DECEMBER 23RD

The Gulf churns around and sometimes
over the jumbled rocks. On hands and knees
I inch the slippery surface
to the last flat boulder where I stand
cold, wet, exhilarated.
Later on I will notice the sky

is the blue of Mama's Depression dishes
and the moon is a white brush stroke.
Angry gulls argue the loss of their roost
and across the inlet a neon sign flashes
BUD AND ALLIE'S, BUD AND ALLIE'S.

But now on the jetty I shout to the sky
that the sun and I have made it another year.
I bless the water and the earth as if,
claiming kinship, I have the right.
And perhaps I do. My outstretched hand
has something to do with tides
and slow burning fires. It has everything
to do with being earthbound, mortal,
        and alive.

Liza Schafer

ON FAIRNESS

"Life is not fair"
my even-keeled mother
first said,
when I was ten
and pointing out
that Dad paid us
far less attention
than Boots-the-cat.

After that,
it became her mission
to season our chats
with the same phrase
until a day came:
she'd simply say "life"
and I'd begin to nod.
(In school we hadn't yet studied
Pavlov's dog.)

And so
we neatly got through things:
Dad's leaving,
his long-legged new wife,
and the two karat ring
he bought her
with all the money in our nest egg.
Mom had an inkling
we'd been sent down
to the bush league,
but it was *sportsmanship*
that counted.

So in 1976, neutral as Swiss,
we sold the home for a trailer,
welcoming our fate
as some backwoods kin.
(Hate, was not a word
in *our* vocabulary.)

Now, as a waitress,
Mom holds her own
at The Crows Rest.
There,
she lectures the regulars
saying "Life is not fair,"
whether they complain
of cold coffee
or uncomfortable chairs.

Ralph Hammond

TETHERED LOVE

So little time to feel warm slant of sun,
to hear sweet medley song of mockingbird,
for out beyond low edge of western sky
the darkness lingers with its final fold
of curtain wrap. In brevity of days
still left, I face the far Atlantic shelf
that cues initial light of breaking day
and learn to cope with least of light or yet
the most of ominous and darkened shroud.

In dark and light I know you're always there,
the memory never fading from the times
we sat beneath the midnight clock and shared
the tiny secrets of our tethered hearts.
And though you've gone into the lasting dark,
your voice remains a constant flow of words
that speak to me again and yet again
when grieving heart recalls the love we pledged
as nectared roses burst in fullest bloom.

Lyn Lifshin

BIRCHES TANGLE

in pines   woodsmoke
crab apple   plum
and honey suckle dis
solve in a red blurring
like sounds when you
take too much aspirin.
Tuesday, ankle deep
in leaves on the way
to my car six years
since the walnuts
turned ragged bark
when I slammed home
from Putman Valley
afraid to touch the
answering machine
for what wouldn't
be there. David's
children old enough
to have their own.
The leaves, like my
Science Project on
the Eye, scream
at me, wild light
that wouldn't stay.
Blood berries, smell
of night on yellow
birch leaves. October
like a wound some
succulents put out
to bear fruit
and be healed

Rita Dove

GRAPE SHERBET

The day? Memorial.
After the grill
Dad appears with his masterpiece—
swirled snow, gelled light.
We cheer. The recipe's
a secret and he fights
a smile, his cap turned up
so the bib resembles a duck.

That morning we galloped
through the grassed-over mounds
and named each stone
for a lost milk tooth. Each dollop
of sherbet, later,
is a miracle,
like salt on a melon that makes it sweeter.

Everyone agrees—it's wonderful!
It's just how we imagined lavender
would taste. The diabetic grandmother
stares from the porch,
a torch
of pure refusal.

We thought no one was lying
there under our feet,
we thought it
was a joke. I've been trying
to remember the taste,
but it doesn't exist.
Now I see why
you bothered,
father.

Rita Dove

ANTI-FATHER

Contrary to
tales you told us

summer nights when
the air conditioner

broke—the stars
are not far

apart. Rather
they draw

closer together
with years.

And houses
shrivel, un-lost,

and porches sag;
neighbors phone

to report cracks
in the cellar floor,

roots of the willow
coming up. Stars

speak to a child
The past

is silent....
Just between

me and you,
woman to man,

outer space is
inconceivably

intimate.

Jim Simmerman

WHATEVER IT IS

Near the end we'll travel as two old men
Leaning lightly on one another for support—
One of us gone a little milky-eyed,
The other a little deaf.

We'll pack what we need in a cheap valise,
Taking turns so it's not too heavy.
When one of us tires, we'll stop awhile
And build a fire to warm our hands.

You'll have then to describe to me
The woods' deep green, the cobalt sky.
I'll point you where the nighthawk calls
So that you see what I hear, so we know ...

Whatever it is we come to,
We'll travel toward together.
So when we're knocked apart at last
Something of each will go with the other.

Two old men hunched to the curve of the earth
And biding a little time between them—
Here is my shoulder steady for you,
Even this long since we started the journey.

B.A. St. Andrews

"RED MEDICINE: SILKO'S *CEREMONY*"

Every issue of the *New England Journal of Medicine* bombards Western medical practice and its practitioners with new techniques and theories. Oddly enough, many of these theories involve ancient beliefs, anthropological ideas, and cross-cultural practices. While practitioners try to absorb these abstract theories, they are also busy serving real and varied populations that incorporate these various beliefs.

That is, a person in the medical community coming from an Irish Catholic ethnic heritage and serving a Native American patient—or vice versa—attempts quite honestly to be aware of and considerate of another's ethnicity. We are all "ethnic"; that is the nature of the American experience. And, not surprisingly, these different ethnicities consider medicine differently. Understanding, therefore, how a culture group defines healing could, quite obviously, aid the medical team in serving a patient's needs more quickly and accurately.

But how is the already harried health professional to assess and incorporate the patient's belief system into the healing process? Who has time, even with an honest interest, to study anthropological treatises on the various "tribes" that *are* contemporary America?

Quite honestly, none of us. The answer, therefore, must be to build a strong, short, sturdy bridge between cultures; books are that bridge, as they have been since time immemorial.

For example, Leslie Marmon Silko's book, *Ceremony,* studies the combat between health and illness. In so doing, she not only introduces the Western, traditionally trained doctor to the subtleties of the Native American patient's belief system but also offers some constructive criticism of "red" and "white" medicines' attempts to heal the hero.

And, in the process of all this quiet medical commentary, she tells a gripping story of many a war veteran's quiet heroism upon returning home.

Silko's plot is simple and timeless: the hero, Tayo, returns from World War II broken in mind and spirit. He constantly weeps; he experiences continuing nausea; he cannot rest. His treatment in Western hospitals has cured nothing. Yet, as the classical hero, he must somehow return to health and, in turn, heal the rift between the Earth deity and her children who have been caught up by "the witchery" of war and drunkenness.

But healing the hero, for any ethnic group, is no easy task. American Indian philosophy simply (or not so simply) insists that every rock, tree, creature, and wind has a metaphysical as well as a physical dimension. Healing—given this profound definition of matter—is a complex and powerful notion. The essence of healing is harmony: that is, right thinking and right speaking can create wholeness, health, and goodness. Wrong thinking and wrong speaking can summon up what Amer-Indians call the "the witchery": illness, fragmentation, and evil.

Since, in Amer-Indian cosmology, everything is connected, one isolated part cannot be healed; the whole must be healed. The medical task seems, therefore, formidable to say the least. First, the mind and body of the sick person, Tayo in this case, can be cured only by simultaneously healing the spirit. Second, the drought on the reservation, caused by "the witchery," must be cured. Third, the illness of one tribal member involves the whole tribe, so the cure must be all-inclusive. As the old medicine man explains it, "I'm afraid of what will happen to all of us if you...don't get well" (Silko, 1977, p. 39).

In "red medicine," the patient must take on this obligation to heal. He must actively participate in the cure, a concept diametrically opposed to Western medicine. Tayo remembers his treatment in the white hospitals: "even while the white doctors had yelled at him—that he had to think only of himself, and not about the others, that he would never get well as long as he used words like "we" and "us"... he had known ... medicine didn't work that way, because the world didn't work that way. His sickness was only part of something larger, and his cure could be found only in something great and inclusive of everything" (Silko, 1977, p. 32).

Given the dimension of this health problem, any self-respecting healer—whether physician, shaman, or mystic—might as well ask where to begin? For all these healers, pinpointing the etiology of the disease is essential. What causes Tayo's nausea and flashbacks? Sound, practical causes satisfy the Western mind: he has survived the Bataan Death March; he has witnessed there the death of his half-brother, Rocky. But, on the metaphysical level which they do *not* understand, he has seen, in the slaughtered faces of the Japanese soldiers, the faces of his own people.

The Western doctors correctly diagnose that he's suffering from battle fatigue, malaria, and hallucinations, but that's too one-dimensional to be of much use to Tayo. While American Indian medicine is based on holistic thought and inter-connectedness, the Western diagnosis is too often stuck in the strict dualism of Cartesian thought. To diagnose, therefore, will not necessarily be to cure. This philosophical dualism, this mind/body schizophrenia, has presented a continuing problem for Western medicine.

Simply put, once the physical aspects of malaria and fatigue have been drug controlled, why do the psychological symptoms persist? If the disease is psychosomatic, how can the mind be encouraged to heal in harmony with the body? Since, in "white medicine," the body remains under the jurisdiction of the physician and the mind belongs to the psychiatrist, how can the patient find two gifted healers willing to expend equal energies and understandings on the patient's behalf?

Mild-mannered heretics in the Western medical community have been trying to heal this schizophrenia since the 1960's. They've introduced new, more gestalt methodologies like clinical bio-feedback. But these efforts are often dismissed by the traditional, Western medical community with slightly tainted terms like "pseudo-medical," "holistic," and "trendy."

Given these entrenched positions, *Ceremony* understandably takes a pretty dim view of "white medicine's" abilities to cure. When Tayo mentions returning to the psychiatric hospital, the medicine man is blunt: "In that hospital they don't bury the dead, they keep them in rooms and talk to them" (Silko, 1977, p. 129). Tayo recalls the drugs prescribed there: "Their medicine drained memory out of his thin arms and replaced it with a twilight cloud behind his eyes. It was not possible to cry on the remote and foggy mountain. If they had not dressed him and led him to the car, he would still be there, drifting along the north wall, invisible in the grey twilight" (Silko, 1977, p. 15).

The rift between "red" and "white" medicine is clear: the curative ceremonies in Native American medicine insist on memory as a personal and a cultural obligation and insist, further, upon active healing. Western medicine, conversely, too often imposes forgetfulness and encourages passivity.

That Western medicine needs to heal itself has been increasingly cited by sources other than Silko's powerful book. For example, in a Commentary offered in the widely-read *Journal of the American Medical Association*, Dr. Morgan Martin (1981, pp. 141-143) praised the "psychosocial approach" of Navajo medicine and questioned Western medicine's exclusively biomedical approach to healing, an approach which ignores cultural values and support groups for the patient. A small, invaluable corrective to this problem would involve working "with patient and family to maintain the balance of this small ecological system."

An article in the *Journal of Family Practice* also scrutinized Western medicine's tendency to keep the patient passive and dependent on drugs and physicians. Too often, according to Dr. John L. Coulehan (1980, pp. 55-61), "physicians are taught that *they* do the healing" and barely credit the body's homeostatic mechanisms. More effective healers in the Western medical community are cognizant that "all patients have certain beliefs about health and illness, and these beliefs do not come from medical textbooks."

Another idea currently bringing American-Indian medicine and the need for change in Western approaches to the front is, oddly enough, quantum physics. Quantum theory has, wittingly or unwittingly, advanced an holistic medical approach. Essentially, Heisenberg's "uncertainly principle," built on Einstein's paradox formulated in 1935, says that two particles hit, fly off, and are influenced by what happens to each despite the distance between them.

This, as Patricia Flynn (1980, p. 5) insists in *Holistic Health: The Art and Science of Care*, "puts consciousness into quantum physics" by advancing "a new notion of unbroken wholeness which denies the classical idea of analyzability of the world into separately and independently existing parts." The new scientific premise does more than undercut the sometimes simplistic "cause and effect" principle of Western thought; it also heals the mind/body duality.

All is connected, quantum theory asserts; the unseen, in turn, exists and affects everything in this "age of atoms" with a certainty it couldn't achieve during the "age of angels." So, the round world of connections that the American Indians have always celebrated is the *real* world to Western scientists, at last.

Western medicine is, in turn, finally admitting that "illness is not value-free or meaning-free" and is beginning to insist that the physician "collect data about patient's beliefs just as he or she collects other relevant data" (Coulehan, 1980, p. 58). As Jerome Frank puts it in his introduction in Ari Kiev's fascinating book, *Magic, Faith, and Healing*, the healer's role combines those of physician, magician, priest, moral arbiter, representative of the group's world view, and agent of social control. "The physician's success," Frank insists, "may often depend more on (an) ability to mobilize the patient's hopes, restore his morale, and gain his reacceptance by his group than on (the physician's) pharmacopeia."

Silko's insistence on the validity of the sophisticated curing system that is "red medicine" also echoes proclamations by famous anthropological minds like Franz Boas and Claude Levi-Strauss who have stressed the utility of "primitive" medicine. Silko's book praises native medicine's specific curative ceremonies: a "Scalp Ceremony" to put benevolently to rest the spirits of American and Japanese soldiers; herbal lore that proudly emphasizes the extensive pharmacopiae of the native healer. She offers examples, too, of medical practices as simple as the sweat lodge and fasting, as complex as the exquisite and highly symbolic medical art known as "sand painting." All of these medical means help to restore the hero.

But *Ceremony* is more than a smug treatise on the superiority of "red medicine." Silko insists that modern healing must be a cooperative venture. This book deals, therefore, with unity among all *tribes*, with oneness as the path to health and to right living in our world. To stress this idea of world healing, Silko sets the novel's final scene in a dramatic place: in the desert where the first atomic bombs were tested.

Thus the ancient healing connects with the modern age. "The witchery" is conquered *here* as the hero stops blaming the war, the whites, the liquor. The hero affirms a vision of wellness in *Ceremony* which unites him with all time and all tribes. His healing is collective and individual; it is physical and metaphysical. The drought, too, is ended; the land receives rain.

Silko's *Ceremony* is a trans-cultural handbook about human values. The world is, as the old medicine man insists, "fragile," and its health depends upon our recognition that spirit coexists with matter as a fundamental medical fact of life. Such harmony can overcome "the witchery" around and within us.

Shaman, psychiatrist, surgeon, or witch-doctor recognizes the same foe called by many names; everyone in the healing arts fights "the witchery." Perhaps everyone involved in this fight needs to combine the best of Western medicine's technology and of native medicine's holistic philosophy.

REFERENCES

Coulehan, J.L. (1980) Navajo Indian medicine: Implications for healing. *Journal of Family Practice, 10* (10), 55-61.

Flynn, P.A.R. (1980). *Holistic health: The art and science of care.* Bowie, Maryland: Robert J. Brady Company.

Kniep-Hardy, M., & Burkhardt, M.A. (1977) Nursing the Navajo. *American Journal of Nursing. 77* (1), 95-96.

Levi-Strauss, C. "The structure of myth." *Critical Essays on North American Literature*. Ed. Andrew Wiget Boston: G.K. Hall & Company, 51-56.

Martin, M. (1981). Native American medicine: Thoughts for Post Traditional healers. *Journal of American Medicine*. 245 (2), 141-143.

Porvasnik, J. (1967). Traditional Navajo medicine. *General Practitioner, 36* (4), 179-182.

Primeaux, M. (1977). Caring for the American Indian patient. *American Journal of Nursing*, 77 (1), 91-94.

Sandner, D.F. (1979). Navajo Indian medicine and medicine men. *Ways of Health: Holistic Approaches to Ancient and Contemporary Medicine*. New York: Harcourt, Brace, Jovanovich, 117-146.

Silko, L.M. (1977). *Ceremony*, New York: Viking Press.

_____(1981). *Storyteller*. New York: Seaver Books.

Evelyn Roehl

PRAYER-SONG OF REGENERATION

Like the leaves of a tree
    I shall grow back anew
Like the grass on the lawn
    I shall grow back anew
Like the blossom of a flower
    I shall grow back anew
Like mushrooms in a forest
    I shall grow back anew
Like algae in a pond
    I shall grow back anew
Like the roots of a carrot
    I shall grow back anew
Like a transplanted tomato
    I shall grow back anew
Like a patch of asparagus
    I shall grow back anew
Like the feathers of a bird
    I shall grow back anew
Like the antlers of a deer
    I shall grow back anew
Like the fins of a fish
    I shall grow back anew
Like the body of an earthworm
    I shall grow back anew
Like the skin of a snake
    I shall grow back anew
Like the arms of a starfish
    I shall grow back anew
Like organs of a sea cucumber
    I shall grow back anew
Like the waves of the tide
    I shall grow back anew
Like the waxing moon
    I shall grow back anew
Like the power of the sun
    I shall grow back anew

The hair on my head
    shall grow back anew
The skin on my body
    shall grow back anew
The nails on my fingers
    shall grow back anew
The cells in my blood
    shall grow back anew
The song in my heart
    shall grow back anew
The spirit within me
    shall grow back anew
My love of living
    shall grow back anew
My belief in the good
    shall grow back anew
My concern for the earth
    shall grow back anew
My concern for humanity
    shall grow back anew
My desire to create
    shall grow back anew
My hunger to learn
    shall grow back anew
My acceptance of change
    shall grow back anew
My willingness to change
    shall grow back anew
My respect for diversity
    shall grow back anew
My patience and kindness
    shall grow back anew
My happiness and joy
    shall grow back anew

David Ignatow

WITH THE DOOR OPEN

Something I want to communicate to you,
I keep my door open between us.
I am unable to say it,
I am happy only
with the door open between us.

Peter Cooley

THE LOOM

Unless light be applied to it like a poultice
sex will not heal in us.
It is a wound less scabrous than any.
Therefore, invisible, Vincent set down here
the landlady's daughter, then the widow, then the whore,
within this little gnome upright over a thread
and composed the man in himself he must have lost
to lust for three women in succession hopelessly.
Or did he sit his ghost inside this frame
and spin out Margot who threatened death after he fled?
Whatever, the facts wash off in this clear air,
reduced to a clean Dutch radiance
which sets all things at such rigid angles to each other
they assume the attitude of prayer.
Kneel down, little weaver, in the falling light,
your heart is a bobbin, it cannot stop
thrashing and trembling even if the shuttle stop.
The loom is a cage. Our bodies are another.
The light falls, a man and woman trade their threads in it.
The light fails and they stumble, fall in it.
They move through each other, they touch and separate.
They find themselves raveled in the expanse of a great cloth.

Nan Fry

RIDDLE

We are animal cries,
groans the body makes,
the shrill keening of grief,
pain and rage howled out,
grunts of satisfaction,
someone crooning to her young.
We're animal cries becoming
human, five daughters
of your mother tongue.

(Vowels)

CHAPTER V

Satisfaction of love
nourishes the body
and makes it receptive to the healing
processes that follow naturally.

memory

M.F.K. Fisher - "At the table"

M.F.K. Fisher

AT THE TABLE

It feels very strange to me that I have spent so many years changing truisms into banalities, although that seems to be the case. One truism that I had discovered for myself early on was that hunger for love is a form of healing. Satisfaction of love nourishes the body and makes it receptive to the healing processes that follow naturally. The three hungers of life (for food, love, and warmth and protection) are basic, and of them all, hunger comes first, for without it we cannot attain the others. Of course, I'm not the first one to figure this out, but it seems some sixty or seventy years later I have belabored the point until it has turned into a great banality. The odd thing is that it is still a truism in the best sense of the word and it always will be.

I was about five when I began to notice the difference in my family's behavior, a general easiness of the spirit that descended like a beneficent cloud around us whenever Grandmother was absent from the table. When she was there, there was always a kind of constipation of the spirit, and then when she went away on her various trips to religious conventions or the Battlecreek Sanitarium, we relaxed into a less formal pattern of behavior. I suppose this extended into other parts of our lives, but it was always plainest to me at the table.

When Grandmother was with us, the conversation was stiff and always courteous, and my younger sister Anne and I never spoke unless spoken to, and then we replied politely and correctly. When Grandmother was away, Father and Mother addressed us oftener and spoke to us as if we were people, not apart from them as children. We ate differently, too, in a slower way, and often sat at the table after dinner when Father had a free evening, and we did not have to leave to our bedrooms at 7:30.

Of course, much later we began to enter into the conversation itself, but it was fine practice to listen to our parents talk in a relaxed way about things that were not mentioned when Grandmother was there...politics of both the church and the state, and money, and even sex were touched on after dinner, and our early listening laid the foundation for good talks later when we grew up.

I began early to believe that this freedom was caused primarily by the difference in the food that was served when Grandmother was not at the table. For instance, we could eat rare steaks served on a plank as Father believed they should be. And he made blotters of the good bread for Anne and for me from the juices that ran down the runnels, carved in the plank itself, that collected in a little puddle at the base of the runnels.

The steaks were thick and rare but they were cut diagonally into thin pieces. They seemed very delicious to us because Father and Mother enjoyed them so much, in an open way that was impossible when Grandmother's stern presence was sitting always at Mother's right hand. And always with the rare steaks we ate watercress, which we gathered that afternoon from the banks of the Rio Hondo in a special place up north of the County bridge, just past the ruins where Pio Pico had lived until the adobe house crumbled.

We never ate watercress except when Grandmother was gone away, for two reasons. One was that Pico was a "dirty old Mexican," and an ignorant native who spent his last days cursing the Americanos, who had invaded his county and who had robbed him of his governorship. Grandmother heard nothing good about him and resented any interest my Father showed in this last of the governors of California. She also had mixed with this strange destestion of dark-skinned Mexicans, a fear of anything they liked to eat, and watercress that came from the land that once belonged to Pio Pico was doubly disgusting to her. Everyone knew, of course, that the Mexicans let their cows stand in the shallow waters of the Rio Hondo, which meant that they also peed and defecated into the water. All in all therefore, watercress was anathema to Grandmother and was therefore served only when she was far away.

It was magic always then to see the change in Father's and Mother's behavior at the table when Grandmother was gone. They were relaxed and easy and they slumped in their chairs as the meal progressed. Mother would lean one elbow on the table and let her hand fall toward Father, and he would lean back in his chair and smile. And if by chance my sister or I said something, they both listened to us. In other words, we were a happy family, bathed in a rare warmth around the table.

The next meal perhaps when Grandmother had returned again from Battlecreek or from one of her religious conventions, we would all sit once more without batting an eye, into the more decorous pattern of behavior she expected and therefore got from us all. Anne and I did not speak unless spoken to and we sat with our elbows close to our sides and kept our left hands in our laps unless we were cutting meat. We were well-behaved children once again, from then on and forever as needed in our long futures.

I think that I have been unfair to my Grandmother. I realize now that what I've written about her has made many people think of her as hard and severe. She was neither. She was never a stranger in our house and she taught me how to read and write, and I accepted her presence in my life as if she were a great protective tree. This went on until she died when I was twelve years old. I felt no sorrow for her leaving, but I missed her and all my life I have felt some of her self-discipline and strength when I needed it.

She taught me unconsciously one of the prime facts: hunger itself is the basis for all life. First comes hunger for food, then for love and warmth and protection, despite what one is told about hunger for love being the primary instinct. We cannot satisfy it without having some nourishment within us. Warmth and/or protection will follow, but first one must eat. This is one of the great truisms of life and it is a pity that it has become a banality.

Maggie Anderson

THE THING YOU MUST REMEMBER

The thing you must remember is how, as a child,
you worked hours in the art room, the teacher's
hands over yours, molding the little clay dog.
You must remember how nothing mattered
but the imagined dog's fur, the shape of his ears
and his paws. The gray clay felt dangerous,
your small hands were pressing what you couldn't
say with your limited words. When the dog's back
stiffened, then cracked to white shards
in the kiln, you learned how the beautiful
suffers from too much attention, how clumsy
a single vision can grow, and fragile
with trying too hard. The thing you must
remember is the art teacher's capable
hands: large, rough and grainy,
over yours, holding on.

Gloria G. Brame

THE VIDEO TAPE
For Jud Jerome

There was once great, amazing hope for me, serious hope that was like a brilliant shining star in the great night of Brooklyn; as if a miraculous hand had drawn a glittering path of light through the drab brown streets of the borough. It was effortless, it was cream, really, Edenic, like love before commitment. Somewhere above my mother's fat bloated belly a brilliant nova exploded and its magic dust entered her womb. This is how my parents acted, full of prideful anxious hope, when I was three. This is what my father told me recently.

One likes to think it happens this way: two beaming, handsome young people cooing over a lace-trimmed crib; one small, pacific cherub, easily comforted, always smiling, always dry.

Is this worth it? And picking only one year? Isn't that too facile?

The summer I was three, we went to a bungalow colony in the Catskills: HyLo's, which was short for Hyman and Lois Cohen, co-proprietors and co-agonizers. They were charged with the tasks of herding high-spirited, husbandless women through the weekday stultification of country living, and then diverting the beleaguered, exhausted men who crawled into the colony on Friday nights.

I remember the drive up to HyLo's. Leaving Brooklyn's cramped, gray vistas and claustrophobic streets, and everyone I knew far behind, excited me. I remember thinking we were already upstate when I saw the lush trees of Riverdale. As we drove along the Parkway which divided its arbors, my parents sang Yiddish songs with my sister and me.

I remember my small thighs sweatily sticking to the plastic liner of the back seat of my father's red and white '55 Chevy. I remember stopping at the Red Apple Rest for a boiled frankfurter. When we cruised by the Motel-on-the-Mountain, I wished we could stop and I could live there forever. I thought that I would be able to see everything that everyone in the world was doing from the hillside windows of that motel. I wanted to see what everyone in the world did. But my father didn't slow down.

When we reached HyLo's, a boy was waiting beside the road for newcomers. He had a tiny little hand, more like a flipper, where his elbow should have been. My mother had always warned me not to get my arm caught in the car window when I rolled it up. When I saw this boy's arm, I realized that his mother had never warned him about car windows. It shocked me.

I remember falling down a flight of stairs and busting my lip. *Here's the scar. It's part of the map of my face that some mortician will reconstruct. Here's the Street of Measles. Here's the Valley of Numerous Regrets. Get a close-up of that one.* I was climbing down a green, wooden stairway. I stared so hard at my mother, who was reading a magazine across the lawn, that I lost track of my steps. I somersaulted down the hard stairs, bomp, bomp, bomp. People shouted and ran to catch me. I watched them run as I fell toward them, women with their hands thrown up in the air and their mouths wide open, running toward me as I watched.

My father lived with us only on weekends that summer. His absence was a dark, impenetrable shadow over that first exhilarating voyage. On Fridays, I waited in a state of anguished impatience for him to drive up from the city. I was never sure that he would come back to us until he arrived. I remember when he hoisted me onto a small stage in the cantine. I sang "I'm a Little Teapot." *Every child in America probably has that memory, which may disqualify it from personal experience: it's more like institutional experience.* My father lifted me off the stage and into an embrace. This was my favorite part of the performance. Then he told me that I was the prettiest child at the colony. I didn't believe him. That's why I remember it so distinctly: it was the first time I didn't believe my father.

I learned to distrust adults that summer. I wanted to play with the older kids, but you had to be five years old to go to the colony's day camp. My mother sent me to Lois alone to ask if I could join anyway. Perhaps my mother thought that if I proved adequately articulate to ask for the privilege, I would be granted the privilege. But Lois explained I was too young and, instead, gave me a bag of potato chips and sent me away. I remember thinking, "You think you can buy me off with these chips. You think because I'm little I don't understand, and that I'll eat the chips and forget what I really want." But I ate the chips anyway, and they were very good.

There was one adult I liked. He used to visit the bungalow colony; he was someone's brother-in-law or cousin. He always laughed when he saw me and picked me up over his head. I waited for him eagerly as his own relatives did. I loved when he picked me up. His hands were big. He never wore a shirt, and he had a tremendously hairy chest. I liked the forests of curls and the gold medallion that glittered on the black background as he swung me toward the sky.

But many things worried me. One night, my mother emerged from the bedroom dressed in my father's clothes. She had painted a mustache above her lips and wore an old hat. A few minutes later my father appeared, a baby bonnet on his head and one of my bottles stuck in his mouth. My sister giggled and pretended to be my mother's wife and called my mother Alfred. My father, the real Alfred, climbed into a baby carriage and curled up his legs. My mother pushed him around the cottage like an infant. He even cried a little, in husky meows. I couldn't fathom what they were all up to. I didn't like to see my father cry. I cried. Years later, I found out that they took first prize in the masquerade contest.

I also remember escaping from bed in the middle of a night-terror and searching desperately for my mother. I was all alone in the bungalow. I fled down the treacherous long stairs, half-blind with panic. Crowds of women were seated at narrow tables. Bright bulbs hung from a tree. Shapes were submerged into one large blur of noise and light. When I found my mother, she didn't seem to mind that I was out of bed. She was winning at Bingo. I sat next to her, shivering in the chill. I listened to the women chattering, their tan and freckled faces like lanterns in the night. Every so often, a high-pitched "Bingo" would ring out amid the cicadas' and crickets' calls. I loved the sound "Bingo." It soothed me and I fell asleep, my mother's warm arm beneath my cold cheek.

Another time, my uncle and his wife visited. There were six of us in the two-room bungalow. My mother and aunt claimed the double bed in the bedroom. My sister and I slept on cots and the men slept on the floor in the main room. I remember waking up and going to the bathroom, hopping carefully over the men's bodies. I stopped to stare into my uncle's gaping mouth and watched the saliva tremble on his tongue; then I examined my sister's motionless hand, which lifelessly hung over the edge of the mattress. She looked as if a giant had thrown her there. The sleepers seemed paralyzed, perhaps even dead. I squatted over my father and leaned my face close to his to make sure that he was breathing. He opened one eye and said, "Are you crazy. Get back to bed on the double."

I didn't understand what "on the double" meant, but I always ran when my father said it and that seemed to satisfy him.

Is that enough? The rest is a book whose pages are glued. I had to dress it up a little to get this far. Stop the camera a minute. It's not that I'm embarrassed about my life. Actually, I'm one of the lucky ones: I can recall my childhood without too much pain. Isn't that why you picked me? I have some happy memories of my parents, some warm memories. But there's something very unnerving about this exercise: it turns my life into a script. At the end, you have to ask yourself: "what happened to that child, what has become of her life?" It raises personal questions that I'm not sure I want answered. Here I am, and what am I? Don't I have better things to do with my time than excavate my childhood for your inquiry? It's as if this script which begins with a few modest answers is doomed to end with a long list of terrible questions.

You can turn the camera on again.

I remember one other thing that happened that year. It occurred a few months after our return from HyLo's. I was lying on my back in my bed at home; it was the middle of the night; the light was so dim that I couldn't see the walls. A strange man stood next to me, looking at his watch, and a woman in a white hat held my hand. Two long tubes, attached to plastic bags, were plugged into small holes in my thighs.

My parents were in the doorway. My mother's face was drawn. My father's face was in shadow. It was dark in the room, darker than any room I've ever seen since. The adults seemed to be standing at the end of a long tunnel. I didn't think they could hear me if I called to them. It didn't matter, because I didn't feel like calling to them anyway. I was feeling calm and curious about this adventure in new territory, this ride along a new highway. I was not afraid of it.

When I think back to that year., my horror at the sight of the malformed boy at the colony seems to have lasted an eternity. I still feel uneasy about car windows, though I know now about Belladonna and what happened to some children my age. But my near-fatal illness in Brooklyn passed quickly, in a dream. I had no idea what was going on, and I have no memory of pain, but my mother's anxious face is an icon that still floats above the scene. It is her fear which lives in my psychology, not my own. I understood that no one could help me, but it didn't matter to me then, and I didn't feel betrayed. I was exploring a new place all alone. It was okay.

Claudia Smith Brinson

I KNOW WHAT I KNOW

I tell them when they ask, and they always do, that I know what I know. I shrug, and I say, "I just know what I know." How can I explain it? Granted, some folks try. They talk about visions or trances or voices of past dear ones from the great beyond or spiritual tour guides or memories of many lives. They take pride in the cards falling as they may or the sticks or the stones, even the power of a book to open to a certain page. Well, not me, which is not to say others don't see things or hear things or find the truth in the random. To each her own, I say. If I can't believe in another's gifts, why should I expect anyone to believe in mine?

So, yes, I can tell you things about yourself nobody knows but you. Or maybe even you don't know or don't dare admit. I can tell you about the shooting. But don't jump so. Secrets are never healthy, although, heaven knows, we all have our share festering and itching inside.The absolute truth is I just look at somebody and I know. That's spooky; I understand that. People would rather believe the magic is in the cards, and they must touch them and shuffle them and cut the deck before knowledge is available. People would rather believe they must hold out their hands, with the lines secretly shifting and swirling into new positions and new fates when no one is looking, and the future passes from their hand into my hand into my brain into my mouth and back to them.

Let me tell you a story about gifts. Fairies reward a man's good deed with an ale cask that is never empty. For years, for generations, the family is supplied with a fine brew from this cask. But how does it work? No one knows, past the answer "magic." Finally, a curious servant removes the cork and peers within. There is nothing to be seen but cobwebs, and when next a glass is put below the spigot, all discover the ale has ceased to flow. The gift, once examined, runs dry.

But you're not here for tales about the danger of examining gifts. No doubt you've run away from your own share of gifted folks, sometimes called artists, sometimes called lunatics, sometimes called witches, sometimes saints. And I'm not here to tell you about the danger of self-consciousness, the loss of magic promised by too many whys. But I do want you to understand that when I say I simply "see" the past, the present, and the future a fog about your body, when that sounds like so much hocus-pocus to you, who must ask, "What does she mean, 'see'? Picture? How does she see? X-ray?" I cannot, will not explain. Just take it as fact that we are all a passel of possibilities, an atomic potion of potentials given surprising spins by great-great-grandma's tale of a lost love, great-grandpa's bad temper, and your blue eyes.

It's those blue eyes that made me look closer, such a blue, like a peacock feather. People used to stop your mother and make a fuss about them trying to name that color. And your older brother—he was always a bit jealous, yes?—would stomp his feet and scowl, and your mother would feel guilty because she believed children should be loved equally, and she would buy him some little present to make up for his brown hair and brown eyes and the grumpy lines beginning between his brows. Ah, but he grew up fine. He's not why you're here.

It's odd how people turn up. A few I invite, like you. I glanced up, after I finished stamping your books—I've gotten in the habit of not really looking at many people, too much information, too much sorrow, too many questions awhirling—and I had to step back to dodge the power of your need. This town is not so small that everyone knows everyone else's business, but a peculiar gift like this, of course it gets around, so people whisper to me as I'm pushing a cart of books through the stacks, they call late at night, they stop me on the street and coax me into a doorway, they're standing in the path of the lawnmower when I pause to wipe the sweat out of my eyes. The funny thing to me is they're almost always embarrassed. They don't want to believe, but then again, they need to know.

So they come; they sit awkward, tense in these rickety chairs. They pick at the scars on this old table, tracing the lines with their fingers so they won't seem scared, just shy. And we talk. Mostly me at first, I've got to be honest and say, until their curiosity is stronger than their fear.

There are many roads to truth. I hold respect for churchgoers, the Baptist, the Buddhist, the Catholic. I hold respect for doctors, the root doctor, the oncologist, the psychologist. This is simply another healing profession, and that's what I saw begging in your eyes, your blue eyes dulled and darkened by this secret. If I could have chosen my gift, if a basket of such oddities as this had been presented me, I would have reached in for healing hands. How much quicker and more satisfying it must be to put hands on pain and soak it up, staunch the pain with the warmth of skin. A physical gift, that's what I would choose. Not this complication of thought and sight and speech, of looking behind and beyond, of naming and labeling.

There is another story I want to tell you about how we spend our gifts. You must carry this one home with you. A poor farmer begs the North Wind, who has destroyed his crops, for help. He is given a box which, when opened, will provide him with whatever food he orders. But after feeding his family, he loses the box to another. He visits the North Wind again and is given a second box with the warning he must not open it unless famished. Otherwise what is inside will not obey him. He opens the box when merely hungry; out jumps a man who clubs the farmer stiff and bruised. At home, he opens the box for his curious wife and children and out jump two men with clubs. In our hunger how we fail our gifts!

Just so was my home harmed by my own gift. As my young husband told me, "A man can hear 'I know' only so many times before he wants to commit murder." For I had taken to honesty with him. He would come home with a smile on his face, his announcement swimming about him, and say, "I got promoted today," and I would say, "I know." I could taste and see his lunch in his hello kiss each evening; I could smell the nights of naked embraces to come the morning before. So, of course, when lunch included the long-nosed brunette teller at our town's one bank where he was an up-and-comer, I could see her shadow draped all over him as he walked in the door.

And when he said, "I have something to tell you," I was so young and I said, "I know." I was a child then and untried. We look back and regret; we look forward and fear.

Sit here in this moment and listen. You are not guilty. Hold that to you. But let's talk of the simple first. It is the proper order: first, the proof in the details, the establishment of trust through the transmission of all I should not know. Then we will deal with the difficult and terrifying, which most often is the past. The present doesn't really exist. It leaves us so quickly, becoming the past before the sneeze is done. Most people come, they think, with questions about the future: Will I marry? How many children will I bear? Will I get the promotion? Will my mother get well? But I want you to understand that it is the past that deserves most of our questions. It is the past—or how we remember it, I should say—that ascertains the future. Take your fondness for quilts, am I right? The only kind of blanket you would sleep under, a child who would never think of picking at a stitch or spilling grape juice on the pie shapes of Dresden Plate. What if it had not slipped to the floor?

Or to get a little more particular, take that scar under your shirt. Yes, excuse me, scars. Brave child, you crept into the closet and found the belt afterward. In that murky crowded light you studied the buckle for spots of your blood. You dreamed of taking it to school and saying to your teacher, "See? See this. My skin, my blood." And she would save you, the beautiful Mrs. Green. Instead, you took it into the woods, and with a kitchen knife, you hacked it up. It took you days and days to carve that heavy leather into shreds.

But now we're to your story, aren't we? You must put your hands on the table, there, palms up. I want to hold your hands, to touch you because it helps me see true. Now, listen carefully, because this is what happened. I know over the years you've told yourself the story worse and better, trying so hard different ways to see it. Let those blue eyes cry, baby, but keep holding my hands. Just let those tears spill. This old pine table will soak up the acid of that time.

He was a bad man. Know that. Say it after me. Yes, he was your daddy, and you loved him. And yes, he was a bad man, and you hated him. But most of all you were scared of him. You were scared he would kill your mama. You would lie in bed and promise yourself that he couldn't really hurt you, and one day you would be big and make him sorry, and one day you would take your mama away to a beautiful house with servants and silence and the scent of roses.

Listen close now. This is how it happened. It was late; he was shouting; he sounded drunk. You were already awake, cold without the quilt, which had fallen to the floor. You heard the thud that meant he probably had knocked your mama down. Your brother woke up, too, but he pulled the pillow over his head. You crept out of your bed, and down the hall, and peeked into that little front room with the TV and the card table. And against the back wall stood your daddy, his shadow thrown up behind him like some giant monster by the lamp he'd knocked to the floor. By the door, so close you could have touched her, knelt your mama, and she was whispering to him, not like she usually did, though. These were angry words. "I hate you. You animal. You pig. You lowdown failure of a human being." And he began coming toward her, stumbling, and you saw the beer bottle in his hand, and you knew he would hit her with that or the lamp or anything else.

That was when you remembered the shoe box you'd found at the back of the closet the time you stole the belt. You had opened the shoe box and seen the heavy black gun. You weren't surprised. He had shot cans off the back fence before. He had said all men can shoot guns; he had said he would teach you to shoot when you were bigger, and now you thought, "Yeah, shoot you. You pig. You lowdown man." And you ran down the hall, not even worried about being heard, and you got the gun, and you came back, and as you stood in the doorway he smashed the bottle against the floor to break the bottom, to cut your mama with those brown ugly edges.

He didn't see you, child. All he saw was his anger and the blackness of himself. Your mama knew you were there, though, and she stood, and she reached for that gun as smooth as could be, as if she knew without looking that you'd been there, gone, and returned, as if she'd sent you, and knew just how low to reach to take it out of your hand. And without ever turning to you, child, without ever saying your name, she shot him. And he fell, and he bled, and he died.

Listen to me. It was the next step. The next step if there were to be life for you, your brother, for her. You did not shoot that gun. You didn't even know if it was loaded. Remember that? All you knew was it looked scary; it would make him stop. She made the decision to shoot that man, and the police and coroner made the decision she had the right to end the terror. Oh, it was a terrible thing for a child to see, but most of all, it was a terrible thing for a child to keep secret. Your brother who did not know, your mother who lied, you were alone.

Remember, now. She carried you back to bed. She told you to be quiet. To shut your eyes and your mouth unless the police shook you and walked you about and told you to talk, and then she told you that you would not talk, you would cry and cry. You would blubber and wail, but you would know nothing. And that is where your pain sits in those blue eyes. No one to talk to; no one to tell. She meant well. She was in the habit of protection and lies. But you hate it that your secret role carries more hurt than his death.

You are not alone now. My gift allowed me to see your secret. I know. That is my gift to you, which will not harm you, will not run dry. You are no longer alone. Say it back to me. Say it out loud and feel yourself lift with lightness. Tell me the story while I watch your blue eyes wash clean. For the nature of a gift is movement. Whatever we are given, we must give away.

Janet Burroway

HOMESICK

In this memory I seem very young and small, but it is crucial that I was able to write a letter, so I will put it at the summer between first and second grades.

I had been left to spend a week with my grandparents in Wilcox. At Gamie's house—it was never spoken of as my grandfather's, Gakie's; I suppose the bank was his place and the home hers—as in California, things were in sharper focus than at home, and in sharper color: the huge black and white squares of the checkerboard kitchen floor, the drawer filled with shining, miniature but real, pots and pans; Weedy the golden Pekingese who spent his waking hours padding across the checkerboard after my grandmother. The grass in the ample backyard was of some vivid apple green that we could not achieve in Phoenix. A black china cat slept on the hearth and a glass-fronted cupboard displayed a whole set of *black* dishes! The ceilings of the bedrooms were plastered in ochre over blue, and the blue shapes could be read as clouds can be, but they did not change, and became familiar: the hatted lady, the pig, the coolie hat. Over my iron bedstead in the guest room Gramma Pierce, Gamie's mother, stared stern and life-sized out of an oval frame, over the window seat and out the window, into the garden at the weeping willow—and I never hear the expression "piercing gaze" without remembering this private etymology.

Every day I walked the half-dozen blocks to the Valley National Bank where my grandfather was manager (it was my first experience of that heady female pleasure, Prestige by Association), and Gakie gave me a shiny dime, which I was then allowed to take to the Vandercamp Emporium and spend at once. Fifteen cents a week was my standard allowance; a dime a day was wealth. No one told me to save a part of it or to spend it wisely. I could buy a little frame, a book of paper dolls, a ball and jacks—anything! Back at Gamie's house I could go next door to the vacant lot and dance on a slab of concrete unaccountably laid as if for my private stage. Or I could poke into the old tool shed, sniff in the musty smell that I never otherwise encountered in my childhood, Arizona being so dry. As I recount this it seems to me a memory of longer ago than the 1940s, and I realize that part of the magic of Gamie's house was that even then, compared to the flat harsh light of home and its boxy houses, Wilcox had the feel of more graceful "olden times."

I loved the place. But one afternoon when I had been there for several days, I was standing at the window seat in "my" bedroom sifting through a box of old Christmas cards. I looked up from the cards, out the window like Gramma Pierce, at the gently tossing ribbons of green willow—and I was struck a blow in the stomach of physical and yet not-physical pain. It was at once empty and lead-heavy, as if emptiness had been made lead-heavy in me. I had never felt anything like it and I could not take in the force of it. I gaped out the window, astonished, immobilized. I stood for a moment trying to breathe, and when I caught my breath I began to cry—not merely from the eyes or nose, but with desperate expulsions as if I could send the thing away, extrude it from my stomach with my breath.

Gamie came to me. "What is it, Dolly?"

I said, gasping astonishment, "I don't *know* ..."

She put her arms around me. "Oh, Dolly, you're homesick."

I believe that my need for words, my anxious and largely misplaced trust in definition, stems from that moment. The pain still choked me but its name had put it in the world. My grandmother knew what it was. It had been before.

My memory does a "cut" to here, to the fold-down writing desk beside the bed. "Dear Mom," I wrote, "I am ..." I asked Gamie to spell the word and I painstakingly wrote it out."... *homesick.*" I was impressed at the length of it. It still sounded alien to my ears. My letters were blurry with tears, and now that I knew the pain was connected with the thought of home, the thought of home brought on the pain. But I knew what it was called and I could write it down. I could define myself by it. I was homesick. It was a mortally grown-up thing to be.

Let me not distort the meaning of this memory to me. The void is very large and the pride is scarcely a pebble. When I have lost a mother, child, marriage, lover, home—"homesick" is how I feel it. When I hurt, it is with that pain I hurt, and thousands of words must be thrown into the void before it begins to contract around them. I have been able to understand the concept of "black hole" only in emotional terms. But if my particular sort of pain took its form in that moment, so did the puny power to face it off.

Angie Estes

POEM IN WINTER

I wanted to remember you the way spring
remembers the dead, the way birds remember
the nests they lived in last winter
while the blue lips of the hyacinth
notched their grip in the dirt.

So I came back to these woods where everything
looks the same, only whiter. How quiet
now that May is done
shouting orders.

In the bluest hour of the night, when the stars finally
lock in their icy sockets and these lids slip
quietly down, over my own
bald moons.

I remember only this:
the narcissus positioning themselves below.
Nothing else imagines the earth with slits
and then makes good on its promise.

Joseph Harris

AT THE WALL

All over America
People come here
And talk to stone.

At the black
granite wall
of war, they
conjure up
the dead to pay
debts and allegiances.

It is the place of
unfinished business,
where the quick
and the dead
barter with silence
and flowers.

In this limbo
between corruption
and incorruptible,
bargains are struck
and vows renewed
with absolution bread.

Guilts are shriven,
expiation is done
here at the wall
of flesh and stone.
World without end.
World without end.

R. David Dahl

A FABLE

There was a man who so hated the world
he was changed into a pig.
In grief and fear he ran
to the medicine-man for help.
The shaman gave him a small drum
and told him to play it until he could
summon a god.

Late at night you can hear that drum
in the suburban or big city distance.
He plays it when the children are in bed
and his wife sleeps with valium.
He plays it until he forgets who he is,
when the hole inside of him yawns.

Only when the god of love comes dancing for him
will he remember who he was before
he changed into a pig.

Mary Sue Koeppel

INSIDE THE SIGN

"Guests permitted
only with permission
of family or doctor."

We are family
and the nurses
buzz us in.

We hear women
yelping in their baths—
the water too hot,
too cold, too lukewarm—
they can't remember
how they wanted
water.

Philip rolls by,
wants to know if
he will ever eat again.
His full lunch tray
sits in his lap.
Janet flips
her birthday cards
over and over and over and
begs the nurse to read
again verses and names.
"Who?"
she asks of each name.

We watch our mother.
"Who are we?"
"Where is she?"
If we can say it right—
one afternoon in November,
or maybe the brown carnation
from December
stirs memories.
We hear her whisper,
"Hello girls."

Barbara Unger

Journey

coming back
from that world
stupid as a sock

I find daisy sheets
smooth
phone wire
limp as a doodle.

no nightmares,
only dreams of flight
trains
busses
planes
journeys beyond sleep.

by morning
Dr. Sanity is tying
my shoelaces
reminding me
not to breathe
names of old lovers,
college romeos
Italian lakes
in the middle
of a desert riddled
with tanks, artillery.

Dr. Sanity opens
venetian blinds,
threatens not to carry out
bedpans, take down diapers.

Rumplestiltskin is
stoned tonight, cannot find
his way home.

Dr. Sanity is our master.
He keeps us cute,

cuddly little girls
never fully ripe.

I study
combination locks,
blueprints of the catacombs
hidden in my shoe.

Diane Wakoski

JUNK JEWELRY

My husband buys me pearls,
the kind I like—freshwater, with their appearance
of gnarling and twisted nacre, but though
my horoscope always says I will love jewels, I
rarely deck myself with these pearls,
and I regularly over the years have lost at least one
and usually and finally the second one of any pair of expensive gold
earrings he buys for me. He knows
I want a wedding ring,
but it is the one jewel he never will
offer. A golden heart necklace for a recent anniversary,
and the next year, a diamond for it. At Christmas, a subdued
and magical pair of antique amber drops to go with
my lucky amber tear necklace on an expensive gold chain he gave me
the year before. He agrees that
a band of emeralds would be nice on my wedding finger,
or a thin line of diamonds, but we both know
that either would cost thousands and we haven't the price.
Still, I would be happy with a plain gold band
handmade by some local jeweler which might only cost
a few hundred dollars, not much more than my longest string
of pearls.

I ask myself many questions
about my many failures,
but one I never ask is why I fail to inspire
Steel Man to buy me a wedding ring.
I couldn't ask this question
because I think I know the answer.
It is no secret
like immortality, or who
will win the lottery. It is simple.
He buys me what no one else has ever
given me, and I had two marriages before this one
both with rings that still glitter with evil memories. Why
should he remind me of the failures of rings.

Our bond is ringless.
Nothing can break it.

Judson Jerome

LIKING WHAT YOU DO

Granted, the circumstances depicted by the containing legend of **Job** are more cataclysmic than most of us ever experience, but the most ordinary households at times experience calamities that might make anyone of a theistic inclination wonder Whose rules governed their lives. A young couple I know were advised that the wife could not bear a second child. They applied for an adoption, and after a three-year wait were told that a baby was waiting for them—premature, six weeks old, weighing five-and-a-half pounds. They were so eager to have the child they went to pick it up sight-unseen. Immediately husband, wife, and first child came down with flu—so serious that the wife had to be hospitalized with respiratory and other complications— just when she wanted to be at home with the new baby. Days later, when she was well enough to come home, the baby got sicker and had to be hospitalized. The doctors are, as I write, making innumerable tests on the infant, whose father is unknown, and one cringes to think they may suspect AIDS. Does one pray under these circumstances? If so, how can one respect the God one prays to?

I mentioned at the beginning that it was the suicide of a friend (along with the appearance of Stephen Mitchell's new translation) that moved me to take up again a long-neglected project—writing a "Job" companion for "Jonah." The parents of the adopted infant I mentioned are not in despair, but the woman who committed suicide was chronically so—with no discernible objective reason. Suffering can become a habit. The term *depression* is most often applied to those who suffer without apparent cause. Those subjected to genuine tragedy are likely to cling to life desperately—to affirm even in the depths of calamity.

Job of the legend had a simple-minded, covenantal conception of God. If I am loyal and obey His laws, he believed, He is obliged to protect me. Many of us grow up with such a puerile view of life, and most of us are sooner or later taken from it by a recognition that Nature has no obligations. We figure out how to cope with life on these new terms. Job is unable to cope throughout most of the poem, and, as I have discussed, the ending is ambiguous. The legend depicts a restoration of the convenantal relationship with God, but a more sophisticated reading sees him as liberated by this confrontation with Nature to a realm of free choice, and a love not so much of God as of life. That seems to me to be mental health—apparently unattainable by those who are chronically depressed. One explanation may be that though they have abandoned— or even never experienced—a theistic view of life, they retain some childlike expectation of justice from the universe.

I have pondered long how affirmation of life could be revived in those who seem no longer capable of it—and I reflected on my own rare bouts of despair. I can remember the moment I made my first important discovery about the matter. I was 55, warming my derriere against the space-heater in our log-cabin in the Alleghenies, and realized that for some days I had been depressed. There was no particular reason for it. Our lives were busy and fulfilling. I had achieved as much as I could reasonably expect to, and there was no prospect that the future held any less for me than continued achievement. We were as materially secure as we could expect to be—considering I had "dropped out" from Academia ten years before to start the rural commune where we were living. Secure enough, I told myself, reviewing all this . . . I was in good health. My sex life was good. Our kids, all grown and on their own, were doing well and loved us dearly.

Why, then, depression? I knew that depression was a disease that sometimes afflicts people, especially as they get older, for no known reason. There are drugs to deal with it. Did I need drugs? Suddenly I straightened my shoulders and left the cocoon of the stove, put on my coat and gloves to go out and put chains on the tires so I could make it up our icy, steep drive and leave our mountain haven for a trip to town for groceries. Depression sucks! I had decided.

Well, actually, it wasn't all that simple. Putting on chains, for example, wasn't that simple. I had cataracts, one of them seriously "ripe," and my depth perception was poor. Lying in the snow under the car, trying to get the blamed hook in the blamed eye and slide the lock into place took minutes—and I could work on it only seconds at a time with my gloves off (poor circulation—a life of smoking). When I finally made it the half mile up to the road, got the chains off again, and drove to town, sloshed in my boots through the slush into several stores to complete my errands, I saw the sign of the realtor and instantly knew that I would never spend another winter at Downhill Farm. I went in to list our property for sale.

That spring I had my ripe cataract replaced with a plastic lens—and, to my amazement, could read the writing on the TV screen in the living room from my office in the loft. By fall we were back in "civilization," the little village of Yellow Springs, Ohio, where I had taught for twenty years at Antioch College before the social and academic upheavals of the Vietnam era drove me into premature "retirement" in 1972. But since that day at the stove I have successfully resisted depression.

In myself, that is. But I seem to spend a lot of energy coping with the depression of others. I was only twenty-five when I started teaching at Antioch, the youngest member of the faculty, and so colleagues and friends in Yellow Springs who remained there after we left for our communal sojourn are mostly older than my wife Marty and I are. They are mostly retired, while, having given up all retirement benefits, we are still busily occupied. I am a freelance writer and editor, and Marty has a small craft business, so our days are full. Part of what fills them, though, is not our work, which we love, but dealing with our depressed friends.

Recently Mary found one of them, Jeannette, dead in her home, having successfully committed suicide. Her husband had died the year before, and that might, on the face of it, seem sufficient reason for depression, but her response to her husband's death was not grief but primarily anger—for his having left her. It was one of those paradoxical marriages of continually bickering upon which the couple become dependent. They were miserable in one another's company, and were most content when they ignored one another, but, of course, she had gotten used to it and though she knew that in a sense she was better off without him—psychologically—she also felt a pointlessness and purposelessness in her life that she had not felt before. We and her other friends (she had many) did what we could to cheer her up, distract her (she went with Marty and me on a tour of China), help her find a new direction, but nothing was working. She had recently returned from a mental hospital, where she had checked herself in because she was feeling suicidal. Again. She had attempted suicide a month before, was rescued and taken to the hospital, endured shock therapy, and was more-or-less under our care after she was released, staying in our guest room until she felt she was strong enough to return to her own home. That lasted a few days. She went back into the hospital for another series of shock treatments. After a couple of weeks of that she returned home, but it was apparent that she was no better. One night, after carefully putting her affairs in order and leaving a loving note for her son, she apparently took every pill in the house. When we could not reach her by phone the next morning we knew what must have happened.

Marty and I were discussing Jeannette's situation before she died with a friend of hers and ours. Henry was repairing our electric stove. A retired engineer, he busies himself doing the odd jobs his friends can't handle. He works for an absurdly low hourly rate because the amount he can earn in a year without losing tax benefits is limited, and he wants to be occupied with work he loves. The stove was pulled out into the room. Behind it squatted Henry—happy as a clam testing wires and switches with his voltmeter, his hands black with the stove's accumulated grease. We thought Jeannette needed an occupation. A tax accountant, she had as much work as she wanted, but she couldn't keep her mind on her work when she was depressed. She did some volunteer work. She had many friends, and a good relationship with her married son, who lives in a distant city, and with his wife and small children. But she didn't want to live with—or nearer to—his family.

Either Henry or I said, "She needs something to do," and we looked at one another in amusement. Neither of us can imagine needing something to do. "I don't have time to read!" said Henry. "After the eleven o'clock news is when I begin reading. I never get to sleep before one or two." Personally, I zonk after the news, so I envy him his couple of hours of reading each night.

And now she is gone—a brilliant woman with, apparently, everything to live for. Among the many complex emotions that flood her friends and family is a large measure of relief. Dealing with Jeannette was depressing. Increasingly, as the year since her husband's death wore on (her suicide was just a few short days short of the anniversary of that event), distance grew between Jeannette and her friends. There was nothing one could do. The main topic of conversation with her was her depression. It was an obsessive topic—like the conversations between Job and his comforters. And, in the last weeks, when all became aware of her unsuccessful suicide attempt, and all saw how little positive effect shock therapy was having, there was a growing recognition of the inevitability of suicide. "She has a right to check out when she pleases," I told her distant son on the telephone. That was a fact all acknowledged, and none could live with comfortably. For days after she made her choice, and the word traveled the telephone network through our little village and to her family and friends in other places, the conversations were guarded, muted. Grief wasn't a warranted response. Nor was elation. Uneasy acceptance. Relief.

Our friends fall into two categories that seem never to overlap: depressed or not depressed. And it is difficult to see the reasons for the difference. The depressed ones talk about being bored. I can't remember ever being bored. The closest I have come to that state was one marvelous afternoon when I was in my thirties. The eye doctor had dilated my eyes to examine my enlarging cataracts, and for a half hour I was free and could not read. When one is free, one reads. What else can one do? I decided to take a stroll through our little town, and it was as though I had stumbled into a Wonderland. It seemed as though for years I had looked at nothing larger than print. People's faces! Signs! Cars! I had a banana split at the drugstore and listened to conversations around me. I was a bit sorry—though not depressed—when my half-hour was up, and I had to go back for my examination.

In between other writing projects I am working these days on a sex manual. It may never see the light of publication because it is in iambic pentameter, but it is unlike any sex manual I have seen in other ways as well. It is really about love. Our fortieth anniversary caused me to give the matter of love a lot of thought. This isn't changing the subject, by the way, because if there is a common thread in the stories of our friends who are depressed it is that they have no love—and sex—in their lives. Recently a psychologist spoke at the local Unitarian church on "Depression and Aging." She said one of her clients in her eighties told her she was worried about her husband of the same age. "He wants sex only about three times a week," she said. "I think he may be depressed." The psychologist talked to the husband. His wife was right.

In my sex manual I say, "Important learning always is conversion." (Iambic pentameter, see?) It comes suddenly. You kick the habit of depression—the only way I know of that any habit is ever broken. Suddenly, as though turning a corner into a new world, you see life differently. I remember the first Shirley Temple movie to use technicolor. It was all in black and white until the final minutes when Shirley went up to Heaven to visit her little brother who had died. There, before eyes accustomed to seeing only black and white on the screen, suddenly spread the miracle of the rainbow. In just such fashion does one overcome depression.

I am speaking of dramatically contrasting views of life. One, labeled Johanine by theologians (after John, the author of five books of the New Testament) is apocalyptic, one might say orgasmic. ("Orgasm is surrender, not a victory." More pentameter.) Belief comes suddenly. Change is instantaneous, transforming, total—as when one is born again. Such salvation is what Frost called an abruption. One sees the light. One falls in love. The other view (Pauline, after St. Paul) is more historical. There are no revelations. One arrives at truth or understanding through a slow process of accumulation of evidence, reasoning, experience. Depression is an affliction of those with this second view. Both Jonah and Job are of this stripe.

I have a friend in his eighties, Dave, who is rather definitive of this view of life. A retired librarian, Dave told me he is a member of the Hemlock Club—a group supporting suicide. After Sam (another friend) and I had a particularly depressing dinner with Dave at a restaurant, Sam and I walked him home, and then walked on together. Sam mused, "Isn't it too bad that the library, Western Civilization, and Dave's life are all coming to an end at the same time!"

His depression seemed terminal until he had cataract surgery. Suddenly he could read fine print again and, even more miraculously, see colors vividly. His mood picked up for weeks, but then slipped back into the habit of seeing life for what it is if you look at nothing but facts and logic—hopeless. This lasted until he fell in love a couple of years later. Now he and his girl friend (in her 70s) seems to have found a cure for depression.

One humors friends like Dave and Jeannette, but humor gets on their nerves. One cannot give the most relevant and obvious advice: fall in love, enhance your sex life. Not only can one not say such things to friends of age, status, and dignity, but to do so would be pointless anyway. If they were capable of the contrasting views of life they would already have fallen in love and enhanced their sex lives. There were a number of attractive, intelligent older women who were interested in Dave (before he found his present girl friend), who went so far as to hint as much to him, but when we talked about that he dismissed each one derogatorily—more, I think, for fear of venturing than lack of interest.

They would already have so much to do, so much purpose, so many obligations, they wouldn't have time to read until after the evening news. Speaking of obligations, it is always those who have seen the light who tend to and take care of those who haven't. That is part of our joy and purpose. Our depressed friends worry about themselves so much they haven't much attention for the needs of others, and, indeed, those who are not depressed have fewer needs.

Love and sex, of course, are merely metaphors for love of and engagement with life. Another octogenarian friend, Robert, has never married and seems never to have had a very active sex life. Recently he had a cancer of the bowels removed and a temporary colostomy, which has now been reversed. That left him temporarily without sphincter control, so his life required constant and unpleasant attention to his toilet needs. Marty and I had a conversation with him about this and we all had a good laugh. Did his situation depress him? No. It made him furious. He had angry epithets for the medical profession, nature, age, food, diapers, and anything else he could think of related to his condition. Anger soon spilled over into humor. It was an absurd condition in an absurd world. Some people might interpret lack of sphincter control as a plague God forgot to inflict upon Job, but, though he complained bitterly, Robert wouldn't let his bowels get him down. Recovered from that, he became blind, and that put him out of sorts for a few months. But he started dictating a novel into a tape recorder. He wanted to get back to work—writing—so he was impatient with physical disability of any kind, and because he could see the humor in his situation, he was indomitable.

What makes the difference? How can a person of the second type convert to the first? Or is one simply born into one category or the other irremediably? According to Jung and many subsequent psychologists there are such things as congenital character types and individual change from one to another of such types is rare. I have talked this question over quite explicitly with the depressed friends I have mentioned. They do not disagree with me, and they do not know the answers to those questions any more than I do. They try reasoning from there to here, but reason and evidence in this matter are of no avail. They envy me and may at times resent me. I report to them simple truth: that since I turned sixty, I have written more poetry than in any time of my life (and much prose besides). I have traveled more, been busier in general, and happier than ever before. How can they endure such news? Is it cruel to tell them that? Or will the shock help them achieve conversions?

Or do they even want conversion? Depression is a self-fulfilling prophecy. One needs one's gloom to prove one's dim predictions, to validate one's frail self-esteem. The depressed people I know have many close friends—more than I have. They are much loved, and, when not depressed, more sociable than I am. They are professionally successful, financially secure, in good health. They are not drinkers—like me. Their lives are orderly—unlike my own. Though they have many scattered friends and family, they write few letters. (I am constantly writing long letters, often to people I hardly know or have never met.) They read mystery novels. Could that be it?

I don't mean to make light of their plight, but it does at times seem willful. Count your blessings, I want to say. Learn to love yourself. Reaccess your values. I remember myself as a driven professor-writer, in my thirties, obsessed by what I called "my work." I must confess than even when I got married one thought in my mind was that I wouldn't have to spend so much time on the el traveling from the north side to the south side of Chicago to spend time with Marty. I would have more time for my work. And now there I was, married a dozen years, spending most of my waking hours in my garage study, scrabbling for some dim image of "achievement," when I happened to step outside into the spring sun. The kids were playing in the yard. Marty was hanging out the laundry. Flowers were blooming.

And suddenly my life turned inside out. Somehow I had let myself believe that all this—a house, a yard, a wife, children, flowers—were supports for my work. But in that spring instant I saw that my work was for all this. Certainly the work had value in itself, certainly it was one of the things that made life worthwhile. But one does not do one thing in order to do something else. There is no way "to get ahead." There is no place to arrive. One is already there. Enjoy. Even my work, I realized, was pleasure, indulgence, done for its own sake.

"You said something in the Fifties that shocked me," an alumnus told me recently. "What was that?" I asked. "You said, 'Life is more important than art.'" I had forgotten what heresy that was in those days, along with a corollary belief: it is infinitely more important to be a good person than to be a good writer. I have to keep relearning those lessons. They come freshly to me in many forms. I went out to wash our car one sunny Saturday in March. It was the good weather that tempted me from my desk, but I soon found it was chillier than it looked, and, the job half done, I was miserable, washing with cold water from the hose, my knuckles barking on edges. "Look Jud," I stopped to say to myself, "either do what you like, or like what you do."

I went in and got a bucket of warm water. Why hadn't I thought of that before? I was rushing too much, trying to get the chore done so I could get back to work. I turned on the radio in the car and opened the doors so I could hear the symphony. I began appreciating the clean painted surfaces, the shining chrome emerging under my sponge. When the washing was finished, I dried the car lovingly. I saw that it could do with a coat of wax. I waxed it. I vacuumed the interior and polished the inside surfaces. How wonderful to have a car! How wonderful to have a *clean* car! What a lovely house—and such wonderful people living there! Look, buds are appearing on the trees and bushes!

Neither gloom nor joy is entirely a matter of will, but will can nudge them. Smile. You can do that deliberately, and if you hold the smile a while, joy often follows. You'll find more things amusing. You can deliberately recall happy moments, dear friends, family members you love. I remember waking one morning in recent years with an almost mystical sense of euphoria. No doubt I had been dreaming; I was gloriously, achingly tumid. But I could remember no dreams. My mind was blank. But I felt as though I had welled up into consciousness on some effulgent cushion of goodness. I had a physical sense that I was a good person in a good world. The experience transformed the day. I even relished brushing my teeth that morning. We can't deliberately have such experiences, but we *can* deliberately summon them to mind, and even to remember them has a transforming effect.

Richard Eberhart

THE REAL AND THE UNREAL

I was sitting in my study on June 22, the longest day of the year, looking out on garden flowers at their summer height in yellow, blue, and white. They were perfectly beautiful. I use the cliché on purpose. There was no need to invent a new term since nature was universal; this was an ordinary but impressive sight. And clichés are built on repetitions. One day later the days would become shorter by mathematical, inevitable regression. Fall would come, winter, the increase of spring, another summer with remorseless certainty.

But what of man?

He has his rise, his stay, his fall, as inevitably as that of nature. How real is the nature we see? It seemed completely real. The flowers could be seen in their full appearance.

Then I looked in my study to a day-bed. It too was real, a piece of furniture, a fine wicker piece, with mattress covered with green and a scatter of same-toned pillows.

Then I thought, what if I were not here? What if it were the year 2000? Supposedly, if the garden were tended, the flowers would look the same on another summer solstice.

When I looked on the bed I had deep feelings from memory. It was on this very bed, about which I wrote a poem entitled "The Day-Bed," that my mother suffered months-long excruciating pain from the fall of 1921 to her death from cancer of the lung (she never smoked) on June 22, 1922. On that day I was eighteen and she was forty-eight. I stayed out of college a year to help take care of her. It was probably the most profound experience of my life, one that begot my poetry, an experience of depth that was inexpressible.

I can see this bed as an object today. But it means much more. If another sat here and saw this object, he would have no other context. So what is reality? What is real? What is unreal?

What is real for me is not real for another. The day-bed seen by a casual viewer could not evoke the passions invoked in me my memory. But only by memory. I kept looking at the bed as a real object. My mother's form, face, and animation were invisible. They were not there. They could not be there. I saw her on that bed fifty-five years ago. She would now be one hundred and three. It all became absurd to total up. What would she be like at one hundred and three? My great dream of her was when she was forty-eight.

But then, what is the meaning of memory? What is the use of it? Why is it so deeply ingrained in mankind? And why is it one of the sources of poetry?

I looked out to the garden again, to the flowers at their height of one summer. I thought of the seasons of the earth, of centuries, of millennia.

I looked at the day-bed, a real thing, a piece of furniture. If it were not for the deep and stirring reality of my memories of pain and suffering and a strange joy of love when I was young, I could believe in the reality of the objective world. Then I thought, even memory is in a sense false, because what if one were thirty instead of eighteen and had a similar experience with some other being on this bed? Would one make sense out of possibilities? The facts might be similar, but the feelings would be different and could not be calculated. A young man of eighteen would not react as a man of thirty, and vice versa. What is real? What is unreal?

What we see, perhaps, is not what is true. What we see may be illusion. I always had a sense that this was true. Visible appearance is illusory. If the day-bed means more to me than an object, an example of the objective world, why, by analogy, do I assume finality or final reality in anything I see? An extension of the day-bed could be, in a sense, any historical monument, say the Parthenon, or Chartres, or the Taj Mahal, where by looking, because these are famous examples of man's work, one immediately thinks of the actual life lived in these places, the human events and situations.

Then, and one approaches this gingerly, afraid of too much logic, why is not the entire world and all life of mankind not something more than appearance? What seems substantial, insubstantial? What seems real, unreal? Why is not all life and nature not an expression of God? We live a short, allotted span on this planet. Time is mysterious, beginning and ending all the time. We can dimly sense a greatness beyond man's mind. Spinoza saw a watch in the mud. He posited a human maker. He looked at the earth, knew man could not make it, and posited God as the maker of the universe.

The facts of death and life are real, the facts of suffering and joy are real, but the whole enterprise of galaxies, the universe, is beyond us and in a sense seems unreal.

What is the meaning of my mother's suffering when I was eighteen, of my other kind of suffering with her? Is memory an enrichment given to man and, if so, why? If mankind has a collective memory, embedded in the unconscious, why should this be so? For what purpose? If we had a choice, would it be better to live in the so-called real world or in a so-called unreal world? Do we have a choice as to memory? Can one live only for the instant? Memory seems to be built into us. And from it, as part of the mystery of creation, flow poetry and music, manifold works of the imagination. If man can imagine God, God could imagine man. If man has to suffer, he also has to enjoy.

W.C. Gosnell

ANSWER

For Janet

I wish I could tell you
what all this means,
why some dreams and memories
appear without warning
out of nowhere
like a band of wandering nomads
from some white desert
of crackling bones.

I wish I could tell you
why I love your cheek
pressing against mine,
why we must grow old,
whether it is together
or apart,
why everything that is
thrown into the world by birth
must weather many hard lessons
and then fade away.

CHAPTER VI

Rituals & Remedies

"... *all cures are derived from their patients' beliefs in them.*"

Peter Wild - "Good Physicians"

Joseph Bruchac, III

THE REMEDIES

Half on the earth, half in the heart,
the remedies for all the things
which grieve us wait for those who know
the words to use to find them.

Penobscot people used to make
a medicine for cancer from Mayapple
and South American people knew
the quinine cure for malaria
a thousand years ago.

But it is not just in the roots,
the stems, the leaves,
the thousand flowers
that healing lies.
Half of it lives within the words
the healer speaks.
And when the final time has come
for one to leave this Earth
there are no cures,
for Death is only
part of Life, not a disease.
Half on the Earth, half in the heart,
the remedies for all our pains
wait for the songs of healing.

Jack Coulehan

MEDICINE STONE

This stone I picked at a medicine dance
on a cold June day near Wounded Knee.

In my bare feet, I carried this stone
into the circle of those with need.

A sun dancer danced in front of me
and touched my shoulder with a sprig of sage.

A sun dancer chanted in front of me
and blessed me with his medicine pipe.

Here in the city, the sky is brilliant.
I carry this stone in a buckskin pouch.

Here in the city, we suffer in private
and each of us stands at the circle alone.

This stone is an aspect of soul that lasts.
This stone is a remnant of no account.

Here in the hospital, coyote is dead.
This small stone is of no account.

Wolves, spiders, moles, snakes, ants are dead.
This spherical stone is of no account.

Eagles, hummingbirds, ravens, bats are dead.
This stone is a remnant of no account.

Only the voices of suffering live,
the skin, and what happens beneath the skin.

Still, I carry this buckskin pouch
and a small stone wrapped in a wad of sage.

This stone is an aspect of soul that lasts.
I call it my friend, my black stone friend.

Alice B. Fogel

PLEASE

Hold closely the red, round, sleek,
solid sphere of apple, perfect
in its vulnerability to earth and air.
Inside, seeds and flesh
lurk in secret slumber, as if waiting.
But not waiting. something could grow
out of this, something could burst it apart
from what it seems. Each seed
has a story to tell that it will never tell,
that it hasn't yet lived or learned.

The body is a globe, whole,
contained and fragile.
What it doesn't know is more immense.
You can't surprise it with predictions.
Right now something inside may be swelling,
reaching outward, working
on its own small life.
Maybe one dark seed
snaps open against your fear—
a sudden awakening into night.

You could die of knowing
or of not knowing, or—
smooth the skin against your palm,
slide your nail along its continuous curve,
its utter sheen, while your own hand
trembles and dares to go on.
Smell its apple smell of wine
and earth and bowl, get its wet envelope
everywhere in your mouth,
such a dangerous delight.

You have to let in the small wonder
of apple, you have to let please
whatever can please you, hold it
skin to skin, dearly, so the wholeness
of its life passes through yours,
healing as it breaks its way
between the walls of cells.

Nan Fry

FROM PERSEPHONE'S LETTERS TO DEMETER

1.

You've got it all wrong, Mother,
flaunting your grief,
stripping the sycamore
down to a ghost tree.
We revel in skeletons,
find the clean lines
sensuous and economical.
The dead sing us songs
I'm learning to answer.

I'm learning new words
Like *pomegranate*,
a word you can suck on:
pom—thick and round, a bittersweet
bulge, *e*—the one you slide over
to get to *gran*—a slow swelling,
cancer or the rose, it doesn't matter,
then *granate*—a stone stopping
you hard and cold.
Pomegranate—a word you spit out,
the snick of seeds
against your teeth.

2.

I remember planting, the small furrows.
and the coat of rabbit pelts
you wore. When I was small
I'd sit beside you and blow into the fur.

I remember dusk
stitching the tulips shut
and throngs of azaleas,
their white throats
open to the moon.

I remember the peach
spattered with red,
furred yellow sun,
all that juice

let loose on my tongue,
and the pit, its secret
bloody mouth at the center.

3.

I want to learn the language of return.
Re is a reel pulling me back,
The hook in the mouth,
the bud on the rose. *Turn*
is the worm biting,
smooth swell of the belly,
the detour that brings us home.

I want the ice to melt,
the slow dripping that feels like loss
and is a loosening, a letting go.
The sluggish floes will crack and heave,
the river stretch like a snake in the sun.
Then the floods of summer, the dense
green banks, the sun pumping
juice through the peach, the earth
furred with a pelt of grain.

That dance you taught us—
I'll learn its language in my body:
lift and flail to beat the grain
from the husk, remembering to save
some to return to you, remembering
that I will return here, a seed.

Joseph Harris

HERBAL

Sweet basil for the bowel,
Hyssop for the breath;
Of all medicines in leaf,
None can cancel death.

But find the virile mandrake,
And get with child a wife;
Visions of death will pass,
And Eros rise to life.

Penny Harter

DREAM TIME

*In Australia the totemic Ancestors walked across
the land leaving words and musical notes in their
footprints. The aboriginals read the country as a
musical score.*

In the Dream Time,
the ancestors went underground,
Honey-Ant here, Wallaby there,
after their magic feet
had planted song in the dust,

and by these songs, the people
learned each totem path,
singing the holy hillock, scared spring,
and burning bush of their clan;
mapping kinship where the tongue shifted
but the song continued,
humming up from the underworld
like the first rivers.

When I listen to the whales
calling deep sea currents alive,
their repeating melodies answered
across great distances;
when I hear the wolves, the birds—
all the tribes descended from the Ancestors
learning the planet by ear,
defining it by song
as the wind does each tree,
I do what I can,
throwing this song out from my house
like a rope in search of water
through the fire.

Nancy Peters Hastings

BY CANDLELIGHT

A woman with raven hair
stirs almond oil and marigold
with a wooden spoon, simmering
past magic with chemistry.
A flash flood creeps under
the glass door, power lines
fall into place as so many
hexameter I Ching sticks
yielding what might be.

Everywhere she goes she finds
her toes gripping the difficult
heat of cement, the soft
contour of canyon riddled
with rock and prickly pear.
Her feet take everything in.
Just as tonight she takes
whatever grows wild into mind,
harvests the soft parts
of a rose to heal with honey.
Tonight she makes rain
as much in her pot as this
cloud confusion troubled
by lightning, stirred by wind.

Wendy Hesford

SONG

In all our acts and words
Let us be all as one
—Pueblo Healing Song

I looked for the oceans of sugar
for the blood of the silver   cut leaf
and red maple
anything to make my life fluid
but everything had turned
to stone
to onyx   to soapstone   to bone
everything had turned
to the marrow of the earth's body.

Everything had turned
to her
to the body of my sister
to the freshly cut rudbeckia
to the body of us all
everyone turned to the gold-flecked flames
the lapis lazuli bed
the fire that kept rising
to the crystalline sky.

Still her life runs
like an unbroken flame
like wind that doesn't heed
her life comes
through the steam of tea leaves
the soft glow of honey
the syllables   the seasons
the stars
they don't ask for forgiveness
they don't ask for sympathy
they know they will become
the stones of the sky
they know they are
all as one.

433

Wilma Elizabeth McDaniel

GOOD MEDICINE IS WHATEVER CURES FOLKS

I was at Mama's heels when we entered the tiny post office of Big Muddy.

Mrs. Knolls was just ahead of us at the window. She tore open the end of an envelope and read something. She appeared to sway and grabbed onto the window ledge in front of her. The envelope fell off onto the floor.

Mama reached out and steadied her. "Are you alright, Mrs. Knolls?" "Did you receive some bad news from your family?"

Mrs. Knolls said almost mechanically, "It must be real bad news. Hattie has give up her job in Tulsa. She feels so poorly that she is coming home next Tuesday." She still held the one-page letter in her hand.

I picked up the fallen envelope and gave it to her.

It was Mama's turn to be shocked. "Why, Mrs. Knolls, I *am* surprised that Hattie would leave her fine job. I do not mean to alarm you but I agree that Hattie would not leave it for any trifling reason."

Mrs. Knolls said somberly, "I know my daughter. She wouldn't walk away from no twenty-five dollar a week job in this Great Depression unless she was bad sick with something. No, ma'am." She stepped aside and made a place for Mama at the window.

News traveled like wildfire in Big Muddy Township. By afternoon practically everyone had heard that Hattie Knolls had quit her job and was coming home. All agreed that only the gravest reason would have caused her to do so.

Hattie took a Greyhound bus from Tulsa and got off at the crossroads in front of Wilhoite's general store.

Mama and several neighbors had waited with Mrs. Knolls for Hattie's arrival. I had tagged along, school being out.

The bus was at least a half hour late. We craned our necks and scanned the state road to the east. Then someone said, "There it comes."

The driver jumped out and began to unload Hattie's luggage before she got off the bus. He brought out three large suitcases and a foot locker and several big cardboard boxes and placed them beside the loading zone.

Mrs. Knolls was standing close to Mama. I heard her saying in a low voice, "Lord, it skeers me to see all of that luggage piled up there. It sure looks to me like Hattie don't think she will ever be going back to Tulsa."

About that time Hattie came slowly down the steps of the bus. The driver helped her off on the ground.

I had not seen her for two years, not since my near Christmas birthday which we shared. She was not the same Hattie. She was so thin! Her ruddy complexion was a paste color and she walked bent forward as if to favor her right side. She embraced her mother and said "Hello" to the rest of us in a weak voice. I thought her eyes looked like what two burned holes in a blanket must resemble.

Mr. Wilhoite loaded Hattie's luggage into his old Model T and took Hattie and Mrs. Knolls to their home.

Mama and I walked across the meadow home. She was silent for a few minutes, then she confided in me, "Poor Hattie has something seriously wrong with her. She can't straighten up and her lips are parched as if she is running a temperature."

The community didn't glimpse Hattie often the first month that she was home, but Mrs. Knolls relayed day-to-day accounts of her condition, especially to my mother.

She said, "I sure am glad that Hattie came home, job or no job. She should have confided in me and come home earlier. She said when she started to get sick, she went to the best doctors. They tested and X-rayed and done everything they knowed what to do except operate on her. She said that if they didn't know what was wrong with her, she didn't aim to let them experiment on her. She told me that if she had to die, she wanted to come home and be with her own kinfolks and neighbors."

Mama asked, "Can she eat anything? She is so thin."

Mrs. Knolls said, "*If anything is ripe tomatoes,* she can eat it. She gets up in the morning with a light fever and goes out in the garden barefoot with a salt shaker. She picks two or three of the biggest, ripest tomatoes and eats them right there with juice running down her chin. That's been going on for ten days. It worries me for fear that she will thin her blood dangerous low without no meat or solid food, but she don't want nothing else."

Mama told her, "Maybe Hattie's system is telling her what it craves right now. Her appetite may return when she gets straightened out."

The twelfth day after Hattie's return, Mama went early to Mrs. Knolls' place to help her pick beans. I had to sign up at the school for special summer classes and missed going with her.

She reported, "Hattie came out to the garden where we were picking beans. She was barefoot in an old wrapper. She carried a salt shaker and picked a big ripe tomato. She ate it as if she was starving, then pulled up a green onion and ate it with a small piece of cornbread that she had in her wrapper pocket. It seemed like a rather unusual breakfast, but it was what she had an appetite for."

I remembered something about Hattie's stooped posture. "Does her side still hurt her so much? She couldn't stand up straight."

Mama said, "Yes, she told me that she still has a pain in her right side about the size of a silver dollar. It feels like a boil, but her appetite is coming back."

Through the next two weeks we received almost daily dietary reports on Hattie. "Today, she ate a four-inch square piece of cornbread with fine leaves of new lettuce and a green onion, along with her tomatoes in the garden."

Early cucumbers came on. "Today she ate a bowl of sliced cucumbers and tomatoes. This is the first time she has eaten tomatoes inside the house instead of out in the garden."

Beets and crookneck squash came on.

Mrs. Knolls confessed to Mama, "I worry a little bit over Hattie eating them beet tops and that squash grated raw. You know that roughage might be too harsh for her side, but she wolfs it down."

Mama said, "Well, you remember that she did not want *anything* to eat when she first came home."

"Yes, that's true. She would have died of pure starvation if she had kept on like that. I know some folks think this rabbit food diet is loony, but Hattie is filling out a teeny bit and I see hope in her eyes. All this fresh produce is like a medicine to her, and good medicine is whatever cures folks."

"Amen."

The next week we received word that Papa's sister had broken her leg. She had four small children and her husband was alone with them at the height of the farming season. Mama took me to the community where they lived, to care for the family. We stayed there for nearly two months.

About the first thing we heard after we arrived back in Big Muddy was "You won't believe this, but Hattie Knolls can stand up straight now. She even walks to the post office for the mail. She has graduated. Eats new boiled potatoes with butter, English peas, watermelon, and even a poached egg for breakfast."

Quickly I asked, "Has she quit her tomatoes?"

"Oh, no, She still eats about three a day."

Mrs. Knolls cried when she met Mama again. "Mrs. Mac, my girl is getting well. I believe it now."

Her words proved prophetic. Hattie's vigor and strength slowly returned. After five months she went to Tulsa for an interview about her old job. The boss was so relieved that he wanted her to begin work that afternoon, said work was piled up.

Hattie told him, "No, not until tomorrow. My mother has never been to a movie. I'm going to take her to a matinee. Jean Harlow and Clark Gable are playing in Red Dust."

Peter Meinke

THE GURU

The guru's eyes were sleepy-wise, so calm
you thought no shark could shock them; no
hurting child close them in grief. Or no bomb
make him protest: let the world go.

And the guru said, "The circle of love
is without limit; we shall hold hands
and keep nothing back, for he who expands
his relationships is one with the tiger and the dove."

I said, "Relationships are like hemorrhoids;
I'd like to shrink them, put them on ice:
most people aren't nice, they should be punched out,
and love like a rubber band gets thin as it expands."

But the guru said, "You are the unhappy creature
of your limited sense-awareness; I reach out
to your isolation: I shall be your teacher."
And he stretched forth his pudgy little hand.

Katrina Roberts

THE PILL

Reason being, it often come to this. So that
at least at last she may shake down her hair,
let it fall like a curtain of dark water across her face, and see herself
as much in the shadowed *there*
as in that which most bounces off
each single strand in myriad shining ways, and finally swallow such
quiet knowledge, gracefully.

Bright-stream-through-the-purple-heather,
Bird-in-the-hand-worth-two, Merry-go-round-with-the-high-up-ring-
teased-by-flocks-of-liquid-gold-as-in-old-Mister-Doctor's-grin,

Pla-ce-bo.
Bolus, beadlette smooth and hard, small
enough to swallow. Nothing
is so simple. If I am
able, being reasonable, I shall please …

***

It has something to do with the vertical language of rain, if I say to you
the pill is a country, or that every person you know
resembles you in more ways than there are
flecks of powder
in the one tiny tablet in your hand. Doppelgangers,
all. No sure-fire way to attain the smallest possible particle
seems to exist,
so you keep on crushing it. The action
is palliative, but still
the pill's innermost core *is* impenetrable. Lie
down here in my mare's-nest for a short while—just one more time.
How we could
believe the farthest-fetched notions
about the machine we had invented together ever
actually demonstrating perpetual motion in any manner.
Taking two of anything necessitates a bit of quick thinking
when a third party calls next morning. Tell yourself: I will never
drink in excess again? Better,
save yourself for the *creme de la creme*, then drink in.

Leave the pill out in another storm like that and the whole song
will be lost for translation.

***

For all practical purposes, call it a device. Like vision,
sometimes it makes you believe
that alleviation of pain is imminent. X and therefore Y.

Why not *always*, you ask. Well, consider, for example
the X on a gunner's sight. And therefore? Let me suggest
that side-effects can be rain
on any parade. That is, if Y = death, will you take it.
The potential is what's most persuasive and dangerous.
Walk through the streets with your hands
in your pockets; which pedestrians take notice? Now,
make the same trip, on your hands. Blood rushes to fill your ears.
Gravel-grit under the nails. You're blushing, merely recalling
the staggering gait of the lovesick boy you used
to be. Head over heels and all that spinning.

The pill rolls over the table most evenly, its many faces
being fairly uniform. Little white coats are coming,
becoming. To the faithful, the pill promises wings
regardless of its silent content.

If sufficient, the idea of it all snug in the tooth-sized
nacreous box of her mind, certainly
we must honor such reason to please. This penchant
for pearl-handled revolvers, for exquisite
parasols with ivory spokes, for marching bands whose cymbals
dash all care from her brain. Un-der-stand.

She tells herself, yes I *do* feel better, wringing her
hands, though, unintentionally of course, she's neglected
the fact that she hasn't yet taken the pill. What's inside.

***

Imagine, if you will, that practical worldly information
could be gained in one quick gulp of the pill—whole
dialects, complex formulas, long-forgotten
lyrics, complete volumes of romantic verse by heart,
cajun recipes using jumbo shrimp … and all
at tongue-tip waiting to unfold and scintillate! Each white powder
coded to explode—like innards of fireworks

439

in an unsuspectedly dazzling array of chrysanthemum blooms,
squiggly ribbons of cobalt, umber, and puce, high
above waves lapping hills which rim them in some distant reach
of the brain. Unnatural brilliance taken for granted?
The sun's eclipse like the unspoken name of a parent. Anodyne
for pain gained through ignorance. What you don't know, then, might.
The pill instructs us as to the ways of the world when our cleverness
dwindles? Talk to me. Appallingly meek, daringly modest,
that prim chalk panacea nevertheless tempts the rebel in us all.

***

So, let me at least try to set things as straight as possible.

Multifaceted, but with no corners in which to conceal—the pill
appears in fact to be single-surfaced. Look closely. How many
smoothed-off angles actually reveal themselves when you press
your nose right to it. That is, for lack of example, if I say green,
what color comes to mind? Herbage, patina, envy, emerald …

The trickiest thing is—unless you quickly nick the sugar-coat,
you'll lose track of which face you addressed just moments ago.
It might then be a wise idea, when you meet the pill, to record
certain facts to help you, if caught in the lurch, recall identities …
Mr. Parotic-mole, Madame-space-between-her-teeth, Miss Cleavage.

Inside, the pill hides its multifarious elements, though they too
are indistinguishable until one becomes well acquainted with their
subtle differences and vastly varied abilities. All white powder
isn't sugar. We revel in the obvious. Ka-boom.

***

Reason being, sometimes when the pill leaves town it's a veritable
relief. So smug, so happy with its wholeness. And something
by which to be forgiven, is missing.

That, or simply the knowledge that our lives cannot entirely be
shared—unless one of us is crushed or consumed. Take me
with you? Its appealing qualities are in essence most addictive:
easy transport to exotic spots, erotic play all night, sweet
mangoes with cream, an entire world of engaging opportunity …
Agreeable, and deadly.

Because, both cure and cause. Something taken, something
given. And all quite interchangeable.

***

Finally, it comes back to this, the shaking and shaking
out. Each piece tumbling into place. Each piece
falling away like restraint itself. Every strand—moving water
across which the light moves. Downward. It all spills down
around her face. Her face, glowing. Her arms still
over her head, as though lifting a feverish child
—as if to lift a child over the hats of a row of people in front,
hushed and embarrassed, all witnesses to an elaborate
ritual, all shifting with curious desire, watching
the two huge dark shapes, their slow and precise lumbering,
heavy loins shuddering in the heavy heat,
two shadows, trying to give entirely, to abandon entirely
their cages of bones and skin, to climb into
each other, to erase the difference *between*,
mystery merging completely with the *this, here,* this *being*
the mystery, this becoming of something
it was always meant to be, a potential. The child,
laughing, and sniffling, the child wide-eyed and lifting
her small dampened fingers up, straining into the dizzy
air, sifting its particles, the thrum *inside*
her head, a tiny muffled voice which begins where you can't
see it ever, which begins deep down somewhere, which keeps rising

Lamont B. Steptoe

PARTS

We saw
people
fragile as brown sticks
in black silk skin
living under
the shells of hats

We saw
rice paddies
We saw
water buffalo
We saw
snakes

I am
part snake
I am
part water buffalo
I am
part rice paddy

I am
part black silk skin
brown stick
living under
the shell of a hat

I am
the rainy season
I am
the dry season
I am
the red dust of the moon

Dorothy Sutton

SHAMAN

We
hold together
edges of the gaping places,
drop healing words
like
soldier ants
directly into the wound
where
they bite down
on the flesh
lock their jaws
seal and suture the cut
We
clip away
thorax and the tail. Heads remain
in place
for several days
until
the words have done their work
bridges across
the pain
then only jaws
ingrained, vague traces of a scar.

Tom Timmins

ACUPUNCTURE AND NATURAL HEALING

Fly and Scatter *

Two hours of talk!
I think about
my new doctor
every day now!

Prince's Grandson

It is the return of spring
that gives me these dreams
every night
of beautiful women
leading me to their beds?

Little Rushing In

I look into the mirror
to tie my tie.
Who is that boy
with a moustache
looking at me?

Palace of Weariness

Is that real pain
in your eyes
when you stab the needles
into my palms?

Joining the Valleys

I told her I was
falling in love
with her.
"Don't worry," she said.
"You'll get used to it.
It's just the absence of pain."

Palace of Weariness

Lazy, mindless
under the potted palm
by her eastern window,

my body warms itself
like a garter snake among
the hollyhocks of August.

Outer Frontier Gate

On the drive home,
blinding white light
pierces the green haze
blossoming over
a raucous stand of
budding maple.

Great Enveloping

If I wear my watch
upside down
on the other wrist,
will I be protected
in the world
as I am in this purple iris
of her treatment room
where I wear
no watch,
no shoes.

Rushing the Inner Frontier

I remember my brother's note.
"The hundred year old elms
that lined our childhood street
have all been cut down, Tom."

Inner Frontier Gate

I ripped weeds out
of the overgrown hillside
as we climbed searching for
the "self-heal" herb.
"I think you've found it,"
she said, nodding at
the green stalks in my hands.

The Ultimate Source

"Some people come here
to talk about their toes

others
reveal their souls."

Wind Pond

"What can I
do to keep well?"
I asked.
Going out the door,
she turned back.
"Why don't you learn
to ride the waves."

The titles of the sections are names of acupuncture points used in different sessions.

Peter Wild

GOOD PHYSICIANS

Your family will be awed
    when they see you nights
        assembled in the kitchen,
  a telegrapher's green visor on,
a prince among the heap of his treasures,
   with protractor and compass and slide rule,
              a carpenter's
    #1 flat pencil stuck behind your ear,
teeth between tongue working out
        among the maple leaves
  of the roadmaps that have just fallen to the table
the precise route you'll all take this summer.
       And so months later it *does* work out
   just as they dreamed of,
         just as you calculated.
In the Rocky Mountains each day is filled
  with black bears hauling picnic coolers across the road,
    stopping to wave once before
       they disappear into the bushes,
and in Iowa, appreciating the Great Plains
       for what they are,
  after enjoying sodas in a small-town drugstore,
rounding a corner—
     there's a movie star!
  just as you all read about.
And at night, the sun down now,
   putting a few more miles on,
  everyone quiet, bonded
      in the hymn after the sermon,
    driving toward the innkeeper
       who over the telephone
  said he'd leave the porch light on for you,
  and finding it as it should be, precisely there,
    as a navigator does, all day
      in his head steering toward a lighthouse,
and proving once again
     what all good physicians know,
  that all cures are derived
    from their patients' belief in them.

Rodney Jones

CURIOSITY

What does a tomato know?
Dangling between the nineteenth and twentieth centuries
on a vine with weak knees,
it has avoided the hoe and hailstone
and carries secretly
a balm for the hangover, a pungent sauce
to embellish the full
and indolent body of linguine.

I sit on the pot and read James Joyce
and then a little Robinson Jeffers
before thinking of my great-grandfather,
Andrew Jackson Jones,
who read almost nothing
and believed people could die
of tomatoes.

Imagine coming out of a black locust grove
on a cool late summer morning
in Alabama ninety years ago
to pick the first tomato in that part of the world.
My great-grandfather must have meditated
a long time on the unprecedented taste
of that tomato. I think
he believed poison was an indescribably smooth skin
covering a soft heart. I think he did not know
whether to add sugar or salt
to tame the wild taste of that tomato.

What did my great-grandfather know?
Turning the earth of the nineteenth century
over into the twentieth,
he had already followed the streaked hams of horses
for thirty years
and had a right to his distrust and ignorance.

What do any of us know
of the infinite possibilities
of tomatoes?

CHAPTER VII

WHITE FLAGS FROM SILENT CAMPS

"One by one, the words give themselves up, white flags dispatched from a silent camp."

Rita Dove - "Reading Hölderlin
On The Patio
With The Aid Of A Dictionary"

Rita Dove

ONE VOLUME MISSING

Green sludge of a riverbank,
swirled and blotched,
as if a tree above him were shuffling
cards.
     Who would have thought
the binding of a "Standard Work
of Reference in the Arts,
Science, History, Discovery
and Invention" could bring back

slow afternoons with a line and bent nail

here, his wingtips balanced
on a scuffed linoleum square
at the basement rummage sale
of the A.M.E. Zion Church?

He opens *Motherwell-Orion* and finds
orchids on the frontispiece
overlain with tissue,
fever-specked and drooping
their enflamed penises.

Werner's Encyclopedia,
Akron, Ohio, 1909:
Complete in Twenty-Five Volumes
minus one—

for five bucks
no zebras, no Virginia,
no wars.

Rita Dove

KENTUCKY, 1833

It is Sunday, day of roughhousing. We are let out in the woods. The young boys wrestle and butt their heads together like sheep—a circle forms; claps and shouts fill the air. The women, brown and glossy, gather round the banjo player, or simply lie in the sun, legs and aprons folded. The weather's an odd monkey—any other day he's on our backs, his cotton eye everywhere; today the light sifts down like the finest cornmeal, coating our hands and arms with a dust. God's dust, old woman Acker says. She's the only one who could read to us from the Bible, before Massa forbade it. On Sundays, something hangs in the air, a hallelujah, a skitter of brass, but we can't call it by name and it disappears.

Then Massa and his gentlemen friends come to bet on the boys. They guffaw and shout, taking sides, red-faced on the edge of the boxing ring. There is more kicking, butting, and scuffling—the winner gets a dram of whiskey if he can drink it all in one swig without choking. Jason is bucking and prancing about—Massa said his name reminded him of some sailor, a hero who crossed an ocean, looking for a golden cotton field. Jason thinks he'd been born to great things—a suit with gold threads, vest and all. Now the winner is sprawled out under a tree and the sun, that weary tambourine, hesitates at the rim of the sky's green light. It's a crazy feeling that carries through the night; as if the sky were an omen we could not understand, the book that, if we could read, would change our lives.

Rita Dove

READING HÖLDERLIN ON THE PATIO
WITH THE AID OF A DICTIONARY

One by one, the words
give themselves
up, white flags dispatched
from a silent camp.

When had my shyness returned?

This evening, the sky refused
to lie down. The sun crouched
behind leaves, but the trees
had long since walked away.
The meaning that surfaces

comes to me aslant and
I go to meet it, stepping
out of my body
word for word, until I am

everything at once: the perfume
of the world in which
I go under,
a skindiver
remembering air.

Rita Dove

ROAST POSSUM

The possum's a greasy critter
that lives on persimmons and what
the Bible calls carrion.
So much from the 1909 Werner
Encyclopedia, three rows of deep green
along the wall. A granddaughter
propped on each knee,
Thomas went on with his tale—

but it was from Malcolm, little
Red Delicious, that he invented
embellishments: *We shined that possum*
with a torch and I shinnied up,
being the smallest,
to shake him down. He glared at me,
teeth bared like a shark's
in that torpedo snout.
Man he was tough but no match
for old-time know-how.

Malcolm hung back, studying them
with his gold hawk eyes. When the girls
got restless, Thomas talked horses:
Strolling Jim, who could balance
a glass of water on his back
and trot the village square
without spilling a drop. Who put
Wartrace on the map and was buried
under a stone, like a man.

They like that part.
He could have gone on to tell them
that Werner admitted Negro children
to be intelligent, though briskness
clouded over a puberty, bringing
indirection and laziness. Instead,
he added: *You got to be careful*
with a possum when he's on the ground;
he'll turn on his back and play dead

till you give up looking. That's
what you'd call sullin'.

Malcolm interrupted to ask
who owned Strolling Jim,
and who paid for the tombstone.
They stared each other down
man to man, before Thomas,
as a grandfather, replied:

          Yessir,
we enjoyed that possum. We ate him
real slow, with sweet potatoes.

Michael J. Bugeja

BONES

The first time I felt them
Lying on the floor of my bedroom
For some reason on my back
Running my fingertips too gently
Over my dumbbell body,

I gasped. I had ribs
And could touch them.
This was the fabled melting
Of the babyfat that happens
Without anyone knowing

Like wax candy on a sill.
The timing was perfect: summer,
Girls in the polkadot two-piece
Of yore. You could see them
Sunning like lizards on lawns,

The elegant ankles,
The bridgework of breasts,
The accordion blades of the back
That stretch and release,
Another distraction.

I looked and lost the myriad
Layers of me lean as love,
Fossil beneath, the skeletal
Remains: I had pelvis, pubic,
And I rattled when I walked.

Who knew what was happening?
Nobody called my name
As I loitered out of luck,
Life on the line. Later
I realized my country had

Bones too. Its myths,
its families don't always
Work but it boasts
Perfect timing, beautiful
People with bottomless

Michael J. Bugeja

Appetites and plenty of
Partners to go around.
Some on lawns, on floors,
Some flat on their backs
In the street melting

There in front of you.

Frank Anthony

MEA MAXIMA CULPA

To Robert Penn Warren

He taught me how to sing
By not teaching me anything.
Coming back from the big war
Coming back full of hate
He looked at me with one eye
He looked and said, "It's late."

Something happened inside,
Something simple had died:
He was not knowing and knowing
Whatever I had to do then
Had already been going on,
Waiting for that to start growing.

Roald Hoffmann

LISTEN

Praise, aloud: human sound, scrapes,
stops, frictions forced on the air, the
tactful massage of what had to be breathed
in, depleted of oxygen, and then, lifeless,
in wondrous re-use swept by the vocal cords,
up into resonant cavities of nose and mouth,
there to be shaped by mucous membranes, tuned
in plastic sets of tongue on palate, lips
opening, cheeks; emerging, air, vibrant
in a thousand frequencies and amplitudes;
everyday babble. It's very quiet in a vacuum.

Nadezhda Mandelstam writes: "If nothing
is left, one must scream. Silence
is the real crime against humanity."

We must sing: and those who can't carry
a tune, search, with the reach of longing,
for that perfect resonant shower stall,
the empty stairwell, where a bass is more
than a bass; or, in higher registers, merge
into Elly Ameling's graced hold on the ideal.

But Augustine in Ostia (who can say if it was
a quieter time) tells his mother: the absence
of language, silence, is the meaning of eternal life.

Anne Meisenzahl

THE LONE WOMAN

If she had a son
she would stroke his hair to wake him
now and tell him firmly that
he must never disrespect a woman.
If she had a daughter
she would write her a letter
telling her she must never disrespect herself
and tuck it beneath her pillow.
If she lived in the country she would
drag a sleeping bag behind her onto the lawn
and tell the stars she loves them.
She untangles the sheets
and resolves to sleep.
She dreams of stones and shattered glass
and delayed subways. In the morning
she works again. She calls her friend whose words
are like melted honey at the bottom of a cup
of strong tea.

William Packard

IF WORDS

were
true

we wouldn't
need
poetry

Carol Miller

EVERY DAY

There are flowers
tied in knots,
so many hearts
given, taken away.
The battle of language is clear.
I dive into the bay
to drown the words
in my head's dark.
Later I stand
in the soft sand
my shadow riddled
with doubt,
gently pulling feathers
from my hair.
The wind is a
returning touch.
I pause, breathe
deep.
The battle of language is clear.
I choose my words,
invent a door, kick it
open and
lunge at life.
I am a serious woman.
What I mean is to live.

Margaret Robison

WORDS

The voices of my dead have not
lain down in the grave with the quiet bones.
The voices of my dead have not
knelt in the cathedrals of skulls,
praying silently to the bold,
industrious worms.

Even the hair gives up
its stubborn insistence on life.
But words!
How they return,
persistent as genes,
as if they too were a part
of the blood and bone of ourselves.

Berwyn Moore

THE DEEPNESS OF LEAVES AND LIGHT

They come in to disclaim their lives,
mutter pieces of themselves

that fall across my lap like pared nails.
What they name as sin, they learned

from childhood catechism: *I committed
adultery, Father, I slept with a woman*

whose name I can't recall. And the distance
they set between flesh and word widens

with each day they can say, *I have not
sinned* or *It is forgotten.*

Before I was old, I knew my name
and tried to hide from its sound

in the trees, from its light
that spilled into the shadows

like water. I could not breathe,
could not hear the wind, but only

my name over and over as I fell
into the deepness of leaves and light,

then lay still, until I could hear
once more the hush in the trees.

Now, again, I hear my name
over and over as it becomes

a thousand sins I can never forget,
never disclaim as I circle

towards unresurrected death,
dust visible in this windless half-light.

Berwyn Moore

BOURBON PRAYERS

A letter today. Pray for us:
Emerson's garage has burned
to a heap of soot, arson, they're sure;
Tommy's best friend was struck by a car,
its skid marks still etched
in front of our house;
Karen's cancer
has spread and John wants to divorce her—

just can't deal with it, he says.
You wonder, the letter goes on,
just how much a soul can take.
I sip bourbon in the dark. I'm alone
and wonder if God listens to bourbon prayers.
I think about the words at my son's
twelfth birthday party. One boy said to him:

You can drink from my glass,
I don't have AIDS. They continued
with their video game and laughed
when someone mentioned Roy Orbison.
They knew who he was.
They knew he is dead.
I would like to walk out of this house

and into the cold and dark, imagine
that shadows from winter trees
were the fingers of an unkind
stranger curling around my neck.
I wouldn't scream. I wonder whether I'd
leave a sign—a piece of shirt, a tuft
of hair, a scent, a smear of blood,

and if anyone would notice tomorrow
when the sun graces the branches.
But I stay inside, sip bourbon
in the dark, savor its burn
against my throat. I decide that God
will hear if he wants to and listen
as the pipes clink in the falling dark.

Linda Allardt

STONE TALK

What I wanted to tell you,
how it was with me,
came out apple tree, crabapple,
its bloom crying out rose or deeper.
If you have words for that color, tell me.
When I groped for speech this morning,
it snowed against the window
a storm of petals driven off the cherry.
That will have to do for saying
how far it is between us, how drifting.
As for what comes next,
my hands are still signing.
Trees will die of it.
Then when I stoop for a word
it will skip six times across water,
split into fossil crustaceans,
fit in my palm to throw.
Stone is the hardest language I'm learning.

Harold Witt

MICROBE HUNTERS

Among the stirring paperbacks I bought
one was called *Microbe Hunters*—Paul de Kruif
reading it by the rushing creek I thought
I might enjoy the scientific life,
improve a microscope like Leewenhoek,
discover harming germs as Lister did—
I lay there naked poring through the book.
Oh there were many bugs I had to rid
the ailing world of; fearless as Pasteur
I'd boil the milk; chewed boys would not get rabies,
and also somehow I'd find such a cure
as Ehrlich had—no more disabled babies—
but "When in disgrace—" singing in my head,
I wrote another fourteen lines instead.

Jeffrey Hillard

SAY IT

I could hear the new woman upstairs savor the words,
wrung, at last, from her stomach, that she wanted
to get on with it, *beat me*, as if the person
with her was one of night's dark muscles
which grows stronger with workout,
like a blast of wind where
there's no safe cover.

Whatever happened happened so quickly the right words
couldn't sidestep the fiery drama inside my stomach.
I'll probably never live comfortably on words
like hero, or say anything about this place
more frightening than the two words she
may have found most pleasurable
after saying them.

When I dig deeper for a pillar of adjectives and freeze,
is it fair to say midnight can stare my voice
into a corner like it will a woman
when her smooth legs lose their confines,
drill his eyes hot and watery,
his mind to do strange things?

I was all I could be. I'd walked the same dark alley
between cafes and front door, my throat loaded
with words, ready to launch praise
into the faces of neighbors, imagined
them cupping my words bright
as a bag of lost jewels.

But I've been struck broadside by runts with stunted
vocabularies and moss-colored, dull teeth.
I know what it's like for the body
to limp away and leave the voice
turning bluish, no proud
beggar to speak of.

Tonight, I promised I'd never again turn the stunned blue
of a Wyatt Earp sitting defenselessly in open air,
a marked man, his lips flapping in shame.
Tonight I still hear her leaving.

If only my voice could follow
her out the door,

the words of my life about to slap fear in the face,
rushing to me to finally hear them, syllable
after composed syllable: rise, crushed, rising again.

Andrew Glaze

IT'S HERE!

It's here!
he tells his mouth, here!
Sing!
And it has taken the oath. So it tries.
But the lips
are sewed shut.

It's here!
he tells his knees, here!
Dance!
They crack and crack, dolefully.
But cannot stir
one inch
from the black muck.

Still, something
hears the words.
His heart obeys.
Bravely it flies,
fluttering, and fluttering
just out of reach,
fierce outrageous wings.

A.G. Levine

THE WORD

I quiet the voice dying inside me
And talk to the plants who mutely accept.
They know about pain; plants do not fight back.
Parched, pinched, lacking sun—they stretch toward it still!
When I was a child, the world spoke to me.
Sky, breeze, smell of grass taught me how to live.
You breathe through the sting of scathing, deadly tongues.
Life in a bottle, see it: inside out.
Oh, recovery resonates softly
when at last we can speak of awful things.
No longer wooed by a false death, chanting,
"Can't, no, should, should not, can't, no, should, should not"
Saved by a kind word welling up within
nourishing seed planted eons ago.

William Packard

AFTER THE CLASS

after the class, after that last 11th hour asking
what did you mean by saying so & so
after the traffic of eyes into eyes has passed into air
i go to the window and stare at the lighted windows outside

then back to the desk to stack up my books
screw on the cup top of my steel thermos
pocket my pipe and rewrist my watch
pack everything together into my black leather shoulder bag

then exit into those tall empty halls
wait for the elevator to drop me down to the main floor
where i go out through the double doors to begin
the long walk home on concrete city sidewalks

it is raining words words words
the syllables go dribbling down my beard

Carolyn Kremers

THE NEW STUDENTS

To her they smell comfortable,
like fish, sweat, sleep—
or like soap, fresh
        from the laundromat, where showers
cost six quarters. The little ones
        grab her arms and legs
with sticky hands, take her "downtown,"
        skipping, pull ropes
for water, call out whose house
        is whose. They walk on ice, not scared,
reveal sod ruins and a skull, yes, watching,
        yellow, almost whole.
Boys offer soft black puppies,
        girls braid her hair.
"Will you skate with us?"
        "Will you be back next year?"
They want to know everything;
        she cannot tell them.
Instead , she asks for words.
        Agayuvik, they say, pleased. Church.
Elitnaurvik, school. *Kalikat*, book.
        Aqumi, sit down. *Tengssuun*, plane.
Nayiq, ringed seal. *Usuuq!* Watch out!
        Akutaq, Eskimo ice cream.
Anaq, dog poop. "And humans, too."

"I like you," she says.
Assikamken, they answer, suddenly shy.

They bring wildflowers, fossils, white
        rocks, leave them on the steps
when she's not there. When she is,
        they swing the chain inside the door, bing
the kitchen timer, want to know
        what spices are for, and insurance.
They chew snuff and spit it, grinning
        at her tales of cancer and mouths.
Some eat popcorn with chopsticks,
        watch *2001* in school,

473

and she tries to explain
 that the apes are not real,
what a synthesizer is,
 how it feels to ride a horse,
or pet one. They laugh lots.

She learns
 to speak slowly,
not use big words,
 watch their eyebrows,
try to listen.
 There is too much to hear.
"Don't touch me, bitch!"
 Marjorie hisses,
eyes burning through the desk,
 long black hair. Pregnant,
like a bomb. Not wanting to give up—
 "Happy birthday, Marge"—
one day she comes home from school
 and smells a ghost:
cigarette smoke
 inside the arctic entryway.
This girl could set the house on fire.
 Or does she want to talk?

Daniela Gioseffi

WORD WOUNDS, WATER FLOWERS

I.

Where can mad money be spent
on windless meadows, vaporized forests,
under dusty snow falling forever acid,
when love sucked from bleached bones
in ashes floats in particles of lips,
songs, paintings or poems for eons
on and on to nowhere's nothing ...?
I can't comprehend nothing of nothing
"Non capisco nulla di niente,"
my Italian grandmother said
before she died at sixty-five
of emphesema from her coal stove
burning through the cold
of dark winters like the eternal one to come
exploding from Godhead to warhead
through centuries of silly soft women
powder-puffed and waiting for men
to come and come, and now they may come
no more ... to smell perfumed grasses, or see
breast of velvet blue mountains, red sunsets
or morning's rise after night closes their eyes
forever, Mother Earth, yes, Capitol Earth, I spell you
rich with color, mood and mud.
Slime and beauty beyond mortal words
from which we come with our ears and tongues,
giving ears and tongues to children
and sleek weapons that could demolish us
to metaphorless similes of dust.

II.

Walt Whitman's voice extolled these states and stars
as Democratic Vistas—but they were stolen
from the Redman who reaps cancerous lungs from mined uranium,
and fire water spills from Her green hills,
polluted valleys, fields of waving grain,
full of nitrates, purple mountain's majesty, America, plump woman

born to poison, your cornucopia fills with nuclear barons' oil spills,
distilling carcinogens from landfills full of greed's garbage,
dolphins, seals, and sea otters breed P.C.B.s. Exxons and G.E.s
P.R. lies and missiles labeled "Peacemakers" that can sizzle
billions in an instant, killing all forever fools of nothing,
no
thing,
unimaginable as zero so profound,
all Promethean longings go unbound.

III.

Have you noticed how angry women are between their laughters?
Tears loom among their witches' brooms,
because they feel the end approaching all.
It makes their gonads reel with rage.
Since there's too little love for berries, peaches, melons, mud,
and disillusioned children, women have less hope
about the future as their intuition throbs between their legs
forced open to keep life coming from legislated bodies, gates
to heaven or hell, since Satan fell from grace,
into Eden's apple trees and Eve fell on her knees
before him in male mythologies of misogynistic verse.
Earth, so little loved and cursed, She'll explode
with manufactured greed for plastic fruits and flowers, polymers,
poisonous whims of monolithic powers, money mad with mad money
grabbed by Morgan, Bechtel, whose name rhymes with hell, Grumman, Hughes,
who help hold the fuse, AT&T who owns me and thee, down to our bones.
Executives profits for motifs and motives
to please the very rich with more riches, and mutants,
birth defects of agent orange or irradiating bomb tests—
as astrophysicists describe a black hole sucking everything to
entropy—and a gap in the ozone layer of climatology
widens as acid rain kills lakes and forests and aflotoxins
like alien enemies, biological warfare agents rain
back down on us. All poisonous greed can't be flushed
away in a Rabelaisian toilet of the universe,
as it comes back to curse our children, poor or rich in one
uni-
verse
all that matters us into matters beyond us
and our separated nations
as each child of us, comes in innocence, dumb with beauty
and the notion of all motion, centrifugal force,

unites nations, flagged by the same photo of Earth
from outer space, mother of an entire race of one
blessed or cursed Earth, Mother of All,
oceanic womb-
man to all children
and we are one in all and only all in one is won.

IV

There's no exotic enemy!
No "them" and "we."
Just ourselves, deep in "us"
a fascination with the exotic other—
dwells in dark sentiment—this passion
with the blood of the other
stains our hands and tongues.
We poke at the fruit, to see
its juices run on the ground,
tear the rose from its stem, scatter petals to the wind,
pluck the butterfly's wings for the microscope's lens,
plunge a fist into a teetering tower of bricks,
watch the debris sail, explode fireworks
until all crumbles to dust and is undone, open
to the curious eye. Does this or that creature die as I die,
cry as I cry, writhe as I would if my guts were ripped
from the walls of my flesh, my ripe heart eaten alive?
The probing questions of sacred exploration,
as if science can progress
without empathy. Does a penis feel as a clitoris feels?
Do slanted eyes see as I see? Is a white or black skin
or sin the same as a red one; is it like me? Does it burn,
does it peel, does it boil in oil or reel in pain?
The obsession to possess the other so completely
that his blood fills the mouth and you eat of her flesh
from its bones and then know if she, if he, feels as you feel
if your world is real.

V.

These are the word wounds,
roots of mushroom clouds to rise
from the pockmarked earth:
Guinea, dago, spick, nigger, polack, wasp, mick,

chink, jap, frog, kraut, russkie, red bastard, kike,
bitch, macho pig, gimp, fag, dike—
word wounds to make stench of flesh follow
sprayed dust of children's eyes
melted from wondering sockets, animal skin, thighs,
men's hands, women's sighs
roasted in a final feast of fire
beasts caught like lemmings
in a leap to Armageddon's
false resurrection.
Word wounds rise from visions of charred lips,
burnt books, paper ashes, crumbled libraries, stones
under which plastic pens
and computers are fried amid the last cried
words, smoke to pay lip service—
as Orphic light rages
against the dying of the light
and all dust into dust returns
to the last words,
sigh of a burning leaf turning: "Life live,
leaf live, love life leaf live …"

VI

There are those mornings
when the spirit stretches out of itself,
reaches up from the breast, radiates from the groin
beyond sex into song and sensual delight
in the way light falls on leaves,
growing green glistens with animal sighs
—and the romance of photosynthesis begins
all beginnings.
There are those afternoons
when knowing beyond saying christens the body
with love for its own breath
and being breathes in harmony with leaves.
There are those evenings when the sunsets with red
and blue glory—even over teeming cities
and glass windows blaze wondrous color,
though children rot in slum gutters
or drug themselves out of the pain
of all that's unfair or insane.

You've smelled the familiar wood, mud, fern aroma,
as red and gold leaves spread a cover over
dried grass and whispering wind on water sings
the stupid and stupendous music of an awesome autumn
milk-weed bursts in silk
puffs of seeds and spiders speed
patterning the water mirroring your face
amidst scarlet fringes of a maple flecked with green,
serene skies utterly blue with the lies of our lives.
You've seen, heard, felt such awe and you, too,
know wounds of words can burst into fire.
You tire, too, of trying to speak
the language of leaves as you grow older like me—
lichens blooming on the side of a dead tree.
So, sing a song of peace with me, please,
because death turns to beauty in the dying leaves
and moss is soft and inviting. Tell me, toll me,
please, listen with me to the leaves
aching with eyes and animal sighs
and cries for mercy in the fall from grace
to this quiet, quiet place.

VII.

There are still those days when peace reigns
in desire's mouth and nothing more is longed for
beyond the taste of color, music of hearts and lungs,
sigh of sun, wet of water, touch of the sea, sweet
juice squeezed on the tongue. Then
the body is possessed by light
until the pitcher of sleep fills with milk
poured into the moon and a song of sleep
glows in the throat—giving night its breathy music,
as tortured beasts howl far off in city caverns,
cries from eyes where genitals are plucked flowers
crushed by sadistic curiosity, bled
into troubled sleep. The child
melted by synthetic doom shrieks.
A premeditated alchemic act devised
to sear human flesh, mutates the baby's body
into horror. Brilliantly, germs are bred in laboratories
to foul enemy armies with venereal disease; prostitutes lurk

on the edges of military bases which protect the rich
from the rich—selling flesh like excrement.

VIII.

In civilized rooms,
rich executives wage secret money`wars,
deal drugs for profits—devils disguised by designer clothes
live elegant lives that keep the poor unfed
and laboring in heat—fountains of their sweat
fed to gun lords who want more and more
corpses of untimely death buried in pieces under flowering trees
without eyes, hands, guitars or slippers.
Those who die tortured will scream in all our nightmare dreams
until brutes are bred into angels, and prisons emptied of agony,
workers clothed with more than chains, until
puppet dictators lose their strings,
until sparrows sing like nightingales,
and fly like herons above the war for crumbs,
—until I learn to love you with your different body,
your disposition imperfect as mine,
until then, death will go on wearing the soldier's uniform
of his illustrious career—a salute masks his leer.
Like a bullfighter he carves
the mighty bull, to still the beast
with graceful cunning, his sleek
sword hidden in his silk cape.
His missiles poised in their silos
empty of grain, filled with fires of the final feast
he'll eat with his cavernous mouth, carnivorous teeth.
His masculine chin chews children, spits
their wasted bones into cinders, swallows
their budding bodies, and the honey of their
breath as it expires, drips blood as saliva from his lips,
a blistered grin. In his hand, he juggles
the blue and crystal ball full of swirling waters,
over a steel and concrete gravestone
where all our names are inscribed with Dante,
Mozart, Bach, Beethoven, Lady Murasaki,
Dickinson, Rembrandt, Madam Curie,
Einstein, Luther-King, Chi'u Chin or Ghandi …
fading into dust beyond the last stupendous flash
of life urges into death fireworks,
eternal winter, as names

and the word could become in the space of moments,
syllables to no one and nothing perceives
light or darkness, as you and I, love, caress
each other's eyes before we touch, hand on smile inventing love.
But cold and silent of human song the planets could spin
unknown to anyone or anything—
fragile as our flesh which thrills with love's
impulse, electric touch of empathy's
mysterious imagery, waters flowing mind
which cannot dream "nothing" without thinking "zero" as a perfect something of the algebraic kind.

IX

We are all one human creature
bound by one earth
under one sun—moon mutant nations where all children's ears
hear "Songs of Innocence,"
as corporational apes of toxic wastes
breathe alchemic greed bloated powers bigger
than all our tiny flesh made lives,
or little seeds of giant sequoia trees,
most ancient living things of earth,
older than king's tombs, true cathedrals
of the blue Pacific as she rocks, swirling
melodies with the Atlantic's green currents,
currencies ... rain songs, sounds swell wells,
lakes faucets, brooks' runes, oceans tunes,
mystic drafts of summer wetness, cool drink seeping into thirst,
earth nearly all water of which we are made one human
bound by one wet planet
under one maddening moon,
under one arrogant sun,
under one, pale watery moon,
under one, bright thirsty sun.

Joanne M. Riley

THE WILLOW BRUSH

A letter to the artist from the Chinese painter's wife

I have waited years to tell you
The history of the brush; waited, I suppose,
To see if you were worthy.
Now with these words, I seek some peace.

He died thirty years ago, or more than thirty;
I was his second wife and younger
So I knew I would outlive him, but this long?
We had no sons; our daughter died at twelve.
To you he left his legacy.

He was once an artist in his own right, you know,
But not with much acclaim and he never liked the limelight.
I was young, full of my own beauty
And I could not comprehend an artist's heart.

He had told me he was making a brush.
We wandered through groves, forests, orchards,
Along the riverbank until one day he found
A willow. We sat beneath it and he read me
Haiku of the masters. After awhile
I began to listen.
Then he harvested the perfect twig.
He said it was the shaft
Of a hand without touch.

He began to set traps for rabbits.
This frightened me since he respected living things.
One by one he caught them; if he could, he set them free
After plucking some fur. With it he practiced
The shape of the brush. One day he snared a king hare
Of the purest white, fur graying, barely, at the tips.
From him he gleaned the bristles.

He neglected his work. We moved to the city and opened a shop
Of artists' goods and other Chinese things.
We made poor living.
He used to talk to artists who came in,
To chat for hours, selling nothing. I chafed and chafed.
It was the same with you; I saw him watch your hands.

Then he gave you the willow brush. He GAVE it to you.
Didn't even make you pay.

That night I cried and cried. I raved at him.
He had made that brush to become the painter of painters
And he had given it away. He looked at me with pain.
Yet I could not forgive.
And then he died. We had no savings, so I kept the shop.
Since I was good at business, it prospered.
I studied, traveled, learned what artists want,
And carried only the best supplies, world-wide.
I became famous in my own right.

And I watched you and your hand-painted pottery,
Read all your reviews, visited each exhibit.
Slowly I discovered how the perfect paintbrush
Brings the mind to life. I came to understand
The way a river understands, taking color
Upon itself, moving while never changing place
Like an old riddle. I came to understand
The nature of the hare, becoming the swiftest landscape
Of each season.

I know art. Art and what it needs. Art and how it lives.
So I received the greater gift,
And knowing this, I write to you.
For you will always be divided,
Hung somewhere between your own talent
And what the tool can do

While I am the heart of the brush he loved.
I have sold the shop.
With part of the money, I have purchased
One of your world-famous vases.
I will use it for my ashes.
Burn the brush and place it with them.
I have earned it.

483

Marjorie Power

TUESDAY MORNING

At last, the sun.
I pour on the table
my glass full of stones.
Here comes agates, highly polished,
in browns, golds, greens,
now sea-rounded bits
of granite, now quartz.
Marbles. These could be drops
of sky, fallen to earth
at twilight.

A letter arrives.

I touch *I am here*
at the Baltic, trying
to understand the poetry
trends of your country ...
just read/liked your poem ...
it would be marvelous
to see your book.
Into my palm I gather
the wholeness
of the human nature ...
we'll attempt to recreate
democracy ... the belongingness
of all to the Nature....

A piece of granite
streaked with rust, *Estonia*
sits in my hand.
Sincerely yours....

What's an unknown American poet to do
when a poet she doesn't know
is *waiting for any response*
behind the Iron Curtain?

Dear Indrek, I try.

Wendy Mitchell

HOW WE LIVE

You say you want
the adulation of crowds
that one prayer is not enough

but you see what an armless man
takes from the day

keeps feathers in your eyes
and you can always be a bird

your memories of love
are like to oleander's promise
full of bitterness

walk with petals in your hands
and praise a single tree
until the wind in your hair is breathless

you ask how a painter's dark images
layered on canvas like ash in a fireplace
can possibly speak to you

if you kneel by the side of death
give that cold mouth one last kiss
you will hear how words
find their sound on a page

sing them to me

M.S. Leavitt

OWED TO BETSY SCHOLL POET

-Men's Correctional Center
Windham, Maine 1989

She said her alter-ego talked tough for her
because talking shit
made her seem less obvious.
Her voice was the flutter of spring wind and robins,
or the flowers she was so fond of.
I think she liked mums and daffodils the best
because their yellow souls
could withstand the beatings of the rain
and not fade, or become lost.

She said the poet was supposed to taste
the blood of the seasons and understand the wounds
of growth and dying.

She said daffodils caught the rain in their throats
and did not choke.

The mums just stood silent.

When her soul wasn't looking
her words drifted so softly
that you could hear the timid beating of her heart
as she blended words and tears
with ferocious delicacy,
weaving shawls of mist
and sunrays.

When she came to teach at the jail
she brought us flowers
and read poetry
that sparkled with life from the outside.
She told the story of how a pimp
once saved her life
as her apartment building burned.
She smiled as she talked of her daughter
and I remember how her voice sounded.
She never seemed to notice that we all wore
blue shirts and talked shit

that we wore on our sleeves
like a stolen badge of courage.

In those weeks we talked of poets
and learned to use words
like a child's fingerpaints.
When she read her poems to us
she would fly
and I could hear the soft flutter
of her wings in the rain.
I remember she let me use her shawl to stay dry
and I caught the soft scent of flowers in it.
Daffodils, I think.

She taught me to catch the rain in my throat
without choking.

She also taught me silence.

Judi Kiefer Miles

LEARNING TO SPEAK:
OVERCOMING IMPOTENCE

Judi could either say yes
and do something she did not want to do,
or she could say no
and do something she did want to do.

"No," Judi thought.
Thinking no, Judi could not say it.
Judi would say no if she knew how.
Judi knew not what to do.
If Judi did it, it would be a negative experience.
If Judi knew how to say no, it would be a positive experience.
Saying no is harder for Judi than not saying no.
Judi's mouth could not stretch far enough not to say yes.
Judi would know how to say no if she would only practice.
Judi practiced how not to say yes.
"No," Judi said.

Lila Zeiger

DOUBLE ENTENDRE: COLONY BREAKFAST

Believe me, I did wake up
thinking the word *gonads*.
Believe me, too, I didn't
connect it with balls
or the castration of bulls
or any of that bull
that we throw like a ball
this morning.

Perhaps crotch is better
than crotchety at a colony
breakfast—no silent table
for us as we mount each other
in words, annoying the stable ones
with our giddy yapping.

Understanding everything
at least two ways—
that may be the essence of art.
Can we make nothing of everything?
Can we make something of nothing?

Describe the locus of your pain:
between your thighs, your ears?
The sharpest point is still
defined by twos.
Does it hurt more when you laugh?
More or less when you talk?

We live as at table—
the duplicity of our lips
may rise and fall
above a blinding flatness.
Lean in. At times we touch the edge
of what buries us
almost to the heart.

Charles B. Rodning

IMPELLING WORDS

A word fitly spoken is like apples
of gold in pictures of silver.
Proverbs 25:11

King James Version (1623)
The Holy Bible

For all of the scientific advancements that have occurred within medical science, the practice of surgery remains very much a craft—the application of artistic, humanistic, and scientific skills to the alleviation of fear, pain, and suffering. To that end a surgeon to a great extent must be an authority regarding wound healing. His responsibility is to provide a milieu for this very fundamental biological phenomenon to occur, which I would argue begins even before an incision is made. I would also argue that healing can only occur within a covenantal relationship between patient and surgeon (D'Aunay and Rodning, 1988), and that communication is as important a part of that relationship as the surgical instruments.

A surgeon is a source of many important components of this therapeutic milieu: the proper timing of an operation; the prescription of anesthetic, antiseptic, analgesic, and antibiotic agents; the use of meticulous and expeditious operative technique; the proper application of bandages and splints; the use of nutritional supplements; and the periodic reassessment of a patient during the convalescent phase. Ultimately, however, it is a patient who must heal (OE *hal, haelan,* "whole,") any wound that has been created. At issue in this regard is the imperative that the process of healing begins with dialogue between patient and surgeon, and that it is this dialogue which sets the stage for the whole process to unfold. A bond is established, a commitment is acknowledged, a covenant is created, as a consequence of the images of caring (L. *caritas,* "charity"), helpfulness, and hopefulness conveyed in that setting. If a patient and a surgeon are receptive to the dynamics of this whole biological and psychological process, fear, pain, and suffering will be alleviated and healing will occur (D'Aunay and Rodning, 1988; Marty and Vaux, 1982; Schaffner, 1981; Sodel, 1979).

All ideas, memories, thoughts, and recollections are contemplated, tempered, and communicated by words (OE *wort,* "say") (Richardson, 1950). The events and experiences of previous encounters and the images stimulated by them are contained and stored within words. Progress through all aspects of life can be perceived as a movement, a transition, from one boundary, from one edge, to another, through words and images:

dark - light

morning - night

sleep - wakefulness

sickness -health

life - death

Our awareness is most acute when we are on that boundary or that edge.

Furthermore, ideas, thoughts, and images, have consequences, and individuals become marked (OE *mearc,* "boundary") by them. The *gestalt* that they create stimulates a succession of ideas, thoughts, and images. Consequently, a perpetual and multidimensional sentient cycle prevails within the minds of mankind.

If words are perceived to possess such influence, a *priori* reasoning would suggest that ideas, thoughts, and images could effect healing. Although some might argue that this perspective is unscientific, since it as yet unverifiable employing standardized scientific methodologic principles, the intellectual history of Occidental and Oriental society, particularly the Judeo-Christocentric philosophy, supports this contention (Richardson, 1950).

According to ancient Hebrew linguistic tradition, words were an expression of an individual's will and purpose. If one's entire soul was applied to an expression—poetry, prose, song, speech—those words bore the whole force of one's personality. In addition, thought, word and deed were not three entities or processes, but rather were interdependent components of a single process—an act of volition. *The word and the thing were identical.*

The translated phrase "the Word ... made flesh" originated from this tradition and is exemplary of the power of words. Note the phraseology of the first chapter of the *Gospel According to Saint John:*

> In the beginning was the Word,
> and the Word was with God,
> and the Word was God (verse 1) ...

> And the Word was made flesh,
> and dwelt among us,
> full of grace and truth (Verse 14).

This phrase denotated and implied the creative and redemptive activity of a Creator, especially as manifested by the creation and preservation of the world *in toto* and in acts of salvation and service among men. I acknowledge that this perspective is a *mysterium tremendus*; nevertheless, the Word created, manifested, or transformed what had been made. The imperative of:

> God,
> Father Almighty,
> divine wisdom,
> self-revelation from God to man,
> expressed and manifested mind and will of God,
> gospel,
> *logos,*
>
> became incarnate and dwelled among men.

This image of "the word ... made flesh" also connotated and possessed a power to heal wounds—physical, mental, spiritual—inflicted by illness or injury; "ravaged flesh made whole" by and through the Word. In this setting, the Word transformed—healed—the wound that had been made. Beyond the figurative and symbolic significance of the Word, the Word and the words conveyed became a literal and pragmatic means by which healing was facilitated and ultimately achieved.

It is impossible for me to contemplate or conceptualize a relationship between a patient and surgeon from any other than this metaphysical perspective. Since all human endeavor begins with ideas, such ideas become the means by which rapport is established and empathy is conveyed between patient and surgeon. I do not think it is too far an extrapolation to suggest that a surgeon serves as an intermediary as he communicates a sense of compassion and faith, help and hope, solace and succor to his wounded patient. His words not only establish a bond, a commitment, a convenant between them, they also serve as a source of energy for healing to occur. Without those words a patient's healing process may be protracted or mitigated. In this setting a surgeon's words are as impelling as his scapel.

REFERENCES

D'Aunay, D., Rodning, C.B. (1988). Patient-physician interaction: Healing power of a covenant relationship. *Humane Medicine, 4*, 107-109.

Marty, M.E., & Vaux, K. L. (Eds.) (1982). *Health/medicine and the faith traditions: An inquiry into religion and medicine*. Philadelphia: Fortress.

Richardson, A. (1950). *A theological word book of the Bible*. New York: Macmillian .

Russell, B. (1977). *Wisdom of the west*. New York: Crescent Books.

Schaffner, K.D. (Ed.) (1981). Reductionism and holism in medicine. *Journal of Medical Philosophy, 6, 93-235.*

Sodel, D.S. (Ed.) (1979). *Ways of health: holistic approaches to ancient and contemporary medicine*. New York: Harcourt, Brace, Jovanovich.

Peter Wild

"SHEILAISM," WORDS, AND JOHN C. VAN DYKE

Of course, words can heal; they also can wound, incite to riot, and give instructions for decorating a cake. If they couldn't do such things, we'd be babbling for naught. Words call a dog in from the back yard and tell a satellite thousands of miles out in space when to click pictures and when to stop. They seal marriages, and with words we end them. Churchill, it is said, saved a nation with words—not at all a poetic exaggeration, when you think about it.

Words, then, are a form of power; they're capable of changing things and influencing people. In this respect they're like money, and like money, they can be used for good or ill. And, if the reader will bear with me, this is where I begin to tremble.

For some years now I've been studying the life of John C. Van Dyke, a turn-of-the century writer. In his unpublished autobiography, he offers this passage on his early upbringing:

> At Green Oaks I had been sent to bed each night in the dark. If I met a bear on the stairs-landing, I was to fight him off. In the big Trenton house when called upstairs one evening about dusk and before the lamps were lighted, I bawled back that I couldn't see. The mother's soft voice replied: "Well, feel."
>
> That was the Puritan of it. If I could not do a thing one way then do it another way and under no circumstances lean on anyone.

A somewhat sensitive soul, a vegetarian and a person who scoops floundering crickets out of the dog's water bowl, I was taken aback at the treatment. "The poor kid," I thought. "He's being brutalized by parents who seemed decent, caring people in other respects, but who had this perversion, this power trip at bedtime."

Some weeks later, however, I came upon this little scene in *The Open Spaces*, Van Dyke's collection of reminiscences. John is now about fourteen or fifteen, out West sowing his oats and working as a clerk on a Mississippi steamboat. The captain gets word of a disturbance below and sends his clerk to stop it. John scurries off to the forecastle deck and confronts a drunken raftsman trying to bash open a barrel of whiskey with a poker. When the boy tells him to stop, the raftsman threatens to run him through with the iron pole. John's response: "Instantly I whipped out a small pearl-handled revolver and brought it to bear straight between his eyes."

Yes, young Van Dyke surely suffered a few psychic bruises facing the bears he imagined on the staircase. But better to face them them than to go to pieces when facing real bears later. Trained to independence, though not at all a violent person, he grew up full of pluck. Once out on the Arizona desert he got the drop on five cutthroats bent on killing him just for the fun of it. And we're not talking about a physical maschismo that may have been handy on the rough-and-tumble frontier but is passé in more peaceful times. As one of the most popular travel writers of the day, Van Dyke steeled himself for the lecture circuit though he didn't particularly like speaking before large audiences. In old age, though dying a slow death from cancer, he kept on writing, writing. And there are other things, as we'll shortly see.

Such toughness and sense of personal responsibility have not outlived their usefulness, either to individuals or to society.

By now you see where we're going, and it will have everything to do with our use and misuse of words.

Consider. A few years ago I knew a seemingly normal young man who had a curious modus operandi when it came to women. After a first date, he'd ask the young lady to go for counseling with him, to see if they were "compatible" and to work out their "hangups." The amazing thing was how many of the women went along with the suggestion.

One can hear Van Dyke snorting at that. Goodness only knows what he'd make of Sheila. Along with a good many other Americans, she's had her share of therapy. Lost and floating, Sheila wraps herself in a form of cosmic selfhood. When interviewed about her religion by a team of sociologists for *Habits of the Heart,* a study of individualism and commitment in the nation's life, she responded that she believes in "Sheilaism": "I believe in God. I'm not a religious fanatic. I can't remember the last time I went to church. My faith has carried me a long way. It's Sheilaism. Just my own little voice." One doesn't know whether to laugh or weep at such goopy nonthought.

I rush to say that politics is not the issue here. Quite the contrary. People across the political spectrum should be disturbed by a feel-good society that masks the real issues with cotton candy rather than confront them. Sorry folks. Whatever your politics, everything is not beautiful in its own way, as the song would have us believe. Life comes with its ugliness, no matter how we'd like to pretend otherwise. Starving children are not beautiful. The pollution of our air is not beautiful. Certainly war is not beautiful. Yet if we insist on dealing with such problems by launching balloons for peace or gathering at night to light candles and send them floating off down rivers, we're in for a big fall, as my mother could have told us long ago.

The problem in a mass culture is that when such sloppy nonthought gets loose, it starts oozing into every aspect of our lives. And here we're getting to the nub of things as concerns words and their potential to heal. While visiting a large university recently, I happened to open its catalog to a course called "Poetry Therapy." The idea was that in the process of writing poetry students would bring their innermost troubles to the surface, where they could be dealt with. That's fine with me. If people have troubles, they should be addressed, and if it takes such a course to do it, all to the better. But what might make good therapy does not necessarily make good art. Revealing our innermost feelings doesn't automatically create a decent poem. Yet in the current mindset proclaiming that everything is beautiful in its own way, we lack discrimination, and the danger of confusing the two acts, of therapy and writing a poem—of saying, "I felt it; therefore, it's good"—is all too real. Still stuck in the 60's swamp of "relevance," we've perverted words to our own self-absorbed ends; we measure their worth only as they have something immediately to do with us. In a society that validates self-absorption, anything else becomes irrelevant. Whether reading Harlequin novels or writing poetry, our culture seems hellbent-for-leather to delude itself.

Cynics will leap forward to point out that every society in the world does that, deludes itself one way or another. They're right. The Romans had a ludicrous hodgepodge of gods, yet they managed to run an empire. The Indians I lived with once had a charmingly Alice-in-Wonderland mythology about how plants and animals came to be. The difference between the illusions of those two groups and ours is that theirs had little to do with their day-to-day lives. In contrast, we've moved our delusions to the very center of our lives and try to live according to them. The Good Lord only knows how many people long for a real-life love affair à la their favorite soap opera, how many are trying to "discover" themselves through writing poetry.

Perhaps we can get some perspective on this by considering what anthropologist Margaret Mead said in an essay of some time back—you know, back in the '50s when we were discovering that each of us was an anxiety-ridden glob of Jell-O shaken by a heartless system, back when we were discovering that it was chic to be a victim. Yes, she says in "One Vote for This Age of Anxiety," we do live in times of constant stress and frustration, with bills to pay, appointments to keep, etc. But compare that with some poor woodcutter out in the jungle, worried that at any moment a tiger will jump out from behind and tear him limb from limb while he screams his life away. Or the uncounted families in the Third World who each day wake to another day of hunger. By comparison our worries about picking up the shirts from the laundry after work are trifles indeed. Mead's message: Stop your belly aching and get on with what's important in your life.

But we don't *want* to stop our bellyaching. It feels so good. And we've enlisted words to massage us in our sloughs of post-industrial despair. By necessity our evidence is anecdotal, but pick up just about any literary magazine and you'll find poem after poem, short story after short story, at turns bitching and dejected, written in the hypermenorrhoeic mode, as if they're messages to the world from individuals in their private asylums. I think words deserve better than that. I think we as human beings deserve better than that, but we've been sorely misled, we've bought a bill of goods and believe that our bitches and gripes should be the proper stuff of art, the pivot of the universe.

Such fey thinking comes about because of a confusion. Early in Tom Robbins' *Another Roadside Attraction,* if I remember correctly, winsome Amanda approaches an old Navajo man making a sand painting. Their conversation goes something like this:

"What's the purpose of art?" she asks him.

The reply: "The purpose of art is to give us what life does not."

Ah, wisdom. Contrary to what we've been told from creative-writing units in the second grade on, the purpose of art is not self-expression, not to get stuck on ourselves, but the hard work of getting out of ourselves and exploring what's beyond. "But I'll lose my individuality. I'll lose my voice," come the protests. Nonsense. Your individuality will come through well enough all by itself. And it'll be improved!

In contemporary poetry, take a David Kirby or an X.J. Kennedy. Yes, their work sometimes draws on their personal lives. They, too, have woes and joys often appearing in their poems. But it's what they do with them that counts. In their poems they make something of them, make more of them than what they are in life. And so such poems triumph. And so, I'd argue, such use of words represents real healing, a real rescue of emotions for a better purpose. But examples from contemporary poetry are hard to come by. By the tens of thousands we've been taught that writing poetry is the easiest art possible. Anybody can do it. Just pick up a pen and tell us how you feel.

Things start looking brighter if we turn to nature essays. True, the field has its share of folks who step into the woods looking on nature as a grand psychiatrist. But nature writers have what poets often do not, or at least, don't recognize. They have a subject out there before them. And some of them have the smarts to realize that they have to study it, to know something about it, before they start gushing words. And—let's click our heels!—the list of such writers is long. John McPhee, Faith McNulty, Robert Wallace come immediately to mind, and they're only a small part of a long line going back to John Muir, Mary Austin, and Aldo Leopold.

For a brief example, let's take a look at Ann Zwinger, a Colorado housewife turned nature writer who prides herself on being a largely self-taught scholar. Pack strapped to her back, she wanders alone through an isolated canyon in the desert of southeastern Utah. She's intensely alert, open to what's around her. In *Wind in the Rock*, she pauses before a great sandstone cliff and later writes of the "massive dignity about sandstone beds that tell of a past long before human breathing, that bear the patterns of ancient winds and water in their cross-beddings." What does that tell us about Zwinger? Nothing. In fact, she's reduced the human element to a speck in time. But it gives us more than what her personality probably would have. It gives us what life does not, hers or ours. It charges us with wonder, attaches us to forces outside ourselves. Yet for those worrying about losing individuality, her life indeed is there, behind every word, a life of study and much thought, and, no doubt, personal turmoil, all that pushing behind her before she comes to the insight. But it's the insight that counts. And that's where the healing is, for her and for us.

In this context, let's swing back to wanderer John C. Van Dyke. We find him around the century's turn doing an extraordinary thing for the times. In those days, people despised the deserts of the American Southwest as useless stretches of cactus and rocks, as God's mistakes in shaping Creation. They feared the hot and nearly waterless expanses as sinkholes for humanity. People wandered off into them and never returned—victims of thirst, howling wolves, and bandits. So at least it was widely believed. Then what's Van Dyke doing out there alone, traveling on horseback for thousands of miles, deep into Mexico, over into Texas and into Arizona? He's just looking around.

By now he has become an art critic. In fact one of the best-known art critics of his day. And when he looks at this strange land of surreal heat and contorted thorn bushes he sees it in a new way, not as a bleak place, but as a realm of astonishingly beautiful forms and colors, a realm of mystery. Then he writes *The Desert,* the first book to praise America's arid sweeps. For him they are ever-changing tapestries of subtle forms and colors, lands of "indigo lizards," of "misshapen," orange-hued moons, lands where the sand dunes flow in waves "as graceful as the lines of running water."

We know from other sources that he had a horrendous time of it out there trying to survive. At times he couldn't find water; sometimes he had no idea where he was. He was attacked by wolves, Indians menaced him in Mexico, and outlaws almost riddled him with bullets. Not to mention that he was sick with a respiratory ailment and at times close to death. And, oh, I almost forgot. He probably also had malaria.

What a thriller, what a cliffhanger he could have written!

But there's almost nary a mention of any of this in the pages of *The Desert.* There's not a person in the book—not one of the Indians, cowboys, desperados, or crazed Mexican revolutionaries he surely met and that the public was slavering to read about. Instead, as does Zwinger, Van Dyke keeps his celebration focussed on the vast and thrilling galleries of nature all around him. And in so doing, Van Dyke creates one of the most individualistic works via his particular use of imagery. He must have done something right. *The Desert* is the most highly celebrated book of its kind ever published, almost a cult book for desert lovers, and after nearly a hundred years still in print. Call such a hard-won and well-worked volume one of those rare triumphs that art enjoys now and then, call it real healing for the pleasure it continues to give us.

Well, I don't suppose it makes much sense to get over-wrought about our culture's massive counter-tug of self-absorption. Maybe, unlike Van Dyke, those of us who grew up in the nearly unbroken good times since the Second World War are spoiled; saddled with the high expectations learned in America's longest period of prosperity, we believe that things will get better and better as life goes on, and when they don't, when we suffer setbacks and disappointments, we go belly up and get sulky. Maybe every affluent society eventually lapses into that. Maybe the various fads in art that come and go every few years are in the hands of the gods, in the stars, follow the turns of the stock market, whatever, and we as individuals can't do a great deal to change them. Yet as individual writers, being aware of the situation gives us strength; it gives us the long view of the values we're pursuing, and then we can decide—damn the torpedoes!—what we'll write and how we'll write it. The deep commitment to words, the larger work we've cut out for ourselves that Sheila probably couldn't imagine, brings its own sense of wholeness.

Allen Woodman

THE CHRISTIAN VENTRILOQUIST

Even as a child, my lips were rigid. My entire body was very still. I used to sit for hours, not moving, not speaking. My father was embarrassed to bring his friends home for lunch. He called me Dummy. My mother longed for possibilities. She thought my silence bred some kind of genius.

She would take me to the music stores and set me on piano stools and place French horns and clarinets in my hands, but still my fingers did not decorously flex, my mouth remained frozen.

It was when my mother had only one aspirin left in the bottle in the medicine cabinet over the kitchen sink, after my father had long since left over the purchase of expensive art supplies, that her inspiration came. She borrowed a TV from Uncle Hoot. She had him fix an antenna onto a pole for better reception. She set me on a little blue bathroom rug in front of the television all day long. She felt the technology would help. Every few minutes she would stop her housework and walk into the room to see what was showing on the screen and see if the sight of it had changed my posture or expression.

Her wish for shape and purpose in my life turned to despair when my hands did not tremble before the visions of Lawrence Welk or Liberace. But then my throat betrayed me.

During an Edgar Bergen movie, as Bergen made his ventriloquist doll, Charlie McCarthy, talk, my throat began to vibrate. It was a cough or a vowel sound, I've never been quite sure which, but my mother came running, and there I was with my jaw and lips rigid, and my throat making ugly sounds that held for her so much beauty and hope.

Then we were in the car driving to Eastbrook Shopping Center, to Woolworth's, and the Dixie Rexall. Then we were whirling down aisles, my mother's hands disappearing under stacks of Mr. Potato Head sets and Barbie Doll Dream Houses.

The druggist at the Rexall sold my mother a special device from a rack of colorful gimmicks. It was in a plastic pouch right next to the finger-snapper pack of gum and the plastic dog poop.

The paper inside the pouch showed a workman carrying a steamer trunk on his back, startled by a voice coming from inside saying, "Let me out of here." It was a mechanism for "Throwing Your Voice." My mother bought it, and, back in the car, she made me put the small whistle, the sole contents of the pouch, in my mouth.

I could not throw my voice to another place or even speak a word. I could only make the sounds of a high-pitched whistle. My mother threw the disc out the window like a tiny, silver bird.

At Toyland, her search ended. There in the back of the store, next to the model kits of the Knights of the Round Table, was a genuine Charlie McCarthy ventriloquist doll, dressed in his familiar black tuxedo, top hat, and monocle.

At home we found the string that operated his mouth. It came from a tiny hole in the back of his neck.

For the next two weeks, my mother would read the pamphlet that came with the doll to me and help me with the exercises. She would put me in front of her makeup mirror, on her knee, and I would put Charlie McCarthy on my knee. She would help me recite the alphabet, and when my lips lost their tight control, she would pinch me on the arm with her long red fingernails. We left out six letters: B, F, M, P, V, and W. My mother said the instructions told how we would learn the substitute sounds for these labials and plosives later. She worked at night coming up with words and phrases that didn't use them.

For days the words came with violence or vanished without a trace or sometimes my lips would bend down out of their fixed smile and my breath would heave like a pigeon's breast. And still my mother would hold me and remind my skin of my mouth's imperfect murmurings. Until, one by one, the letters came and then the words and phrases. Until, with each breath, I could faultlessly hiss, "She sells sea shells Sunday at the seashore."

She sewed a tuxedo for me that looked just like Charlie McCarthy's. She made a monocle for me out of a broken pair of eyeglasses. She had to buy a top hat at a dance supply store.

Next, we were standing in the Garden Club Room in the back of Flink's City Florist. The women all wore the same dust colored dresses. Each held in her hand her favorite variety of daffodil. There were trumpet and large-cupped blooms and a sprinkling of doubles and short-cups in cluster types. The flowers ranged in color from deep gold to pure white.

I was billed as Little Ed and Charlie Jr., and, after a short script my mother had borrowed from an old Shari Lewis TV show, my finale arrived.

My mother had driven to Atlanta and spent almost ten dollars at a magic shop for a trick glass that appeared to make milk vanish. It only took a small amount of liquid to make the glass look full, and an inner chamber caught the liquid when the glass was tilted and spread it out so that it looked as if I were actually drinking the milk. My mouth was freed up behind the glass to form even the toughest of sounds.

As I held the glass to my lips and pretended to drink, I recited a Wordsworth poem, "I wandered lonely as a cloud that floats on high o'er vales and hills...." I made my Adam's apple bob up and down as if I were drinking. "When all at once I saw a crowd, a host of golden daffodils ..." And as I continued reciting, the ladies in the group stood up in unison and thrust their prized flowers in the air and began to sway vigorously absorbed in the landscape of blooms.

"And then my heart with pleasure fills, and dances with the daffodils," I finished. My mother thanked the ladies and added that it was a special pleasure to be there today since it was also my seventh birthday. I had already had my seventh birthday two months before, but just the thought of it brought the ladies marching forward to embrace me against their thick white necks and still larger chests and press a dollar each into my tiny hand.

For eight years my mother kept me in the public eye with bookings at nursing homes, American Legion posts, and Elk's Clubs in Mobile, Dothan, Selma, and Montgomery. She developed a fancy anti-smoking script where Charlie Jr. appears to blow out my match every time I tried to light up a cigarette. The PTA loved the idea and we were invited to almost every elementary school in Alabama and Georgia.

When I was sixteen, my mother met a man who owned three doughnut shops in Birmingham. We were the guest act at the grand opening of his fourth store. After the show, he took us back to his house for dinner.

Charlie Jr., and I sat in the dirty kitchen. I ate a box of day-old crullers. My mother and the man watched TV in the living room.

My mother kept making this loud laugh. It sounded like a crow. I peeked out the kitchen door. My mother had her dress pulled up. She was sitting on the man's knee. He kept whispering something to her, something he wanted her to say.

I sat back down at the kitchen table. Charlie Jr., sat in the chair next to me. We were still dressed exactly alike in our matching tuxedos, except I had taken my hat and monocle off and left them in the man's car.

I started to eat some chocolate twists, but my eyes kept looking at Charlie Jr. He seemed to keep getting smaller and smaller, or maybe it was just that I felt like I was getting bigger and bigger.

I walked out the back door of the house to get some air. The stars over the trees and houses in the neighborhood seemed so tiny. I kept walking.

Dressed in the black tuxedo, I had no trouble catching rides. Truckers would stop just to rib me about how I must have gotten lost from my senior prom.

I headed south for Gulf Shores. Once, Mom and I had stopped for gas there on our way from Pensacola to Mobile. It was a beautiful little place along the coast of Alabama with the whitest sand I had ever seen. And towering above the sand, just under the bright sky, were golden yellow beach houses stuck up proudly on pylons. I wanted to stand very still in the sand and look out into the green water of the Gulf of Mexico and know that silence was the best language ever spoken, but we were on a schedule and due in two hours at a women's club tea room in Mobile.

I arrived at Gulf Shores at dawn. I walked out beside the Pink Pony Pub and the Sea Horse Motel to where the water met the jagged creosote poles of a decaying fishing pier.

The water moved towards me in graceful ripples that reminded me of the way a magician's silk scarf might flow in front of him just before it changes colors between his huge palms. I did not think about what I would do the rest of the day or the next. I did not think about how odd I would appear dressed in formal wear, standing perfectly still in the white sand when the others arrived with their coolers and Hang Ten towels and Frisbees. The beauty of the Gulf carried no overwhelming need of thought.

I stayed on the beach all day, sometimes standing, sometimes sitting, hoping that the sun would fade away the black fabric of my clothes and hoping that the salt would corrode the leather and brass of my shoes; but by evening all I could feel changed was the exposed skin on my face and hands. As the night closed in, I took my shoes and socks off and dug my toes into the giving sand, unconcerned with what life lay beneath it, the sand crabs and spiders. I looked into the moving water, my eyesight failing, searching for the dark outline of boats moving beyond the sandbar.

I wondered if people out on those boats would be able to see me sitting so motionless on the shore. And then I heard whistling. It was not the metallic sound of my first ventriloquist whistle. It was the sweet human sound of air pressed between lips. At first, I could only see the glint of something silver, something barely the size of a woman's slip showing beneath a hemline. Then, as the figure approached, the silvery form revealed itself as the aluminum leg of a summer lawn chair.

A young woman carrying the chair unfolded it next to me as if I were invisible. She pulled a beer off of a plastic ring that retained two others. She wore a one-piece bathing suit with a sweater tied around her thin waist. Her legs were as white as a pearl against the dark air.

She began whistling again in between sips of beer. The tune meant nothing. Then she stopped and wet her lips with her tongue. I looked down at her feet. Her toes were long and beautiful. I wanted to form some words to say to her. I thought of phrases that would be easy to say. But I feared if I opened my mouth only a stream of air brighter than the aluminum of her chair, whiter than her legs, would come out, arching between us, breaking the perfect silence.

She turned towards me and offered me one of the two remaining cans of beer. Her well-formed mouth invited me with a smile. I took the can and opened the pop-top and watched the beer foam through the small opening. I held the beer up in a kind of a toast. "To the Gulf," I said, "that swallows up everything." Then she tried to speak, but her lovely face twisted and jerked and tried to catch that receding tide of language. Her labor for vowels and consonants told me of her drunkenness.

She could not tie words together to ask of my attire or name. But just her look, past speech, asked me to return with her, carrying the lawn chair back to the only brick cabin on the beach. And there on the bed, under a wooden ceiling fan, she communicated with her breath and tongue against my skin, stopping only to turn the dial of a portable radio that hung from the bedpost by a strap to suitable music.

I awoke to catch the sun at every window. She was lying quietly on top of the sheets.

Then I showered and used a large red beach towel to dry up the water I'd splashed onto the bathroom tile. I looked through her cabinets for some deodorant. I used her toothbrush. I wanted to wake her up with kisses for her eyes and mouth. I wanted to tell her things about why I was on the beach in a tuxedo and ask her about her own night vigil. I wanted to ask her name so I could blow the word sweetly back to her over a generous breakfast of fresh peaches and figs. I wanted to wrap us both in words like soft animal skins. But the telephone rang in the other room.

I opened the bathroom door to see her standing naked, lit in silhouette by the white-lighted window. Her face struggled again to conquer simple words. Her "hello" and "yes" fought their way from her mouth like air from a drowning man's lungs. One side of her mouth pulled tightly while the other side seemed to stretch wide enough to swallow an egg. It brought back the violence of my first struggle, my imperfect words.

It had not been drunkenness the night before but something else.

She hung up the black phone. She wrapped the sheet around her. I dressed and explained that I was going out to look for a job, that I would be back later, but her eyes could see my invention.

She turned and toyed with the radio. It seemed harder to get the right station during the day.

After that, I lived for awhile over the Mother of Pearl Dry Cleaners in Mobile. I found a job service that would send me out about three days a week. On the days I didn't work, I just stayed in my room and listened to the steam presses below until I felt too sweaty and stiff to move.

The service had me fill out a list of interests and hobbies, but the jobs never seemed to match them. For several weeks I worked in an ice house shucking oysters and cleaning crabs, and then I worked a few days emptying trash cans and sorting mail at the newspaper office.

One morning the phone rang. A man from the service asked me to stop by the main office. He called it the *main office*, but I knew they only had one room in a building down on Magnolia Street.

When I arrived the man had my list of interests and hobbies laying in front of him on his desk. He picked it up and fanned his big face with it. He told me how the service prided itself on placing applicants with the right jobs. His lips seemed to move too much for the few words he was saying. It was almost like his words were dubbed.

He smiled and asked me if I wanted coffee. He said the job would last for at least six weeks. He chewed a bit on the end of his pen. He wanted to make sure that I planned to stay in town on the job. There would a bonus at the end if I did. He gave me the address card.

It was the largest church in Mobile. The banner out front read "Summer Christian Youth Festival." The reverend took me down a long hall to my classroom. Along the way, he informed me of words and subjects he didn't want me to use in front of the children. He took great delight in going through his mental list as if he had recited it over to himself many times before in private. He also told me he'd be happy to go over the routines and dialogue that I planned to use later for the final Christian Youth Recital.

In the room, I was surrounded by children, all between the ages of six and eight. In each of their laps they held the innocent dummies. The dummies were all fashioned after religious models. Most of the boys had small fiberglass figures of Jesus sitting on their knees, and the girls had been given Virgin Mary dolls. On the instructor's desk in front of the room were other costumed forms of angels, wise men, and even a special baby Jesus in a basket figure. It was my first class in Christian Ventriloquism.

I slipped my hand inside the baby Jesus figure and found the metal levers that controlled his eyes, mouth, and head movements. The inside of the dummy felt hard like a seashell empty of its soft mollusk.

As I cradled the basket in my lap, I told the boys and girls how to find the control levers in the back of their dummies. They practiced manipulating them.

The cow-eyes of the dummies winked. The heads turned. One of the girls had a more expensive figure than the rest. She could get her Mary doll to wiggle her ears. All of the children wanted to trade with her.

The children laughed and laughed. Then it was time to give them voice. I told them how to hold their jaws rigid. I taught them how to smile and keep their teeth slightly parted. I had them all repeat the simplest of sounds, the sounds made without the use of lips.

I looked around the room and saw the children smiling and heard their droning noises seemingly coming from the sacred figures swaying on their knees. "Ay," I said. Then they mimicked the sound through clinched lips and teeth. "EE," I cried. Again, they repeated it. "EYE ... OH ... YOU."

Then phrases returned from my youth, "She sells sea shells Sunday by the seashore." The skin on their small faces tightened and strained as I forced them to form harder and still harder sounds and phrases, faster and faster, and in louder voices. "Satan sell sea shells Sunday by the seashore."

Their mouths became ugly machines, twisting up and transforming air into sound into life for their faithful dummies. Their struggling faces reminded me of the woman on the beach. Their gasping for the consummate voice, her gasping, my gasping. "Kum Ba Yah," my baby Jesus shouted for them to sing. "Kum Ba Yah," it shouted and shouted. And the girl with the fancy Virgin Mary began to cry and one of the others ran out of the room trampling over his fallen figure of Jesus as he ran to get the reverend back, and my lungs felt like they were going to explode and send my heart pounding into the engulfing past.

I'd scare you if I told you any more. I'll only say that after the service let me go, I tried to call my mother. Every time she answered the phone, I couldn't speak. It was too painful. All I could do was listen. She kept shouting, "Speak up! Speak up!"

I thought of going back to the woman on the beach, but I knew it would never work with two dummies. There was only one alternative left.

I'd once read about how in the sixth century before Christ there was a temple built in a place called Delphi. Sometimes the priests there would stand very still and listen for strained sounds to come out of their stomachs. Words would form, but their lips would not move. Then one of the priests would try to interpret the belly-noise for someone who had come to them seeking the advice of the gods. But one day all of the oracles fell silent.

And now, sitting in my small room over the dry cleaners, I wait for their return because I know that memory and loss are just mirrors and time itself comes back like a reflection. And circumspect, I will wait for that tiny private voice within to articulate all possible things, and I will generously listen so quietly and so still that I will hardly be here at all.

E. P. Bollier

AFTER TALKING ABOUT POETRY
for William Greenway

How to explain, even to myself,
why at midnight I write a poem,
or try to write what I hope is a poem,
when I have nothing to say except

I hope. Hope is enough, you said,
to justify writing, hope that something
will jell into words, and words, meaning.
But what if meaning at dawn is left

behind like cracker crumbs in the bed
from which I rise to face tomorrow
with yesterday's beard in morning's mirror
to concentrate the intellect

on other losses? Do not regret,
you said, poems are made from losses—
why even the morning's stubble proposes
a metaphor to say the unsaid.

Of course, you're right. Loss is less
if out of it comes something creative.
So I'll sit here, contemplating
until dawn. Nevertheless....

Leon V. Driskell

READING NAMES AT THE MUSEUM

The woman before me grieved for a son.
So did the woman who followed me.
Both of them about my age, one black
and one white. The last name the woman
before me read was her son's name.
Keep the love alive, she said to me.
She indicated the column of names where
I should start reading. In front of me
hung parts of the quilt. Beside certain
panels, stood mothers, sisters, maybe lovers.
They wore lavender ribbons like mine.
The visitors moved slow; they stood to read
the names, some penciled, some stencilled,
some embroidered, or appliqued on the quilt.

Scott's Mom tells him death's not so bad;
it's as if he has gone into another room,
but she can talk to him still. About some
of the dead, placards tell more.
A mother and grandmother, age sixty-seven,
opened her heart to everyone—choirs on tour,
refugees, foreign students ate her food, slept
in her home. Nephews and nieces tell Uncle Gregg
that they miss him. Hospice recalls Willard,
whom no one else would take. They say they learned
from Willard, learned about love. An automotive
worker, stricken in Toledo, took refuge
in his sister's home to die. He knew antiques
and glassware; she feared what the neighbors
would do should they know her house
harbored somebody with AIDS.

I am reading aloud some
of the names, small print, several columns per page.
Each name needs to be sounded, given its time,
said distinctly. Some names are complete with titles
and middle initials. (Thus, I discover one
long-time-ago friend I did not know had died.)
Others are reduced to initials, some to nicknames.

I am reading the names that begin with M.
Maria. Little Maria. Maldonado—many with this name.
Someone began reading the names that begin with A
four hours ago. **Martin** (many of them). **Mendez.**
Sue tells me enough have died to populate a city.

My voice rises above the talk of the visitors
standing before the quilt. Others watch and listen
to TV monitors and perhaps recognize a name.
Maybe they hear the name they came to hear.
I read **Mapplethorpe,** a name deserving honors,
recognized now perhaps because of the hate his art
unleashed. Others I name doubtless were artists.
Our friend Barbara designed a quilt, blueprinted
photographs on it: **I have my friends to keep me warm.**
I sleep under a quilt my almost-blind aunt made.
Her note, accompanying the gift, says that the Amish
put flaws in their quilts as a reminder that only
God is perfect. She says she couldn't **help** her flaws.

A woman's hand touches my shoulder.
I place my finger on the column of names
where I stop and she begins. She starts
strong: **I read in memory of my precious son.**
Her daughter watches, ready to take over and read
the names should her mother falter.

          I move into the group
looking at the quilt, and hug my former student—
Loretta's daughter. **Yes, she's lost many friends,
her fiance last May.** She's glad I read.
Another young friend waits to speak. I feel
the softness of her Afro when we hug. Stewart
gives me a message from his mother.
It seems we are all family here.

I buy a t-shirt and buttons commemorating
The Names Project. I pin a button to my lapel.
See the Quilt, it reads, **and understand.**
I return to the panel with Scott's Mom's message.
I have seen part of the quilt, but do not understand.
I have not today read my sons' names, or my daughters'.
They are alive, my daughters and sons.

The woman who reads after me had finished now.
She is talking to the woman who read before me.

Keep the love alive, they say.
A man reads now. We are scarcely into the N's.
At the museum revolving door, a volunteer
tells me it's too pretty a day to spend inside.

I walk into the first day of September.

Eugene Walter

HEALING AND POETRY

It is only, relatively speaking, a few seconds of time since Logic was enthroned and her three grandmothers, the three Eyes, were sent off to their various St. Helenas, Siberias, and Washington, DCs. The three I's—Instinct, Imagination, Intuition—had ruled since the Cave Age, not as primitive a period in human history as some would have it. Time was a parabola then, sustained by the Three Eyes, not a nervous shudder sustained by the so-called Fact, so-called Statistics and so-called Order.

The three Eyes are in the head, the navel, and the crotch. Logic lives in the back of the neck.

Every single sound employed by humans to communicate contains some secret pun, or joke. Fact spelled backwards is Tcaf, and giving the "tc" a Russian pronunciation you get "chaff." Statistics is Scitsitats which becomes "Skittish Cats" and Order is nothing but "redro" which is "retro."

The word "heal" is the same as "hale" and "whole"; "poetry" in its Old French and Latin roots means first of all "Art" and then words with rhythm, or meter, or patting your foot in time.

Colors, music/poetry, laughter have been considered healing agents since the human creature stood up on its hind legs and grunted an *oom-pah-pah*.

Some very distinguished British scientists have come to consider that much cancer is a result of hidden boredom.

Since time immemorial South American Indians have successfully used an intensely-purple-blue flower as a remedy for headache. All you do is stare intently at the bloom while a repeated three-note motive is played on the flute.

***

"In the beginning was the word ..." We all know that phrase in its usual context: Christian. But in every culture, every country, every era, there is the eternally repeated idea that in giving something its correct name, in precisely identifying anything at all, one learns its complete function and destroys its power to harm. Look at Rumpelstiltskin, Tom-Tit-Tot, etc.

Since analytical measures have taken over, everything is geared to digging in the subconscious; when are we all going up into the attic—the sopra-conscious—and see what's stored in those old trunks, hat-boxes, and cardboard cartons? And only poets know that there is a sub-subconscious—a sub-cellar where countless dictionaries of forgotten words are stored along with Medusa's false-teeth, horseshoes for centaurs, and Bette Davis' first mascara pot. Woe to the family that hasn't kept spare horse-shoes for its centaurs: things *will* get trampled!

When a doctor identifies an ailment and calls it by the name doctors call it by, the patients, if not altogether too far gone, seize on the name and consult the three eyes, those I's, and thereby all the mechanics they employ to identify the ailment for themselves.

I mean, to find his name for it, and their own cure. I mean, we all have a strange and wonderful system, *not yet named or defined*, inside each and every one of us, which can heal: I mean that is-it-subconscious, is-it-sopraconscious blend of folklore, poetry, family history in the veins, which sets the system in function in that highly personal individual three-eye, three-I computer, data bank, microwave, fax, word processor, music box, alarm clock, cuckoo clock, xerox, churn, mixmaster, pencil-sharpener, shoe-brush complex inside us which still has no name!

I mean the vast, universal yet personal not-yet-understood complex of electrical impulses, selective memories, portable plumbing, real world and unreal even-more-real world we carry inside us.

Laughing, patting your foot, finding the right word is the beginning of all healing.

Logic spelled backwards is "cigol" which is "cigale" another name for the great grasshopper. So hop, friend, hop and sing, pat your foot, take a year off and consider the real facts of life as shown by the three I's and study the worlds of the cats and the monkeys and indeed all our mammal cousins struggling as are we with the mythology of the real and the reality of the myth.

***

The doctor can suggest a remedy but only individual patients can find inside themselves the authentic name for the malady.

FIND THE WORD!

The greatest minds are able to change the word, thereby change the coloration of their problems, even find the energy to cure or at least stall indefinitely the uneasiness, the dis-easiness.

***

So find the Word. Out of all. Not the Tower of Babel but the Power of Able.

***

> Words like gadflies fan the brain,
> Will change their forms and fly again:
> For Pain is Chain and Chain is Chide,
> And Chide is Hide and Hide is Hoard,
> And Hoard is Bored and Bored is Lose,
> And Rose is Nose and Pear is Pose,
> And Rare is Pear and Ruse is Rose,
> And Roar is Fear and Fear is Prose,
> So, SING, Sillies All, till the Sun is done!

Richard Moore

WORDS AND HEALING:
WHAT'S IN IT FOR THE POET?

Aristotle is perfectly clear about the healing effect he thought the words of tragedy should have on us: "Tragedy... through pity and fear" accomplishes "the proper purgation of those emotions." The great philosopher was a pristine ancient Greek for whom emotions of any kind were a distraction, a nuisance, and in their extreme forms, a sickness. They wounded one's tranquility. It was not that out latter-day obsessions with and indulgence of emotion—as, say, the hot pangs of sensuality and love—were unfamiliar to him. One can even argue that the Greeks must have had such feelings in greater intensity and abundance than we, since emotions— even "good" emotions like "pity"—seem to have been an ever-present annoyance rather than a rare delight.

But if that is the healing effect that poetry should have on its audience, what effect should it have on the poet? What does he or she "get out of it"—or lose to it? Is the poet like the doctor who suffers with his patient—which, in the days before the brisk efficiency of scientific medicine, was about all a doctor could do? Some years ago when my physician and I—in those days when I could still afford one—were discussing the size of his bill, he asserted that members of his profession were not overpaid, as I claimed, because they suffered sympathetically with their patients as part of the healing process: they paid dearly in their own flesh, so to speak, and it was but a poor recompense to pay them mere currency in return. Sometimes poets and our attitudes toward them seem a little like that. There was, for example, the spectacle of Dylan Thomas drinking his way through America, tearing those poems of dark passion, soaked in that rich baritone, out of his bleeding throat. Was he, like my physician (or even like Jesus Himself), suffering, if not to make us well, at least to make us feel better about being sick? Then there were the agonies of Sexton, Berryman, Plath, so thrilling, so exciting, so brilliantly authenticated by their deaths ...

These are, I dare not doubt, wonderful phenomena; but they may not exhaust the possibilities of a poet's relationship to his poems. After all, the majority of poets, including the greatest, seem to have led orderly, even quiet, lives and to have died peacefully in their beds. Could it be that their poems somehow healed them as well as us? There is that well-known dictum of Robert Frost, that a true poem's conclusion must be unforeseen by the poet because, as Frost put it: "no surprise for the poet, no surprise for the reader." This suggests that a poems's effect on the poet may be much like its effect on us. For the present purpose, one may emend Frost's remark to read: "no cure for the poet, no cure for the reader." In place of the Savior who suffers for us all, we may offer instead the equally sacred Pharaoh of ancient Egypt, whose destiny in life (and death) seems to have been *triumph* for us all. It seems to have been enough for the mortal peasants of those dark times that the king alone should journey into eternal life. Indeed, the ideas of holy suffering and holy enjoyment do not always stay neatly distinct. Lucretius, for example, would clearly have regarded the Pharaoh's destiny of eternal life as a terrible burden. The great comfort for Lucretius was that, as he believed, there *was* no eternal life.

If the poet is purging himself of "sick" emotions at the same time that his poem is purging us, then clearly he (or she) is very personally and intimately involved with the poem. This tallies with our untutored feelings when we respond to most good poetry. Shakespeare's great hold on even the sophisticated audiences through the centuries seems to be related to the impression of personal involvement that he gives to each play and poem—even when the plays and poems, taken together, seem to imply a personality too vast and various to fit into a single human being.

But this is naive, it has been the fashion among critics to say. We know virtually nothing about even the "facts" of Shakespeare's life. To take his art as testimony of his emotions belittles the art and distracts us from it. Clearly he was not—certainly not primarily—"expressing himself" at all; he was merely trying to make good plays and poems—that is, verbal structures and scenarios that would work on and gain the approval of this or that audience. There is even some evidence that, if he did use his private emotions "to get the artistic job done," he did so reluctantly and even surreptitiously. He seems, for example, to have kept his sonnets out of the hands of printers for as long as he possibly could, precisely because they were—or seemed to be—more personal than his other poems.

This observation introduces a new twist to our account. If some poets have made "displays" of themselves, others have been unusually furtive in their personal involvements with their poems. Yeats springs to mind in this respect. We remember Richard Ellmann's remark that, in his early poems at least, Yeats conceals far more than he reveals. Sometimes, having confided too much, he even made faintly ridiculous attempts to have his poems misinterpreted—"The Dolls," for example. Yeats' note on the poem is so misleading that we had better carefully read the poem itself before we expose ourselves to the comment.

THE DOLLS

A doll in the doll-maker's house
Looks at the cradle and bawls:
'That is an insult to us.'
But the oldest of all the dolls,
Who had seen, being kept for show,
Generations of his sort,
Out-screams the whole shelf: 'Although
There's not a man can report
Evil of this place,
The man and the woman bring
Hither, to our disgrace,
A noisy and filthy thing.'
Hearing him groan and stretch

> The doll-maker's wife is aware
> Her husband has heard the wretch,
> And crouched by the arm of his chair,
> She murmurs into his ear,
> Head upon shoulder leant:
> 'My dear, my dear, O dear,'
> It was an accident.'

The poem is not really the mystery that it may seem at first glance, but has the character rather of a riddle that becomes immediately clear once the "key" occurs to us. The doll-maker and his dolls, that seem alive but are really just inanimate objects he has made, are like the poet and his poems. And it is equally clear that the "noisy and filthy thing" (because it cries and needs its diapers changed) that resides in a "cradle" is an actual human baby. Yeats was neither the first nor the last artist to feel that the demands of a family threatened his art, and the poem expresses such anxieties and conflicts with grace and exactitude—as when we expect the older doll to speak with wisdom and moderation, as befits age and experience, but hear instead that he "out-screams the whole shelf." The delightfully comic surprise emphasizes the inhumanity of artistic ambition: the dolls in this are like Homer's gods and goddesses, carrying out their heartless little comedy in the heavens. The portrayal of the wife in this situation is fine and touching. She is aware that her husband has heard "the wretch"—her word, but also the husband's word, who is trying, we suppose, to be a good father. Of course, the child is "an accident" in the obvious way that most children are; but the term also has a precise meaning in the Platonic philosophy that Yeats loved: the accidental is all that which merely *happens*—by chance, "hap"—without rhyme or reason in the mess and misery of earthly life—as opposed to the non-happenings, the pure harmonies in the changeless world of art and ideas.

Now let us hear what Yeats has to say:

> The fable for this poem came into my head while I was giving some lectures in Dublin. I had noticed once again how all thought among us is frozen into 'something other than human life.' After I had made the poem, I looked up one day into the blue of the sky, and suddenly imagined, as if lost in the blue of the sky, stiff figures in procession. I remembered that they were the habitual image suggested by blue sky, and looking for a second fable called them 'The Magi,' complementary forms of those enraged dolls.

I don't see how one can escape the conclusion that Yeats is simply covering up the meaning and the true function of this fine and moving poem. He would doubtless have found the public avowal of its evident concerns embarrassing. He had become a solid (and solemn) presence in the literary world and had appearances to keep up. Yet the poem does heal. It reconciles professional ambition and the needs of ordinary life in a basically comic way—another reason why the vatic Yeats, who would own up to no hint of comedy in his poems, would have to deny it.... Why did he write it, then? Clearly because it heals in the way I have suggested. And this is why it remains one of his memorable poems—and why his contemporary, Thomas Hardy, who was free of many of Yeats' pretensions and embarrassments, may turn out eventually to have been the greater poet.

But Yeats and the critics are right: art is not life. There is more to it than imitation, than simply making an image—as Aristotle himself said. The image must also be harmonious—since those are the twin instincts in man from which art arises: the child's love of mimicry and the philosopher's need for order and harmony. Yeats' doctrine of the "mask" is in keeping with this distinction. When the lyric poet says "I," it is not the actual poet that is meant, not the poet whose telephone bill is overdue and who likes poached eggs for breakfast, but a generalized, perhaps even an idealized representation of some kind. Yeats even claimed that there was a "mask" and "opposite" to the poet's self somewhere among the mysteries which the poet must wear or become in order to utter his poem. Perhaps we may simplify that to the more obvious statement that we discover something about ourselves in our poems. We discover attitudes we didn't know we had that may frighten us at first but can ultimately enlarge us, resolve inner conflict, and so heal us. That may be the harmony to which Aristotle refers.

But we can sometimes also use this mask idea to defend ourselves—our ordinary, bill-paying selves—against the threat that such discoveries pose. We have just seen Yeats busy at a cover-up, perhaps even from himself. I know a woman who writes excellent poems which imply a brash, racy, thoroughly frank and uninhibited speaker. The woman herself is soft-spoken, shy—all, evidently, that the speaker of her poems is not. "The woman herself," we say and she says; but isn't this a case of a person playing different roles in different situations? How can she say with confidence which person is really her? And does it matter? For her to say, "That person portrayed in my poems is not the real me," is to dismiss the poems—is to say that they are mere "creations," "inventions ." The greatest art is not invention, but discovery. What it finds is really there—just as surely as the Second Law of Thermodynamics is really there.

Permit me to illustrate the complexities of this matter with an example from my own work. My second book is a rather grim or, as I prefer, a grimly comic sonnet sequence about living with my recently married English wife and our very young children in a converted farmhouse previously owned by my father in the hills of Vermont. Living there gave us many problems, the severest of which had to do with my rather unsatisfactory relationship with my parents in Connecticut and the need to make an extended visit to them twice a year. For some reason (or perhaps for no reason, since it was not a matter of reason) those visits moved me uncomfortably close to the edge of my sanity. I discovered to my surprise that writing the sonnets made the relationship much more tolerable. What I said to my parents on the visits and in the letters and phone calls grew milder, became human and acceptable to them, but was nothing at all like what I was saying to them in the sonnets. What was the reality, then? What was the true image of my parents in my mind?

I told myself at the time that in the poems I was exaggerating my feelings of anger in order to reflect certain historical themes, deepen the comic tone, and make a good story. Whether or not that was true, it was also true that our relations on the visits improved because I had begun to feel downright apologetic to my mother and father for the awful things I was saying about them in my poems. The more I think about this, the more I am struck by how utterly impossible it is to say where the "true image" of my parents is to be found. In many ways I was like the duplicitous politician saying different things to different constituencies. But aren't we all such politicians, merely dealing with every situation (getting along with our relatives, writing the best poems we can) with as much honesty *as possible*? (And when we demand more honesty than is possible in a given situation, we become ridiculous, like Moliére's Alceste.)

But surely such sleights of mind and sleazy prevarications will be exposed in the long run! Our parents, if no one else, will find us out—naughty children that we are. My first book had been a great comfort to my mother with the evidence that it provided—its publication, not the book itself—that I might not be addled after all. What would that second book have been for her? We shall never know, for she went to her grave many years later, entirely ignorant of its existence. Marvelous how concealable a book of poems can be! "Count your blessing, dear!" as she herself used to say.

So I escaped, and my devious self-healing and truth-telling went undetected—that time, at least. I was not always to be so lucky. In other stories later, there were descriptions of my own growing family which were understood by all at the time, I thought, to be ridiculous and ghoulish exaggerations. But they became true, as it turned out, and I am left with the scary possibilities, either that I had given a true account without daring to admit it to myself or, worse, that life had imitated art and my descriptions had reshaped human relationships in their image. Poetry, like all healing, can be dangerous. Sometimes the doctor kills the patient.

But doctors and patients, like poets and readers, are part of a pattern of life that we call civilized—a manner of doing things, a style, that is the source of our reality as people. Without such things, we would be—we will be—lost. This is the final healing: to achieve—to accept—an identity among our fellow human beings. We tell a story, as I have said, not primarily to please ourselves, but to bring the joy of laughter and weeping into the lives of others. But to make the story real, we put some part of ourselves into it; and to make it believable, we often dream up surprising versions of ourselves, make ourselves to blame, perhaps—or inept or absurd—and thus utter an otherwise intolerable truth under the pretense of just telling a good, believable story. The pleasure of telling the truth in the form of art mitigates its pain.

Wounding ourselves, we heal ourselves.

Jack Coulehan

ON MEDICINE AND POETRY

I.

I was asked to participate in a Poetry and Medicine workshop held at the Society for Health and Human Values meeting in Chicago, November 1990. The theme of this workshop was to explore the relationships between poetry and medical practice. This theme could be understood in a variety of ways. For example, we might investigate the ways in which physician-poets utilize their practice as a source of inspiration. Or we might suggest that the discipline of writing poetry actually helps physicians by making them more sensitive and empathic. As I thought about the assignment, however, I decided that I wanted to make a more radical claim. I wanted to suggest, in fact, that the healing act performed by a physician and the creative act performed by a poet share some important characteristics.

This suggestion appears radical because in our culture medicine sits quite close to the scientific end of the spectrum of life projects. Doctors are scientists, technicians, warriors, activists, important contributors to our society. Poetry, on the other hand, sits squarely at the artistic end of the spectrum. Poets are hopeless day-dreamers who presumably contribute little to a society that places little value on art. Yet, in many cultures, and for much of its history in Western civilization, medicine was (and is) considered an art, an art that often utilized symbol and ceremony, ritual and poetry, in its practice. In the workshop I wanted to ask, *Despite appearances, does poetry still lie at the core of healing?*

My first attempt to answer this question was to outline two points of conjunction between medicine and poetry. The first conjunction has to do with seeing, visualizing, entering into, and revealing. Like the poet, the physician puts himself or herself into the skin of someone else (or perhaps something else). The skill of empathy is crucial to both diagnosis and treatment. Empathy means being able to understand accurately both the cognitive and affective components of someone else's experience. Empathy is concrete and individualized, rather than a generalized virtue (like compassion) or a feeling (like sympathy). Empathic understanding allows one to see connections and to value connections, rather than to concentrate entirely on isolated fragments of biochemical processes.

Traditionally, physicians viewed the art of medicine as a sort of intuitive creativity in diagnosis and treatment. However, "intuition" suffers from bad press in medicine, and throughout our mechanistic society. Psychologists and philosophers have studied the process through which physicians make diagnostic judgements, and attempted to embody them in algorithms or mathematical models. While these are helpful, they generally serve as *post hoc* rationalizations, rather than as actual models of clinical judgement. This is not to imply that clinical judgement or medical "intuition" is haphazard, unpredictable, or unscientific. It is based, however, upon a foundation of tacit knowledge (to use Michael Polanyi's term), rather than being entirely concerned with explicit knowledge. It requires knowing both explicit content and appropriate steps of reasoning; but the skilled practitioner then integrates these (judgement) in new, insightful ways.

Acknowledgement that the act of *seeing* in medicine bears a family resemblance to the act of *seeing* in poetry (whether it be the poet's initial act, or the creative act of a reader who "sees") is a step toward regaining the concreteness and humanity of medicine. It allows for the development of therapeutic core qualities like empathy, respect, and genuineness. It strengthens the focus on the person-who-is-ill, and helps avoid a fragmented, solely disease-focused approach to medicine.

The second poetry-medicine conjunction has to do with *saying* rather than with *seeing*. Healing arises from saying the right words, from performing the right acts. *Therapy of the word* has existed throughout the history of medicine. *Therapy of the act* has also existed since prehistoric times, but commonly (until quite recent times) the efficacy of healing acts depended almost entirely upon the context in which they took place, and the *meanings* ascribed to them by both patient and healer. Thus, even *therapy of the act* often healed through the word.

Today we tend to view scientific medicine as a radical *therapy of the act* in which personal meanings and values play little role. Only physiological and statistical meanings have importance. While we understand that American Indian ceremonies and religious healing practices are *therapy of the word,* we believe that such symbolic healing is no longer necessary in our enlightened age. We think we live in a world of bodies, yet the human world is a world of symbols. Medicine cannot be stripped of metaphor, image, symbol, meaning, and interpretation. Ill persons experience meaning in their lives and illnesses, they (like all of us) experience themselves as characters in a life narrative, and they find in medicine a vast network of healing symbols. Physicians (like poets) manipulate those culturally important symbols. They speak in metaphor. They tell stories. They conduct ceremonies. Thus, physicians (like poets) systematically influence others to change their experience by using a kind of liturgy of the word.

This perspective raises many questions. How can we better understand the poetry of the body? If a physician believes she is healing only by virtue the body, is she a less effective physician than one who understands that she heals also by virtue of the word? Can physicians who fail to see the meanings of their words and actions, actually harm their patients and cause iatrogenic suffering?

II.

I selected these paragraphs from an essay entitled, "Hard Medicine, Soft Medicine" (1989). In the essay, I characterized as HARD an excessively mechanistic view of medicine that concentrates only on bodies-as-machines and HARD science. I suggested that, to accomplish healing, medical practice must in fact be SOFT as well as HARD, and that a poorly understood softness is actually responsible for much that we (mistakenly) attribute to our technological tools. Among the attributes of SOFT medicine are: careful listening to the patient's story, the establishment of a healing connection, and the use of metaphor and story as therapy. This selection plays around (a little) with some of the metaphorical ways we think about medicine and medical practice.

***

Medicine is Hard. And Hard Medicine seems so natural. It proliferates all around us. The media constantly call attention to its achievements and benefits. Its economic power is enormous. Hard Medicine is based on hard facts. It works. Or so we believe. Yet, if Hard Medicine has become an article of faith in American culture, is it possible that the existence of that faith tends to distort the facts? As a practitioner of Soft Medicine, I believe that our vision is often narrowed rather than broadened by technology. In fact, I believe that unperceived and unexpected Softness accounts for much of the presumed success of Hard Medicine.

Softness means the healing connection, or at least the potential healing connection, at the core of any doctor-patient interaction. Softness is what the medical anthropologist Arthur Kleinman has termed "empathic witnessing." Softness acknowledges that persons live in a world of metaphor and symbol, even though their bodies appear to live in a world of "Just the facts, ma'am." Soft Medicine understands that each person experiences herself or himself not as an abstract biological entity, not as a body in a world of bodies, but as the main character in a life narrative. Soft Medicine understands that illness disrupts or destroys that narrative, and that medicine can heal by helping patients to re-write their fractured stories.

DISEASE-ENEMY and BODY-MACHINE are metaphors. Today it is fashionable to emphasize "hard science" in medicine, yet even this use of the adjective "hard" is metaphorical. I don't mean that medicine is a firm object with solid boundaries, nor that it presents a barrier difficult to penetrate. When "hard" and "soft" are used as approaches to knowledge, they are part of a system of metaphor so deeply embedded in our culture and language that we forget we are thinking and speaking metaphorically. Underlying this system are some core metaphors like THE REAL WORLD CONSISTS OF SEPARATE ENTITIES, REAL ENTITIES HAVE HARD SURFACES, and SCIENCE IS A CONTAINER FOR ENTITIES. In such a system, softness is unscientific, squishy, and vague.

III

Certain phrases and sentences appear frequently in the language of medical care. These statements appear so often because they are shorthand—shall I say, ritualized?— ways of expressing concepts or values that are particularly important in our medical culture. One example is, *I treat all my patients aggressively.* Or, *One thing you can say about him, at least he's aggressive.* In medicine such aggressiveness is considered to be a virtue, one that sometimes compensates (at least in part) for the lack of other qualities, like prudence or compassion. The high value we place on aggressiveness arises from the belief that medical practice is a battle, and that physicians are warriors. In the following paragraphs from "I Treat All My Patients Aggressively" (*Journal of Medical Humanities*, 1990), I discuss PHYSICIAN-WARRIOR as well as some of the other metaphors so embedded in our thinking about medical practice that we often take them to be factual statements, rather than metaphorical descriptions.

***

Medical practice is like a war. Disease is the enemy. The patient is a battleground. In many cases we know that we cannot win the war, nor even the battle, but still it is difficult to retreat. In war, aggressiveness is a primary virtue. Prudence is secondary. And there is little room for compassion.

Such naked aggression would make some sense if medicine were literally a war. In some cultures, the MEDICINE-WAR image is considerably more literal than it is in ours. Shamans in Central Asia and *curanderos* in Central America, for example, believe that much illness is caused by spirit possession. The healer must engage the spirit and vanguish it. If the healer makes a mistake, if he demonstates a weakness of character or a lapse of attention, the shaman might himself be destroyed by the enemy.

MEDICINE-WAR is not the only metaphor embedded in our concepts of medical practice. Images abound in our language describing doctor-patient relationships: physician as parent, teacher, colleague, technician, interpreter, and provider. Each of these images implies a different metaphor for medical practice. If the doctor is a parent, sick persons must be children. If the doctor is an engineer or technician, then the body must be a machine and disease a malfunction or a defective part.

Many physicians prefer to look at their work through the lens of technique—rather than the lens of war. To them, most of medicine is measurement. The PHYSICIAN-EN-GINEER image serves to channel and disguise aggression. It can launder the battle, turn it into a more emotionally neutral contest.

We often confuse medical aggression (or slavish devotion to technique) with paternalism. PHYSICIAN-PARENT (paternalism) gets a bad rap in our culture because we tend to view many traditional medical practices—like lack of truthfulness with patients or neglect of informed consent—as primary manifestations of the parental metaphor. Though our culture rejects this PHYSICIAN-PARENT metaphor, it avidly accepts PHYSICIAN-WARRIOR and PHYSICIAN-TECHNICIAN images. But does a warrior consult with her battleground? Or a technician obtain informed consent from his machine? In completely rejecting the parental image, we lose the light it sheds on medicine, as well as clearing up the shadow. After all, PHYSICIAN-PARENT implies beneficience, listening, gentleness, caring, and nurturing. Parentalism is not the whole truth, but it does reveal some of the truth.

Each of these metaphors is true. Each sheds some light on the doctor-patient relationship, but also casts a shadow. While capturing one characteristic of illness or healing, each metaphor downplays or ignores certain other features. We need several such images to tell us the truth. Sometimes, however, physicians—and patients—forget that their thinking about medicine is embedded in metaphor.

IV

Among the Navajo, healing is poetry and ritual. While Navajo people are quick to accept the benefits of scientific medicine, they find that it provides only partial answers to their questions about illness and suffering. Western medicine often relieves symptoms of illness, but it fails to address the personal and cosmic disharmony that lies at the core of illness. "In Beauty May I Walk" (*Humane Medicine*, 1991) illustrates this need for symbolic healing with the stories of two of my Navajo patients from Lower Greasewood, Arizona. The following paragraphs speak to community and connectedness as central to the healing process.

***

Among the Navajo, serious illness has meaning. Its human significance is paramount. Illness has to make sense in a larger pattern. The Navajo use ghosts and witches in their system of thinking about illness, concepts no more difficult to accept (to those untutored in science) than the notion of invisible animals so small that billions of them can take up residence in your lungs and cause sickness. Underlying the ghosts and witches, though, the Navajo had one unifying belief about illness: suffering resulted from lack of harmony. The sick person had somehow gotten out of harmony with himself, his family, his world. He cannot be healed unless that harmony is first restored.

This was not easy for folk as geographically scattered and as poor as the Lower Greasewood Navajo. A ceremony (or Sing) ranged from three to nine days in duration. It required the presence of the ill person's extended family and other clan members. For the Sing, these people would have to set aside their job and home responsibilities to spend several days in the patient's camp, participating in a series of chants, prayers and dances. During that time, all participants would have to be fed. Sheep would have to be butchered. The *hataali* or Singer and his assistant would have to be paid. While Indians were entitled to free medical care through the United States Public Health Service, it cost several hundred dollars to hire a *hataali* and stage a full nine-day healing ceremony.

In Lower Greasewood I learned that, for the Navajo, penicillin shots and arthritis pills were simply symptomatic treatments. The Navajo were practical people, eager as anyone else for quick relief of their ills. They knew that the doctor's shots were the most efficient way to treat pneumonia. But when fever and cough were gone, an important question would still remain. I could draw diagrams for them. I could explain the mechanisms of disease. But I could not answer the questions, "Why me? What does this illness mean in my life? What does my life mean in the face of this illness?"

V

In autumn of 1989, the movers-and-shakers of our University Medical Center placed videotape displays in a number of lobbies and public spaces. The videotapes were very serious professionally produced paeans to the marvelous health care we provide. They illustrated how serious and scientific we are. In fact, they said, we are delivering medicine of the 21st Century today. The figures on these tapes—machines, health care workers, patients—all appeared wooden, heavy, and self-important. In "The Incredible Lightness" (*Pharos*, 1990) I described a fantasy in which I replaced those orthodox images with images depicting humor, compassion, and poetry in patient care. The following paragraphs consider the role of humor in healing.

***

We think too much. Physicians take themselves far too seriously. If we are doing such a good job curing disease, why don't we shout with joy? Or at least crack a wry smile?

Take Norman Cousins. Cousins, the former editor of *Saturday Review of Literature*, was once quite ill with a mysterious syndrome—fever, malaise, arthritis, a strange constellation of symptoms that left him hospitalized and incapacitated. His doctors diagnosed an unusually severe case of ankylosing spondylitis, one that did not respond to therapy. Suffering greatly and frustrated by his doctors' inability to help, Cousins tried to take his mind off his sickness. He discovered that a few jokes, a little humor, made him feel a little better. When he laughed he felt good. Why not try a little more laughter? He then embarked on a rigorous regimen of vitamins and humor, including a daily dose of Marx Brothers films. His sickness seemed to fade away. He got better. Cousins believed that laughter played a major role in his cure.

When I first read Cousins' experience with humor, I was angry. Where were the qualifiers? His message was too simplistic. Of course, it is important for patients to have a positive attitude. Of course, doctors should listen to what their patients tell them. But laughter as therapy? I thought Cousins was doing a great disservice to humanistic medicine by promoting simplistic answers. He neglected to consider all the other factors that may have been involved, and to warn his readers about the hazards of generalization. Cousins sounded like a quack.

It took me several years to see his point. Take the metaphor, UP IS GOOD, DOWN IS BAD. Laughter is UP. Laughter represents joy and lightness. The serious view of medicine propounded by much of medicine today is DOWN. It represents heaviness. The Czech writer Milan Kundera chose as the name for one of his novels, *The Unbearable Lightness of Being*. I was struck by that phrase, "lightness of being," a phrase that recalls golden late October days just emerging from a trace of fog. The lightness of being is growth and harmony and joy. Lightness is beauty and laughter. Lightness pulls us into the future, while heaviness drags us down and makes us repeat the present.

VI.

I was asked by the editor of *Literature and Medicine* to write an essay considering the relationship of culture to healing and, in particular, cultural aspects of contemporary medicine. Of course, cultures are systems of symbols. I began to explore further my belief that scientific medicine is not only a system of facts and technique, but is also a vast network of symbol and metaphor. "The Word Is an Instrument of Healing"

(*Literature and Medicine*, 1991) describes various aspects of the healer-patient connection through which words and ceremonies contribute to healing.

***

Medical names are powerful symbols. The healing power of a diagnostic word ("You have ...") is well expressed by John Berger in *A Fortunate Man*, a book in which he examines the life of an English country doctor. Berger wrote:

> The illness, as an undefined force, is a potential threat to our very being and we are bound to be highly conscious of the uniqueness of that being. The illness, in other words, shares in our own uniqueness.... That is why patients are inordinately relieved when doctors give their complaint a name ... because it has a name, it has an independent existence from them. They can now struggle or complain against it.

Ordinary biomedical narratives also include the names of procedures or tests. A patient may have heard or read about a new test (e.g. positron emission scanning) that is said to be more accurate than the standard test (e.g. magnetic resonance imaging), and wonders whether the new type of scan would "help" him. While physicians see diagnostic procedures as simply ways of obtaining information, patients may respond as well to their symbolic meaning. In our biomedical culture, a test result may convey more than information; it may evoke a sense of order, understanding, and control. At times a positive test, by endowing an illness with medical "meaning," may facilitate healing even when—as in the case of CFS—no official medical treatment is available.

***

Stories of sickness (texts) are written against the background of culture (context). In *The Illness Narratives,* Arthur Kleinman notes that headaches, dizziness, and weakness receive particular attention in Chinese medicine. He comments that the current epidemic of chronic pain syndromes in the United States might indicate that enduring pain has a special claim to (negative) significance in our highly individualistic and optimistic culture. Such chronic pain does not translate well into strictly biomedical language because it appears to occur in the absence of definable disease, thus violating the empiricist model of clinical reasoning. Consequently, conflict arises between patient and physician. If viewed, however, from the perspective of illness-as-cultural-construction, chronic fatigue syndrome and chronic pain might best be considered cases in which a particular cluster of symptoms has achieved a relatively widespread significance in one culture (the patient's), while at the same time being incoherent or inexplicable in another culture (the physician's).

Medical anthropologists use the term *culture-bound syndrome* to describe folk illnesses that reflect primary dysfunction at a symbolic or cultural level, which then (secondarily) may lead to excess physical disease. *Susto*, a condition observed in certain parts of Latin American and among Hispanic people in the United States, is a well-recognized example of this concept. People of these cultures believe that *susto* (magical fright) occurs when a person's spirit is detached from the body, having been frightened off by a ghost or terrible life experience. The person's body then begins to wither away, and may die unless effective treatment is obtained. *Asustados* complain of weakness, listlessness, aches and pains, restless sleep, and poor appetite, but they also demonstrate an excess of physical problems like anemia, dysentery, and parasitic infections. While a medical doctor might provide temporary relief, only a traditional healer or *curandero* can re-connect the patient's physical and spiritual selves. Some anthropologists believe that patient-perceived inadequacy to meet social role expectations precipitates this culturally-accepted cluster of symptoms. In essence, *susto* is a story through which the patient reveals a certain form of disharmony in his symbolic world. By telling this particular kind of story, the sick person gains the concern and support of his community. A *curandero* then steps into the patient's narrative and ritually "speaks" a new story of healing.

***

I start from the premise that medicine is meaning-centered, and I argue that scientific medicine is a form of cultural healing. Just as symptoms have meanings for patients, the words, rituals, and paraphernalia of medicine also convey meaning and constitute a culturally-designated context of healing. Within this context, physicians "connect" with patients on a symbolic level to facilitate healing. Ideally, this connection includes various strands—I have called them empathic, narrative, and cultural components—that together form a conduit through which words and rituals enter the patient's "lived body" and lead to healing.

VII.

Stories abound in medicine. Some are stories of bodies and machines. Others are human stories, replete with heroes, villains, and unexpected twists of plot. Recently, some writers have developed the metaphor of physician as reader or interpreter of patient texts. But, of course, the physician doesn't merely interpret. She helps tell the tale. She becomes a co-author of the patient's narrative of healing. While a physician-writer or a patient-writer may sometimes capture this feature of healing in an actual story or poem, co-authorship as a metaphor helps us to understand ordinary (verbal) healer-patient relationships. In this selection from "Medical Texts, Medical Stories" (*PLN Newsletter*, 1990) I use a few of my poems about patients as concrete examples of story-telling in medical practice.

***

Most of the stories, tales, vignettes, and anecdotes that fill medicine are actually translations and revisions of original narratives. While they begin as *experiential* texts (personal narratives of sickness and suffering), in order to be clinically useful, they must be translated into *biomedical* texts. Only part of the patient's tale is considered truly important. This is the part that can be translated into a strange new language. The new language contains few verbs. Its nouns avoid complex issues like meaning, suffering, value, and belief. Rather, they name body parts, machines, and processes.

Many tales defy translation. These experiential texts jump-out from the nooks and crannies of medical practice. They simply will not disappear. Take, for example, this elderly woman who brings her painful hand to my office and dumps it on my desk as if the hand were an intransigent villain. "It's worthless," she tells me. No matter how hard I try, I cannot render her invisible. This lady (in "The Knitted Glove") is too opaque, too tough.

You come into my office wearing a blue
knitted glove with a ribbon at the wrist.
You remove the glove slowly, painfully
and dump out the contents, a worthless hand.
What a specimen! It looks much like a regular hand,
warm, pliable, soft. You can move the fingers.

If it's not one thing, it's another.
Last month the fire in your hips had you down,
or up mincing across the room with a cane.
When I ask about the hips today, you pass them off
so I can't tell if only your pain
or the memory is gone. Your knitted hand
is the long and short of it. Pain doesn't exist
in the past any more than this morning does.

This thing, the name for your solitary days,
for the hips, the hand, for the walk of your eyes
away from mine, this thing is coyote, the trickster.
I want to call, *Come out, you son of a dog!*
and wrestle that thing to the ground for you,
I want to take its neck between my hands.
But in this world I don't know how to find
the bastard, so we sit. We talk about the pain.

Yes, a major part of medical practice *is* knowing the trickster's name. Often we view patient narrative as nothing but a source of name-finding. The phrase "taking a history" reflects this view. "Take" evokes an image of aggression. An active doctor takes something from a passive patient. What does she take? A "history," an entity that lies like a black box amid the debris of human foibles and suffering. The doctor—with her special knowledge—can identify and remove this black box, this medical history, while nonmedical persons are misdirected by compassion or confused by irrelevancies. While the patient has many stories to tell, she has only one biomedical text. But where does that leave us when we "don't know how to find the bastard?"

Here is another patient ("Rock of Ages") so covered with coal dust that he resists becoming transparent. Deep in his narrative, I see a man struggling for his life, running from the "ominous figure" that follows him, while on the surface he speaks only about his wife's fears and "the dampness."

This miner comes in
with hardly a story for anything
serious. A little pain
back where he busted his back,
sick to the stomach
since Easter, not enough
not to eat. *Man's got to eat,*
right? When he takes a smoke
his stomach rolls like a room
in Noah's ark. He's plain
apologetic. *It's nothing,*
it's the wife, she's always
looking for the worst.

Blue-black roots around his arms,
he stumbles, coughing,
from the elevator cage
covered with coal from head to foot,
clanging his lunch bucket.
He pulls off his black boots.
His feet are porcelain.
Crystals glisten
at the base of his neck.

I put my hands on his chest.
The skin, granite-like at first,
cracks and crumbles.
Shale! I listen
to his stony breathing,
and hear a man
scrambling the lip of an open mine
and kicking showers of shale
at the ominous figure
that follows him. The man
is running for his life. He's not
fast enough. *It's nothing,*
it's the dampness.... His skin
is translucent, revealing

cold, hard lumps of coal
that endure—I tell him, *Yes,*
you need some tests—

when the rest is gone.

Denial? If I wanted to translate this man's story into a biomedical text, I could begin by using the term, "denial." Defense mechanisms are somewhat outdated, but still reasonably respectable. However, perhaps I simply cannot make this patient transparent and still be an effective healer. Perhaps I must somehow learn to participate in his personal story.

Rosaly DeMaios Roffman

POET AS SHAKER AND HEALER

Vladimir Nabokov once surprised an audience by beginning a textbook in the following way. "This is a Russian grammar book and I am eating a banana." He had a reason for wanting to shock an audience unused to smiling when they started to do homework. He also had the beginning of a poem which could be a way of thinking about Russian grammar, but he did not press on to write a poem. He knew precisely what he was doing and leaves us a competent grammar as well as a memorable first line.

When I sit down to write a poem I am a party to the grammar of witnessing, but I don't always know how it will turn out. And I don't have a contract to write a book. I don't think "grammar." I don't think "bananas." I don't think "sickness" nor "healing," yet I have been thinking intensely about what poets do, and what connection it has to the planet; and I believe it has to do with healing. If I have any integrity, I care about respecting that impulse no matter how frustrated or elated I may be afterwards—after writing the poem. But I try to remember the world never said I had to do it nor did the gods whisper audibly in my ear. I have been ruminating about the intensity that lies behind the impulse which propels the poet forward to write the poem. And I believe it has to do with deep re-creative desires. And they take many forms—perhaps that's why poetry poses so many difficulties for those who read it without fine tuning, without experiencing the poem/poet. Poetry appears to be the unfinished business of the race as well as the poet. To talk about this means inevitably to talk about damage and mending, wounding and healing.

When I was a student in New York City, I had a quiet friend who used to paint in his apartment near the Cloisters. He figured out a way to earn his living so that he could use the best hours of the day to be at home and paint. When the light was poor, he stayed in his apartment and retouched photographs in order to earn just enough money for materials. Friends came to see him, not the paintings which were always there and a part of him—those large canvasses with their own language. Soft-voiced, he took them, like children by the hand, to galleries and returned home knowing he did not associate with the right people. Nothing happened. But then he would come right back to the Cloisters to paint. Well-meaning friends and family were always there to inquire—"Couldn't you get a job in the post office? Don't you feel bad about giving up the conventional creature comforts and amenities (in other words 'things') to paint?" That was decades ago. My friend, quiet and Greek, would say simply, when he would deign to talk or sully the process, that he didn't give up anything, that a person didn't have a choice. He was one of the few artists I ever met who made everything he used. Although he was a painter he taught me what the process was all about. It was the pouring of linseed oil and the grinding of sienna red or cadmium blue. What I remember most vividly was that my friend would become ill if he didn't paint. I like to think of

527

him, all alone, not unhappily painting his primed canvasses still on Academy Street, asking no one except the room for approbation. But the paintings were there—we could see them. It was the paintings that made their little speeches to God. To me he was a kind of witness, and those paintings with their color spoke for us too. Where did they come from?

A second story that insists on being part of the backdrop for this paper on healing has to do with a former teacher, a woman who used to help run Black Mountain College—a maker of poems and pots who gives talks, and writes books with all kinds of offerings and practices on the discipline of centering and crossing points. She is an expert on the subject of separating and connecting in poetry, pottery and living. She has chosen to live in a community with the handicapped and to learn from them.

In 1983, the year she decided to take a sabbatical, she become quite ill. "Energy," she said, "it is a shifting of energy." At that same time she also began to take up singing—the shifting of energy, perhaps a sign of moving into a new arena? Until then, she described herself as visual, tactile, intuitive-thinking; but opening her mouth to make singing noises represented an important turning point. Does she let them in or out? Is her body tuning itself for new melodies?

Just when the new semester (then) at my university began, my teacher called me from Stanford University Sleep Disorder Center to ask in the utter depths of her body's dysfunction and mystery, if I could recommend a myth or a fairy tale—or any story for the purpose of meditation on insomnia and sleeping problems. I thumbed the pages of Stith Thompson's *Folk-Motif Index* and went through my files on the subject, and I did find a few. What she had in mind was the healing rituals of non-Western and preliterate societies—why wouldn't it be worth a try? In certain parts of Siberia and Polynesia (and other places) healing was dependent upon the stories, incantations, dances and prayers that were "worked" upon patients to relieve them of pain. The Hindus frequently give the sick a fairy tale or myth to ponder, knowing the story would be chosen carefully by a shaman or a medicine man from the shaman's or tribe's repertory. In some tribes you had to dance the story or demons out of you (Yoruba). I did discover an insomnia devil in the *Mishnah*, a Hebrew Holy Book. He was a miserable character who stole babies; there were also sleeping songs in some Polynesian tribes prescribed for sleeping maladies.

Finding out that narratives and songs are vital to the healer in different parts of the world—and that in many places the doctor is both priest and singer—makes one wonder about the healing effects of the word, the healing presence of poetry, what the word invokes. We neither study nor teach it this way, but poets are aware of the power, what the word "can do and does," not only for the hearer, but for the writer as well. No one can say for sure what the complex process of writing a poem entails or where the words come from, but a poet often seems to behave as an agent or intermediary between this world and some other. In communities which are less sprawling than ours and where people are closer, there is no question that the poet is a doctor or healer. He is a visionary and speaks for the tribe and the tribe's mysteries (Black Elk). The greater the power of his singing the more complete the healing. Of course I wished as much to find a story to help my teacher as she wished to heal herself. But wouldn't it be even more effective if the entire tribe were engaged in her healing (like the Navajo or Nepalese) and not just a diagnostic clinic?

I thus became inspired to go back—to return to a review of the original poet's impulse to pray, bless, celebrate, to keep the faith, to rearrange the furniture of any room so the world of anyone-who-gets-touched-by-poetry might be moved directly. The poet is a sharer of secrets perhaps like the shaman—of his life and of the race. Then we respond and we ask the poet to do it over again, or we paste poems in journals.

A number of poets in the West transcend consciously that world of the concrete and make us feel sometimes that we are outside of the body as well. If one reads Whitman, Rilke, Kabir, Bly and others, and studies the Japanese poets, one watches a genuine contending with the ghosts and unseen dwellers of the planet. They are ghosts that the poet reckons with. Even at the risk of sounding "schizzie" (which preliterates don't worry about because their brains, categorized as "undifferentiated," respect the voices that come from the other world) I tell myself it is all right to see faces on doorknobs. I tell myself "you owe it to the doorknobs to give them their just due." I try as witness in my poems to think of what I'm doing as an act of discovery, of bringing back or finding the poems that comfort, cajole, give in—poems that extricate poet and reader from difficult places. Like Neruda's phone calls to the dead, we must heal wounds by laying them bare and making ourselves heard as we listen even in silence.

I made the effort to do that in these poems—thinking, "poets are engaged in this work all the time." What is the occasion for the poem? I have had good teachers ... expression is the act of integration. With your first poem you wrestle with the unconscious. I wanted to bring something more forward, even then, but I didn't know what the "more" was. And like many children I thought about religion. My first poem, at the age of thirteen, I can still recite:

> God, give me a little piece of land
> And lend me the seed of my soul
> That I may boldly plant it here
> And boldly watch it grow.
>
> And prove to me, oh God,
> That life is greater than the goal,
> For every weary footstep trod
> Be you the master of my soul.

I don't know what wound inspired the wish or the prayer, but it is implicit in the poem—as is the relief. I think that much poetry has within it the element of prayer—a wish to make things better—or to acknowledge the ghosts as I have called them—even a poem about cups ("A Story of Cups") celebrates a power that enables that to happen. Poetry can't cure or heal in the same sense as a physician—but it can provide balm.

A Story Of Cups: With Appended Prayer

There is one still steaming
in a mountain inn close to a lake.
And I have one that I glued together
that my teacher made with blue weeds
inside, and one with no handle, good
for pencils or sticking your toe in.
Every day I lose one in a coffee room
to someone who doesn't care about sludge
and has the grace to return cups to shelves.

An old woman brought me one
with a teakettle when I sat in a bar
closed for the morning, and my friend
always brings me tea in a thin German one
with a black rim. I have saved a child's broken
one—with a rabbit no one could throw away.

Being drunk or hurt you get a thick one
in Maine. In the basement is a paper one
a soldier, never making it to the garbage.

Let me come into this life a cup,
let me fit myself to fingers
without being weary. Let me celebrate
all these hands, these chapters,
moving through tight corners.

Bless our many heads bending over.

If someone can invest in the intensity of a moment that "takes them out of themselves," a poem has the power to call forth a self that sometimes reader or listener might not have known was there. The reader is startled by how close the poet gets. My students often say "this poetry is speaking to me." When this is done well, the poet like a practitioner may offer a prescription or suggestion for the listener ("While it has you"). Even when this is done not so well, we can still acknowledge the good will and generosity of the Hallmark card (verse) buyer. If only the card shopper had stopped to write a poem.

While it has you
hang onto pain

as it moves
down, way down

a single gypsy bead
on a black chain

rail against it
put it in your mouth
tape it to the wall
down, way down

Then let it
tattoo your chest

become a bright bird

with wings that move
when you're without
good clothing

like outdoor roses

remember, you can't
wash away this bird

this angel for stirrings
your worry bead
turned sparrow—but walk

it says walk
tall and uncovered
that bird

flying those roses
from down, way down

Reading poetry can make anyone feel better. Craft and mystery make this so. Certainly the therapeutic value is not confined to what it has to say. The language used by the poet brings delight, just as nursery rhymes delight the child. Such delight is a form of healing. Hearing and saying is experience. Even corporations realize the joy that comes from singing the words too. As raisins and cigars and bugs croon their messages, I am reminded of a friend whose bright little boy asked her to "tell him a commercial" instead of a story before he went to bed. I think the music of society tells us through the slogans, commercials, and bumper stickers what children know by heart.

Music is primary and, obviously, the response to the chanting and reading of poetry is not based on intellect or reasoned judgment alone, even in a post literate context. Sometimes poems become vehicles that remind us we are not alone in our responses to the world. There is a connection between diverse things. The music of poetry reaches listeners and readers even when they are unaware of it. I remember being stunned by the singing of Dylan Thomas before I ever saw his words on the page. At parties we played his records and everyone stopped to listen to "Do Not Go Gentle" and "A Refusal to Mourn"; his voice was his acoustical guitar; there wasn't any other like it.

Jung reminds us in his essay, "Psychology and Poetry" of how vital the poet is as the voice of a people. He writes:

> The psychic need of the people is fulfilled in the work of the poet, and therefore the work means more to the poet in action and truth than his personal destiny, whether he is conscious of it or not. He is essentially the instrument and he stands below his work, for which reason we should never expect from him an interpretation of his own work. He must leave the interpretation to others and the future. (17)

I think of the poet's personal stake in the process of healing or externalization of inner feelings. In earlier times and even today among Native Americans and peoples of Africa and Polynesia, the persons who perform best are asked to do so on behalf of the community. They memorize the secrets of the tribe and relay them in the songs and stories they tell on behalf of survival. Making contact with the spirit of disease and then learning or absorbing that spirit's power seems to be the principle. The poems I have mentioned here are not mini-term papers; yet, practices and rituals have become the sources for these poems. Still, one of the dangers in writing poems like "Prescriptions," "Arm as Instrument," and "Brief Blues Song" (based on Serbian medicine) is in sounding culturally patronizing. Healing information transcends my awe; but in my poems, what I hope the reader sees or thinks about is the voice that acknowledges. I marvel at healers who appear in every society and are crucial to keeping that community intact:

1. In Northern Luzon (the Philippines), so that people can utilize demon songs and dances for exorcism, a shaman casts a patient into a trance and encourages a fight to vanquish the demon-assailant. The patient then demands a song and dance from the conquered humbled spirit. At this point the shaman ends the trance. The patient follows by singing the song and performing the dance he has learned so that other people can repeat the demon dance.
2. The witch-doctor uses calm music in Yoruba when imploring the spirit of disease to release the possessed patient, but he sings martial music when he fights the unfriendly spirit with a spear.
3. In Mexico the cuandera employs both medicine and prayer to rid the patient's body of evil spirits and, as part of the incantation, he begs the spirits to inhabit another body.
4. The Chippewas believe that the disease-causing spirit must be lured into an appropriate cave and must be sung to after the medicine man has learned its rightful dwelling place and song.

The equivalencies in my own poems have to do with a desire that is re-creative. I try to sing out the harming spirits and then I write my own "Brief Blues" and "Facing the Angels" in hopes of managing those feelings in the poem. The idea is to treat or offer a poetic alternative for the impossible rather than heal the incurable. Of course that can't be done in a literal sense. It is consciousness that heals. In life you sometimes don't have a second chance, but in poetry you have alternatives—many chances to co-create, to do over: to hold someone, to soften blows, to yell or sing, like Orpheus, to rescue someone from hell.

I also try to take on—as poets sometimes do—as Rilke does, in his *Sonnets to Orpheus*, acknowledgement of a circumstance for which I am not responsible. I want to soothe children who get taunted mercilessly by other children ("The Barn Swallows"), stop a therapist from killing herself ("Time to Say Thank You"), thank a doctor for his patience ("Small Gratitude"). For the unspeakable, a poet may find a way to speak. And that is healing.

Small Gratitude

You risk it, take my hand—
and there is a small animal in the holding
which makes its way through your fingers
and surprises all the sleeping creatures,
the knot of toads, the muster of peacocks,
the skulk of foxes, the charm of goldfinches
—all are so stirred by the faint music
that they lead you down the familiar path,
knowing how easy it is for strangers
to stumble along the way, and miss
all the stored up grace in this forest.

Poetry is constantly engaged in the process of transformations; and sometimes these metamorphoses derive their energy from rearranging circumstances so the poet enters the scenario of the poem. He can make wishes come true. The poet becomes then a co-sustainer of the world, a redesigner of fate.

Of course if you are intentionally writing healing poems, you are conscious of wounds and areas of vulnerability, of painful places. Conversely, James Hillman argues in *Healing Fiction* that it is only when a fiction is taken literally that it becomes a lie. Our symptoms and fixations are symbolic constructs.

It is impossible to escape theories of psychosomatic medicine and the effects of the spirit on healing in the reading of history and medicine. My poem, "Prescriptions," tries to address the significance of the believer's faith while participating in his own therapy. Another book by a Jungian develops the idea that glaucoma and other eye diseases are actually manifestations of having to grant oneself new vision. The mind and body are inseparable—and this appears to be the common denominator of belief in non-literate societies. In folk medicine, as practiced in Serbia for example, the healer acknowledges that spirits inhabit parts of the body, while not separate from the soul;

each limb then is entitled to a life of its own. And this information inspired "The Arm as Instrument" in which I tried to imagine the arm as a dancer with its own distinct life.

Also as part of the series, I had planned a number of "Envy" poems. Poets can create and resolve in their poems anything—even the seven deadliest sins, their own. A deliberate basis for these poems is that the object of envy (or any emotion) is not only named, sometimes deliciously, but also becomes useful as a vehicle for projection—even imagined forgiveness. A poem can't talk back but it is essential to pay homage to the feeling attached to the projection—to make room for the demons in order to know and then destroy or work with them. Poetry is that kind of act and enlightenment. The poet is conjurer.

Examples of contest-with-the-demon-envy poems are addressed to two people I never met, a blind woman and a poet who lives in Greece. To re-create such feelings is to offer them a place in your life: to invite them to dinner. In my poem about a blind woman with her "Trust Under the Moon," the enviable is her response to her handicap—her ability to walk courageously and with alacrity down the street without seeing. And her handicap becomes mine—how do I know her? She is a mystery creature—but the poet is everywhere sensing her presence.

Trust Under The Moon

Your dog is leading
and his rhythm is a gift.

You come out of the shadows
past the silence of men and women
who never practice anyone's rhythm.

How lovely it is: trust under the moon,
eyes not knowing where straight ahead is.

At corners storekeepers watch as they turn
down their lights and mothers with children
walk around you. A thousand people talk to you

through their eyes—and you move on
trusting a love that is all ears

never contending with the politics of streets
never confusing trust with blackness.
Everyone knew when to turn around; the old game

to be played; they know when they've passed
the church and the river; when they've vanished

down the next block. But you can't know
unless smell tells you who is close
and your dog has to sort out caring.

Now I've never had a dog nor a time
when getting there was what took me.

Every night I watch the runners go
and the cyclists with flags whipping,
and they're fast but they don't count.

Only your eyes behold the mysteries of streets;
I see a flat sheen moving you out of dreams and on.

Singing and dancing offer comfort through dark times, and many poems provide ways to make it through. To believe in the poem is to believe in the poet and his capacity to alter states. "Coming Back" was written while watching someone struggle in a recovery room. In the "Blue Fairy" the healing agent responds to an old man's request to have his masterpiece brought to life—to make a boy of a marionette. The deed renders life to the maker's dream—a reward for all the love invested in the marionette. Without the woodcarver and the blue-fairy, any block of wood could easily go unnoticed, any face on a doorknob. Bravo blue fairy! Bravo Pinocchio! Bravo Poetry!

Brief Blues For Singing Out the Harming Spirit

Go now:
I embraced you once
and you moved in
and took over,
putting each small piece
of body you borrowed
into a box collection.

I can't feed you,
clothe you,
stand looking at you
in the mirror.
I am on the mend
with the wound
like a corpse
ready for viewing.

How I received you
I don't know;
You make us
feel like pinched buds
come alive when no one
thought it could happen.
With doors open, any demon
can demand to sit at table.

Go now:
and while I'm empty
and able to sing feeble songs
I'll settle for ocean
instead of fever
behind these eyes.

Blue Fairy I
Pinnochio and Gepetto Dialogue,
Blue Fairy Response

Gepetto: Help me to swim
Through the mouth of the whale
My life's work is at stake
Grant us a candle to keep us warm
And forgive the daring of imagination
He was almost alive to the chimes of a universe
Gone mad with the requiem for a suffering
Father.

Pinocchio: Passing through this life
My strings could be broken
My body could sense missing fire
After it had seen the knife
But a kind man intervened
He's willing to chance a tired boy:
Let me not be a child's unhappy puppet.

Blue Fairy: Wishing upon a star
Is not the only way to do it
Being a boy is risky—
I will give you a symphony
For your dance—only the love
Of an old man could spare
The tree—and sprout heart
Where bark would ordinarily be.
Remember to hold your own child
As close to the music as you can.

Prescriptions: listening deeply to the wisdom of the unlicensed

I.

Walking barefoot
while there is still earth
might steady you.
On the soles of feet
is a great map
of body wanting to be
spelled out—
not washed away
without being looked at
and thought beautiful.

II.

For fear of the unknown
sit under a giant aspen,
for stark terror
you'll have to find rockroses,
and for discouragement try gentian;
a Swiss mountain guide preferred
this purple tea, and nothing stopped him;
he could yodel loudest and longest;
but what land will yield vervain
for those who exhaust themselves
in the service of others? An illness
and a person must be studied and understood.
Find it in your heart to seat demons
at table and force them to drink
bitter tea and ginger whiskey.

III.

For your spring cure
cover a basin of raisins
with linen and after two days
eat the fruit and drink the water.
From the grapes you get the sun
in your system, perhaps stars too.

IV.

There is a sleep cure
for sleep debtors and a story
about a famous sleeper—
as a boy he found a mystic cave

and went on dreaming for 57 years.
He awoke fully enlightened and fully Greek.

V.

Every night, after sitting
in meditation, your healer seeks
advice about cords, color and number.
He is told which cords to select
and then weaves them into a bracelet
for pain. Not even the sick may
touch your wrist; and your healer
may only use tongs to remove karma.
Whatever you can do to reduce pain,
do. And only near the end,
hire agents to drum on your behalf.
You will have to pay them with secrets.

VI.

Every morning
like the Cheyenne
upon rising,
dip yourself
in a freezing river. You will
warm to the rest of the day,
and the blue water will
keep you from darkness.

Rosaly DeMaios Roffman

The Arm as an Instrument

In the moonlight
your arm has separate life;
it moves
wanting to say something
on behalf of snowflake light.

It wants to grab hold
and touch the child
in her ceremony
of the crooked limb,
in this clarity of winter.

The soul is dangerously thin,
like a hair; it is tiny
like a pea; it has a thin tongue
of flame; it has feet like an ant
and lives in a woman's heart.
It could do a man's work
but it is also a message
that comes from the other side.

Contending with envy

(for Jack Gilbert who lives when he can in Greece)

Winter—
and more than breathing
I want to be where you are

Stalking the wild gardenias
because my grandfather fought
wild men in these mountains
and my jealousy is
and you are
and I'm not
living in love
and a white house
a who's on first joke.

Jack, grant me forgiveness
for my deadly sin way of saying,
you, making it in the land
of my father, by writing poems
feels like a penny in my throat
Better, if you kiss my other cheek
and rescue me from burning—
you who never asked to be born Greek.

Ask, and I will come and walk the island
with you, and sit under the lemon trees;
and if these same gods are willing
I might bring my son and we three
could break into friends and dance
That would be a better way to manage
spring.

Time To Say "Thank You"

Shaved from the thinnest of abalone shells—
I remember those ivory elephants in your ears,
I remember how your shoes sounded when you came,
how you talked about your childhood in Boston
even though it was my treatment; I remember
how you gave me money and said, "call,
when in trouble," that you would come so fast
and then you said "eat"or you would bring food.

I remember we laughed at what haoles we both were,
and how your clothes were always crying New York,
your sweaters always tied around your shoulders,
how you outlined which white apartment was yours,
one of those beachfront condominium lookalikes,
and then how you described the building we were in,
"This was an old TB sanitorium" you would say,
in a voice that made your life sound more interesting.

And one day you dropped a file on the floor
so I could see the name of a patient who was my friend
who said he met you at one of the drunken parties
he went to—this beautiful blonde man who didn't know
I knew him—who wore big rings given by old ladies
he entertained from Minneapolis and St. Louis—
he said "watch out; that doctor's very hungry."
And I asked you what did he mean by that?
not imagining the unspeakable pain of those fingers
drumming on that metal desk—beneath us, stunted trees.

Years later, I realize you were telling me
he was hurting on purpose; years later,
I realize you are kinder and lonelier
than my own mother; they said—too late,
you had gone to Molokai, were now the sole
doctor for lepers, had no forewarding address.

And suddenly it comes to me, as I rock
the child I brought back for you to see,
—I hear you describe the black blindfold
you wore to banish the Oahu sun from your blue eyes,
I remember you would say "try the blindfold too
if you're not sleeping" —and then "please,"
You would yell—I'll always remember the "Now please,
pack up and get yourself the hell off this island."

Rosaly DeMaios Roffman

The Barn Swallows

You do not have to win prizes.
You do not have to fast in the woods
or have your sins whipped out of you.

You have only to understand how perfect
you are through your own imperfections,

what it means to keep your eyes on eyes,
what it means to let someone
speak to you without speaking.

Tell birds your sorrow and they'll tell theirs;
while the old moon and low mists
travel over the mountains; beach-plums
form new patches near the ocean,
barn swallows hang on wires overhead.

No matter how secret you are,
the world has room for your shadow,
for breathing, for the tree whispering—
whoever you may be this morning
pour yourself into a gold vessel
think of yourself as a barn swallow
making perfect circles above the mimosa.

Coming Back

Morphine on your doorstep,
I said, "you are very brave,"
You said, "sure, but I can't
stand constant pain." I thought
about the demons, about who
was the first person tortured
then called hero—
why is *that* a man?

You whispered, lids half-shuttered,
"I know where we got it—we
got it from the Indians"
I wanted more from you in your stupor
I leaned closer to your breathing—
You said, "they were first to walk
through fire" and then you passed
through a ring, your palms like small friends
protecting each other; we knew then
the damned were doomed in cages of logic
on the other side, and that brave ancestors
walked through the muscle of thunder
without   speaking.

Facing The Angels

I always wanted a room of them
men with beards, wise faces,
women with thin smiles who listen
as part of a love affair gone brown.
The eyes have never been damaged
but stare down and through terror,
there is Einstein and Shaw,
and Jung and Georgia O'Keeffe,
and Whitman and Rabindranath Tagore.
Let them sit on my porch in Indiana
beside the pear tree that barely
makes it through winter, and talk
not about meaning but about growing old.
Let them tell me what awaits touching
for my body when it becomes a stick,
why longing hasn't killed them.
When I put up their photographs
I will pray for someone to lie down
beside me, as must be their good fortune,
and to whisper in everyone's lined ears:

Come, feed your soul the right food
and your brain will give you the right face.

Sandi Kadlubowski

THE PAIN POTS

You can't plan these things. They have to just happen—come from the gut. It was mid-December and I had just enough time for one more firing before Christmas. I was working very hard, throwing mugs, bowls, platters, vases—all the things I knew would sell. You develop a rhythm when you are doing production work. You draw on all those years of training and practice, and there is a security that happens when you don't have to struggle with technique. It gives you time to think and let your mind wander. My thoughts kept returning to my friend and her months of struggle after her accident. She had once shared with me her poems, her healing poems "Faces on Door Knobs," and her "poet-as-shaker-and-healer" paper. They touched me to the core. I felt privileged to receive them, and I recognized the intimacy that may come upon one with poetry. To see these words—read about pain, other people's pain, overwhelmed me.

Then the accident ... my response to those poems ... and then the knowledge of the pain my friend was experiencing would only take me so far. I wanted to do more—but felt there was nothing I could do or say to make the hurt stop.

It was late at night, and I was to beginning to experience the fatigue of the evening. Time to stop. But I couldn't shake the mood or the thoughts of my friend.

Closed forms started happening. A closed form is a pot that you pull into a completely closed top—trapping air inside. It looks like a ball. You keep teasing the lip of the pot in toward the center of the pot. The lip gets very thin and it is a delicate process. When the lips finally meet, you seal them over, and you have a closed form. I thought of them as wombs—the ultimate container-vessel—a protective place. Rosaly and I are great protectors. Now I am literally throwing wombs to hold her. So there I was sitting in front of these four forms—in my mind, wombs, and I opened them with gentle tears—so she could enter. Then I went to bed.

When I got up the next day I thought—she can't enter these pots, but she can put her words in them.... The rest was calculated. I called her and asked her to write words on slips of paper—whatever came to mind. Of course she was puzzled. But I said "Just do it—There is a reason," and asked her to mail them to me. After Christmas, I glazed and fired the pots. I invited Rosaly to lunch the day after the firing when the kiln would be cool enough to open.

As we ate our bread and soup, I explained to her we were going to have a kiln opening and there was something in the kiln for her. I also told her the whole thing might be a failure because you never know what you'll find when you open a kiln.

Well, we opened the kiln and there they were. They were too hot to touch so we donned insulated gloves and lifted them carefully out. We brought them into the house, and I handed her the envelope containing words. I asked her to drop the slips of paper into the pots and let the pots hold the words and the pain. Let them be a place to which she could transfer the anguish and give herself a chance to heal.

Thus the pain pots were born.

The Words Said Before Viewing the Pots Were:

Prayer
Constant
Blue cold
Near breath
Glass Victory

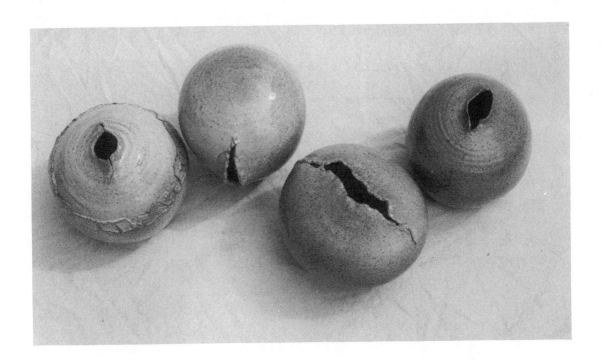

Sue Walker

PATTY CAKES AND POETRY

If I were to walk into the supermarket or a tire store this June summer morning and take a survey on who had read what poem in the last week, I do not have much doubt about what the results would be. If I weren't laughed at or classified "deranged," I would be surprised. Certainly I could make no great claims for poetry. A line like "Shall I compare thee to a summer's day" wouldn't be recognized as easily as the Infiniti symbol on their high-tech car or song lyrics by "The Grateful Dead." What use is poetry if it is seldom read, little appreciated, and rarely committed to memory aside from some English teacher's quirky demand that in order to pass American Lit, it is necessary to memorize Frost's "The Road Not Taken."

If I love poetry—and I declare that I do—am I able to make a claim for it? Say that it has some use? Okay, I want to try, and I guess I should being with my acquaintance with it and assume that what is true for me has some validity for others also.

My earliest memory of poetry is of nursery rhymes. No, I can't say that I remember clapping my hands and reciting "Patty-cake" to my parent's great approbation—though I think that this early memorization of verse is one of the first ways a child earns parental approval and recognizes that this is so. But what I do remember is crying because my father would tease me by inserting a stray poetic line into my recitation. I would start with "Little Miss Muffet sat on a tuffet," and he would add "eating a Christmas pie." I would shriek with rage. That wasn't right, and I knew it. Looking back and considering the significance of the experience, I think it had something to do with a sense of order and rhythm that is a part of life and living like the cyclic turn of winter to spring, of summer edging into fall. It was satisfying to feel the flow of rhythm and meter come from the fit of the right lines of verse. Perhaps it would not be too fantastic a leap to claim that this rhythm simulates the human heart and that my outrage over the disruption of "Jack and Jill went up the hill" with "to sweep the cobwebs off the sky" was kin to the arrhythmic heart that needs a pacemaker to set it right. But let me go on.

I want to speak of another memory connected with poetry, a more concrete and vivid one than the recitation of nursery rhymes and the game my father liked to play. I was five and had just had my tonsils removed. I remember waking after the anesthetic wore off, the pain of my sore throat. I wanted my mother to read to me—in particular, from Robert Louis Stevenson's *A Child's Garden of Verses*. Nothing brought relief like the lines:

> I have a little shadow that goes in and out with me,
> And what can be the use of him is more than I can see.
> He is very like me from the heels up to my head;
> And I can see him jump before me, when I jump into my bed.

Can I maintain that the order and rhythm of Stevenson's verse helped set right the pain and disorder that I was experiencing from the removal of my tonsils? Is it too bold to say that when there is a disruption within the self—pain or fear—that the something within which cries for reparation, for order restored, just may receive it from the balance, the ebb and flow, the rhythm of poetry? I think not.

Let me jump forward some thirty years. this is the June of my father's dying—a time when all the summers I have known have pooled together like a box of Crayolas left in the sun. The green of grass and trees have melted with hibiscus yellow-red, and the world is a splotch of color that seems surreal. People are figures of sticks, and I find it hard to get anything into perspective. Everything revolves around my father lying in a coma in intensive care from a stroke that takes his life and causes the most disruption I have known. Some of the time I weep, but when I try to put the loss, the rage, the confusion into words, I find myself turning to poetry. I try to be stoic, tell myself that, in Yeats' words in "Lapis Lazuli"

> All perform their tragic play,
> there struts Hamlet, there is Lear,
> That's Ophelia, that Cordelia;
> Yet they, should the last scene be there,
> The great stage curtain about to drop,
> If worthy their prominent part in the play
> Do not break up their lines to week.

And I buck up for awhile. Other times when there is silence too deep for tears and I feel more zombie than human kind, I think of Emily Dickinson's "After great pain, a formal feeling comes— / the nerves sit ceremonious, like Tombs—." Then, when a sense of outrage engulfs me because the world goes on when I am racked with sorrow, Auden's "Musée des Beaux Arts" come to mind:

> About suffering they were never wrong,
> The Old Masters: how they understood
> Its human position; how it takes place
> While someone else is eating or opening a window or just walking
>   dully along

And over and over again, I come back to the sustaining power of love, to the lines of a poem I wrote when my father first developed heart trouble over five years ago. It is a poem that asked words to alter the reality of thing—one entitled "Live Old Soldier, Live":

> I refuse to let you die, Dad
> See you suffer, struggle for breath
> Flat on your back in a hospital bed,
> Your life an electrocardiogram.

I'll stage it another way. Listen;
The month is April.
Azaleas blaze with color in Mobile.
I wear the wishbone pin you gave me,
And when you drive up,
We'll lunch at Korbets as we always do;
I'll order shrimp cocktail,
You'll have chicken and dumplings
With a side order of turnip greens.

Old Soldier, your heart is forever
In the sanctity of a moment like this.

I believe that there is a sanctity of poetry that encompasses both life and death and strives for a kind of order and harmony that replicates the music of the spheres. Before the Fall, it was said that humans could hear this music, but because of sin, of human imperfections, their ears were stopped. In Shakespeare's *Merchant of Venice,* Lorenzo tells Jessica that:

Such harmony is in immortal souls;
But whilst this muddy vesture of decay
Doth grossly close it in, we cannot hear it.

It is easy to see how poetry manifests harmony in times of joy, for even lovers who never strive to be poets find themselves writing rhymes to their beloved. It is in its rhythmic effect, the melos of poetry, that its greatest potential lies—both in the exploration of areas of human consciousness and in creating an aesthetic experience. Poetry is the heartbeat, the brain waves of our humanness that represent that represent a harmony and order beyond this world we know. It is a movement from maturity to sanctity that embraces life as a fulfillment of youth, and death as a fulfillment of life. Whether we recognize it or not on a hot June day standing in the check-out line of a supermarket or buying a new right-front tire, poetry is within us—dormant perhaps, but available and ready to be of use.

Robert M. Randolph

THE PATIENT'S NAME STORY

Patients with serious illnesses might feel as though they are being forced to live a life which is not their own. There may seem to be a well self, that is grieved for, and a sick self one is being forced to be that has nothing to do with the patient's deepest sense of identity.

The illness might be seen, in literary terms, as a hiatus in the test of the patient's life. In that situation, a sense of health, well-being, or perhaps even being (or meaning) itself, may seem to have to originate from outside, and the powers of the "inner healer," the body's natural regenerative and creative powers, might have to work against the attitude of the patient.

In biblical terms, the question of identity or self-concept is often related to the question of "name," a person's name being directly connected to their life story. "Abram," for example, becomes "Abraham" when his life changes. That is a useful concept. To patients, the "name" that they call themselves might seem appropriate now that they are seriously ill, and the truer, deeper name may not be presenting itself.

In stating their understanding of their "name" to the doctor, nurse, chaplain, family member, or visitor, patients are telling a story, and the tools of literary criticism can be used to help heal them through the story. The integrity of the story is directly related to the integrity of the patient's self-concept; the "better" the story, the deeper the meanings in it, the truer the "name" would be, and the fuller the sense of identity the patient would have.

Two kinds of stories must be identified and avoided in order to get at a patient's own name-story. The first is the story in the language of the doctor. This is often told by the patient from the third person point of view and is full of articles (the cancer, the femur, through the throat to the spine, the heart) and sometimes an abundance of words from medical texts. The story is really the doctor's story. Patients speak of themselves in this story as a setting for the illness, and the illness is really the central character.

The other kind of story to be steered away from is the simplified plot of guilt/punishment and confession/automatic restoration of health. Although the healing power of confession cannot be doubted, ideally the confession need be as deep as the sense of guilt it addresses, and axiomatically the confession need be genuine. Often, however, the gap between the simplicity of a confession story and the complexity of patients' true stories is too wide to permit the release of creativity and healing from their deeper selves, leaving miracle as the only hope. If the sense of guilt is "truer" than the story of confession and the confession does not, in that case, open the self to healing, the story is too shallowly conceived and actually protective of the evil it wants to confront. In terms of religion, the confession can be seen as insincere; in terms of literature, the story is contrived.

The name-story, on the other hand, is a kind of art described by Martin Buber in *I and Thou:*

> This is the eternal origin of art that a human being confronts a form that wants to become a work through him [or her]. Not a figment of his [or her] soul but something that appears to the soul and demands the soul's creative power. What is required is a deed that a man [a person] does with his [or her] whole being. (60)

Art in this sense is the expression of *being* in a person, the telling of one's "name" in the biblical sense. It can be a conscious story, which patients and visitors can interpret and work on as if they were working on a novel to which the patients would later affix their signatures.

The idea that story and self can be so closely related needs little defense, but the idea that this relationship can be used to help heal is receiving new consideration. In a recent book, *The Living Human Document,* Charles Gerkin writes, "Language constructs world" (30). He adds that in the "dialogical hermeneutical process" that takes place between a patient and a hospital chaplain, "a new set of images emerges that structures a new, less painful and more helpful story" (28). His book argues that hermeneutical approaches are useful in helping heal patients.

Jungian analyst, James Hillman, has developed the idea of treating the patient's story, in a book entitled *Healing Fiction.* Hillman writes:

> Patients say, "It doesn't make any sense; I've wasted the best years of my life. I don't know where I am, or who I am" … The patient is in search of a new story, or of reconnecting with the old one. I believed the story to be the sustaining fiction … but [the patient] had taken her story literally in the clinical language in which it had been told her, a tale of sickness, abuse, wastage of the best years. The story needed to be doctored, not her; it needed reimaging … She was indeed a victim, not of her history, but of the story in which she had put her history" (17).

Although the connection between story and self is newly considered by these writers, the rootedness of the idea in human experience can be suggested from many ancient texts. The biblical story of Job provides one such example.

After telling his name-story, Job receives a new understanding of his identity at the deepest levels of his being. One could well argue that if Job's story had had less integrity (if he had given in to his critics who offered their own "readings" of his life, and had cast his story in their terms) he would not have seen God with his "own eyes," as he finally says he has done. It could be strongly argued that the fuller relationship which silences Job is the effect of Job's telling his name-story as he knows it, and as he himself painfully works it out in dialogue with his critics. It is the story he puts together as truly as he can, his central story, which he can sign with his own "name," that brings him peace. Only after telling that story does Job see God and understand his life's context, which is surely the real restoration of his riches and his sense of well-being. That he struggles with his story as much as he does with his afflictions is incontrovertible, and clearly suggestive of their interconnection.

In the ancient story of Job one encounters the idea that one's true story is the way to true identity, and to a sense of context within the universe, which is synonymous with a sense of one's *being*. God appears finally to instruct Job, but this instruction follows Job's telling of his own story. God's criticism does not downplay the importance of Job's integrity or the integrity of Job's story, but points out that Job is not God and that there is integrity in the structure of the universe of which Job is but a part. Job, Oedipus at Colonus, the Ancient Mariner, and countless others, learn such lessons. They learn that their story is both their own and part of a larger story, the former awareness leading to the latter.

How can this idea help today's patient? Consider an example of a name-story in an actual hospital situation. A chaplain is visiting a patient. The patient is a forty year old man who has been run over by a train and lost one leg just below the knee. He does not remember if he was sleeping or walking on the tracks, because it is "not gone right at the knee", but a bit below. He says he is "lucky because other people get run over and die." He says that there is no infection in his leg and that he will get out of the hospital in a few days and learn how to walk. He says that the local paper has written that he was "drug thirty yards by the train," but he is sure "it wasn't that far." His final statement to the chaplain on the first visit is, "I woke up in some bad trouble, but never nothing like this."

If the chaplain had been listening to the story as a student of literature, the patient would be a hero in not being killed by the train, in not being dragged thirty yards, and, most importantly, in having a speedy recovery. In fact, he is something of a picaresque hero. There is a strong clue, however, to the possibility of incoherence in the story which is expressed in the words, "I woke up in some bad trouble, but never nothing like this."

In talking to a social worker, the chaplain learns that the patient has been living a life full of railroad tracks and drunkenness, that his past is "sketchy," that he has had many jobs and a long history of severed relationships. He is looking at a long-term recovery, including learning to walk again, perhaps considerable frustration, and more likely than not a change in lifestyle. That outlook is not a comfortable setting for a picaresque hero. What the chaplain can do is help the patient revise himself as a major figure, to fit into his current story without loss of his power as the central character of his whole life, because in that thrust lies much potential for healing. By revising his name-story, the patient can revise himself as a hero and come to star in his own actual life, thus encouraging the "inner healer" to have a reason to do its work.

Helpful discussion, criticism, or observation, might go along these lines: What can he learn about himself now? In Aristotelian terms, this could be seen as "recognition." What does the future look like? This is the idea of "plot." How does his new "name" draw from the person he has been? This idea concerns unity of action. Since he might have to start thinking of himself more as a person who does not give up, instead of a person who can move on whenever he wants to, are there instances of his not giving up from his past? This is similar to revising a text and discovering meanings previously missed. In any case, repeating the old story would not help him begin to "write" the new one, the one he is actually starring in. His old "name" is now too shallow, being drawn from a less *complex* story, but it is certainly not lost.

Although the details in this example are unique, the patient may well be representative. Patients who are seeking their "names" are in the grip of incongruity. Their old values and strengths do not necessarily seem applicable to their current situation, which nevertheless demands from them a sense of identity. They could feel that they have fallen from the role of central character in their own lives. In terms of literary analysis these people are experiencing a "reversal" on the way to a new identity, which includes a "recognition," a sort of change from ignorance to knowledge, even if they do not experience the restoration of physical health. They might, in fact, be learning how to be the central character of their own death.

As patients tell their stories, in the flashbacks there may be instances of the newly needed strength. Visitors, as critics, can point those out and help develop those instances into a perspective. They can help turn the lights down, in a sense, on some parts of the story and turn them up on others, thereby highlighting the new useful parts. This results in a "deeper" reading of the patient's life, and the identification of symbols and motifs previously left unexplored. Patients will then know themselves in a way which is both new and nevertheless deep-rooted and familiar. The goal of this process of revision is to achieve something, finally, like what the poet Rilke prays for in his poem translated by Robert Bly:

> O Lord, give each person his own personal death.
> A dying that moves out of the same life he lived,
> In which he had love, and intelligence, and trouble" (34)

And in which, one might add, that patients increasingly sense their inner "names."

The following terms and ideas from literary criticism seem useful in talking with people who are seriously ill.

Title: Is the title of the patient's story, for example, "My Death," or "My Despair," or "My New Understanding," or "My Redemption," or "My Victory?" The title might give a clue to the focus necessary for the integrity of the story.

Structure: Where does the story start? A story starting with an accident two years ago, for example, is not a whole-person story. Do the episodes go from surgery to surgery, from understanding to understanding, or setback to setback? If the movement is from diagnosis to diagnosis, for example, is there a parallel movement from self-definition to self-definition as a central character? The understanding of the episodic structure could show the patient's outlook on the next episode.

Theme: Do patients embody the main idea? If not, what idea do they embody, and what stories are being told around them? Do they feel they are living along side of their own real life?

Point of View: Is it the patient's own story, or the doctor's wife's, husband's, or minister's? Is the patient or the illness the central character? Are patients giving up their rights to their own stories?

Subplot: Do patients do things primarily because others, who are in the "real" plot, ask them to? Have they been responsible for the choices which influenced the plot of the story, as they tell it? What is the story in which the patient has been responsible for the choices? Is the patient's story, and illness, a subplot of somebody else's life as the patient sees it?

Tone: To what audience is the patient telling the story? What does the patient hope to get from the story? Is there a sense of manipulation of the audience involved in the way the patient is telling the story and, if so, is it toward sound artistic effect?

Healing is not necessarily the restoration of physical health, but a sense of integrity of being and interconnectedness with being in a larger sense. The tools of literary criticism can help heal the story of a patient and, in so doing, help heal self-concepts, and possibly, physical bodies as well.

REFERENCES

Buber, Martin. *I and Thou*. Trans. Walter Kaufman. New York: Charles Scribner, 1970.

Bly, Robert. "A Wrong Turning in American Poetry." *Claims for Poetry*. Ed. Donald Hall. Ann Arbor: University of Michigan Press, 1982.

Gerkin, Charles V. *The Living Human Document: Revisioning Pastoral Counseling in a Hermeneutical Mode*. Nashville: Abingdon Press, 1984.

Hillman, James. *Healing Fiction*. Barrytown: Station Hill, 1883.

Gerald Weissmann

THE AGE OF MIRACLES HADN'T PASSED

Native of Pesaro in the Marches of Ancona, Michelina Metelli was married at the age of twelve to Lord Malatesta of the dukes of Rimini. She became a widow at twenty, and shortly afterwards her only child died. She distributed her goods to the poor and, after St. Francis' example, begged her bread and sought humiliations. ... She also devoted herself to the care of lepers, tending and kissing their leprous sores, and sometimes, they say, miraculously restoring them to health.

OMER ENGLEBERT, *The Lives of the Saints*

Eighteen hours after she was rushed to Bellevue Hospital, Dyanne Watrous was miraculously restored to health. She had been admitted in shock, half comatose, and with open sores over much of her body. Her mother told medical residents that Dyanne, now thirty-one, had suffered from "lupus disease" since her late teens in a Harlem high school. The condition had responded to cortisonelike drugs over the years; despite it, Dyanne had been able to do well in high school and secretarial college, to bear a son and hold a job in a Wall Street brokerage house. With pluck, she had survived two miscarriages, an abortion, and bouts of cocaine addiction.

Then, some three months before Dyanne was brought to the hospital, things fell apart. She stopped taking cortisone on the advice of an herbal therapist and soon grew listless; fatigue forced her to give up work. She became progressively more depressed, lethargic, and bedridden; her weight dropped from 120 pounds to 87. On the morning of admission, Dyanne had been suffering from prolonged, shaking chills and could not be roused by her mother.

At Bellevue, an astute medical team quickly sized up the problem. They decided that in addition to her underlying disease—which had affected mainly her skin, joints, and platelets—Ms. Watrous had an acute infection of the bloodstream. She also showed signs of that relative exhaustion of the adrenal glands which follows prolonged treatment with cortisonelike drugs. Many patients with lupus require treatment with these powerful drugs as diabetics require insulin, to make years of normal existence possible. When as a young medical student I saw at first hand the miraculous response of patients with lupus to cortisone, I became an instant convert to rheumatology. The secular orders offer their own epiphanies.

By the time we saw Ms. Watrous in consultation, she had been restored to the land of the living by antibiotics, which fought the bloodstream infection, and by intravenous hydrocortisone, which overcame adrenal insufficiency. Our patient was alert, but understandably tired. She seemed pleased to see a flock of rheumatologists; since high school she had known that her condition fell into our bailiwick. Unwrapping her dressings, we found that her skin bore not only the chronic lesions of lupus but also new scarlet blotches over her shins and the tips of her fingers. These resulted most likely from an unusual reaction (toxic epidermal necrosis) to her bloodstream infection. After we had finished our examination, she sat up primly in bed to face our row of white-coated doctors. Her ebony head was wrapped in a white cotton turban that covered her marred scalp, her chest heaved under a blue hospital gown, red blotches speckled what could be seen of her skin. After we had listened to more of her story, I held her hand and asked her to describe how she felt, overall, in comparison to a few weeks ago.

"Doc," she replied, "never mind weeks. Compared to what was it, Tuesday? It's like a miracle happened!"

Sure enough, I thought. In fact, on that bright spring morning, as sun shone through the windows of 16-East at Bellevue, the entire scene—the primary colors, the spare furnishings, the blotched invalid upright in bed—reminded me of those fourteenth-century predella panels that illustrate a miracle of healing wrought by one or another of the company of saints. Later, away from the bedside, when we discussed the management of Ms. Watrous, the predella image persisted. I wondered out loud whether a panel illustrating her miraculous recovery might be more appropriately dedicated to Alexander Fleming (1881-1955), the discoverer of penicillin, or to Philip Hench (1896-1972), who first treated rheumatic diseases with cortisone. The choice would be a toss-up: certainly both qualify as "heroes without halos"—to borrow a phrase of Phyllis McGinley's. Both were canonized, but at Stockholm rather than Rome, the more common practice nowadays.

A young colleague pointed out how outdated my quandary was: "Simple. It all depends on the DRG that you pick: 416 it's Fleming, 240 it's Hench. Let HCFA decide!"

A briefing is required, lest you think that DRG is a new sports car or that HCFA (pronounced "hickfah") is a ritual bath in the Ozarks. For the last several years, American hospitals have been reimbursed not for what it costs to take care of patients, but according to a complex book of schedules that divides all human maladies into twenty-three major "diagnosis-related groups." These spell out not only who pays how much to whom when and if, but also for how long and for what. As might be expected from a program based on a compound adjective, it is monitored by an agency based on the gerund, the Health Care Financing Administration. Its two aims are noble: the cutting of cost without the cutting of corners. Most would agree that the first has been achieved.

Be that as it may, my choices for Ms. Watrous's patron saint were not made easy by the DRG handbook. Had her primary diagnosis been that of an infection of the bloodstream #416 (*septicemia age > 17*), she would have had 7.4 days in hospital and merit $7,093 reimbursement. On the other hand, a DRG for lupus #240 (*connective tissue disorders with complications*) would have also permitted a stay of 7.3 days but netted a mere $4,262 to the hospital. Since she ran into trouble from adrenal insufficiency, the appropriate DRG might also be #300 (*endocrine disorder with complica-*

tion), with only 6.0 days, and $4,848. An unfriendly QA inspector might accuse us of prolonging her stay had we tagged her with #416 or #240. "QA," by the way, stands for "quality assurance" and means its exact opposite.

All this categorical confusion had diverted the discussion from sainthood, but an item in *The New York Times* (via AP, April 17, 1988) pulled me back to the *The Lives of the Saints*. It seems that the inspector general's office of the Department of Health and Human Services had accused American hospitals of overbilling the Feds by "$2 billion a year." On the basis of a review of old records rather than fresh interviews with either docs or patients, this QA task force concluded that many of the "unnecessary admissions were 'social admissions' such as providing a bed for an elderly person without any other place to stay; admitting someone who really belonged in a nursing home; and in a few cases admitting someone who simply did not need acute medical care.

"The report found the unnecessary admissions tended to be concentrated in five diagnostic groups: back problems, diabetes, bone cancer, digestive disorders and upper respiratory infections."

I stopped worrying over the choice between Fleming and Hench and, in outrage, began to compare my DRG handbook with *The Lives of the Saints*. Both volumes provide detailed schedules of miraculous cures, but the company of saints was not expected to deliver these on demand or anticipate their cost; miracles are priceless in the eyes of God. Surely the saints would have bedded those "without any other place to stay" and admitted those with diabetes or bone cancer!

One wonders what rebuke would have met the Blessed Guy of Cortona (d. 1245) who housed and fed St. Francis of Assisi, then without any other place to stay. After washing St. Francis's feet, Guy said, "When you again need tunics and cloaks, do not hesitate to purchase them; I will pay for them." Would HCFA authorize the payment? Would its accountants refer to St. Audrey (d. 679) if considering patients whose admission for upper respiratory infection is considered "inappropriate"? This saint "wore inconvenient and clumsy clothing; after matins she remained at prayer in the choir until morning. An abscess of the throat from which she died towards the end of her life has made her the patron of those who suffer similar ills." The QA team would certainly reproach a modern administrator who followed the example of Abbot Hugh of Grenoble (1053-1131), by refusing orders to report on the comportment of his Carthusians with the gentle "Why set down faults?" St. Peter himself might be in for reprimand. St. Petronilla (first century) was his particular favorite, yet, "there came the day when, afflicted with paralysis, she was incapable of any work. 'Why don't you cure her?' Titus asked St. Peter. St. Peter answered: 'It is good for her to remain like that.' " The Feds might read it as DRG #17 (*nonspecific cerebrovascular disorder without complication*), or 4.7 days and $2,837. Since "God, however, restored her health," I would interpret St. Peter's admonition as a lesson in patience and faith.

It is depressing to think what guidance medical bureaucrats would draw from these exemplary lives. Englebert's book describes as many of the ills that befell the saints as those they were able to cure. As in the inspector general's report, the major ills of saints are concentrated in a few DRGs. Since many of the blessed were also martyrs, DRGs #444 and #445 are the most common (*multiple trauma, age > 17*), with and without complications. Yielding a hospital stay, short of martyrdom, of 5.3 or 3.7 days and expenses of $3,663 or $2,313, these DRGs describe the deaths of, among others, Sts. Catherine of Alexandria (dates unknown), Barbara (d. 235), Placidus (d. 540), John of God (1495-1550), and Sebastian (d. 288). St. Sebastian miraculously survived multiple wounds from Diocletian's archers (DRG #444), only to be cudgeled to death and thrown in a sewer (DRG #27, *traumatic stupor and coma > 1 hour;* 4.3 days, $6,584). DRG #457 (*extensive burns without operating-room procedures*) would cover Sts. John Before the Latin Gate (d. 95), Justina and Cyprian (d. 304), and Joan of Arc (1412-31). They each would be permitted 4.1 days and $11,299.

DRG #148 (*major small and large bowel procedure, with complications*) is the most generous with respect to length of stay and reimbursement: 14.5 days and $14,449. Into this category fall St. Erasmus (d. 303?), who was eviscerated by means of a windlass, and St. Ernest (d. 1148), whose insides were twined about a stake by his persecutors.

This sort of clinical detail is missing from the DRG handbook: its pages lack the touch of purpose. Better to have stories of devotion and martyrdom written by someone as eloquent and witty as the patron saint of writers, St. Francis de Sales (1567-1622) who might be considered the moral equivalent of Waugh.

Not all saints died as martyrs, nor are all martyrs saints; Dr. William Ober has reminded us that nowadays a martyr is defined as someone who has to live with a saint. Martyr or not, the saints were effective healers. Their cures also cluster in a small number of DRGs. Leprosy and plague were most susceptible: DRG #423 (*other infectious and parasitic diseases diagnoses* [*sic*]) permits 8.0 days in bed and $6,843. St. Peter (d. 64) healed lepers with his shadow, Sts. Romanus (d.463) and Michelina (1300-56) by kissing the lesions, St. Francis of Assisi (1182-1226) with prayer. Plague shares the same DRG with leprosy; its conquerors include St. Roch (d. 1327), Avertanus (d. 1370), Emiliani (d. 1537), and St. Charles Borromeo (d. 1548).

Other DRGs well handled by the saints were #419 (*fever of unknown origin, age > 17;* 5.9 days, $4,364) and #47, blindness (*other disorders of the eye, without complications;* 2.6 days, only $1,612). My favorite saint of this DRG is St. Macarius the Younger (d. 408) who brought back sight to the blind cub of a hyena and who was rewarded the next day by the hyena with the gift of "a magnificent sheepskin." This story touches all but university presidents.

Although *The Lives of the Saints* makes better reading than the DRG handbook, there are miracles in our new schedules that the saints might envy. I would love to read about St. Christiaan of Barnard or St. Michael De Bakey, who have revived more failing hearts, DRG #103 (*heart transplant;* 25.8 days, $53,209) or DRG #104 (*cardiac valve procedure with pump and with cardiac catheterization;* 17.4 days, $32,768), than all the saints in Englebert. Where are Sts. Selman of Waksman (tuberculosis), Max of Theiler (yellow fever), Jonas of Salk (poliomyelitis)? So great are their miracles that the diseases they conquered have all been reduced to DRG #423, alongside plague and leprosy.

The Lives of the Saints treats cures as unique events that testify to the glory of God; the DRG handbook publishes schedules of medical miracles that have become as routine as the Pan Am shuttle. The DRG schedules deprive us of words, of narrative, of secular devotion, of that flutter of delight when a miracle passes. I doubt that anyone is likely to find the healing vocation in the DRG handbook: what we have gained in power, we have lost in glory. Those dreary DRG numbers tell us that social justice makes poor reading.

Making rounds at Bellevue, checking in to see that Ms. Watrous remains improved, I watched a preppie woman resident wrapping her patient's shin. I was reminded of St. Christina the Astonishing (1150-1224), a holy woman who served the poor and sick with extreme devotion, despite her anguish at the stench of unwashed human flesh. "After contact with it, some time was necessary before she could stand her fellow man." She misbehaved at her own funeral: so many of her unwashed devotees crowded about her coffin, that the coffin—with fastidious Christina kicking inside—bounded away to the rafters of the church to escape the smell of humankind. But the saint returned, to mark a sanctuary for the sick. In such a sanctuary, there are no "unnecessary admissions."

John T. Morris

HEALERS AND WORDS

A certain chemical (or virus) invaded the human genome, approximately one million years ago, causing the development of communication by way of speech and altering forever man's relation to man and his environment. This development brought about the art of negotiation, and so the oldest profession was born. Several centuries or millinea later the second oldest profession, the practice of medicine, came about. The two professions have enjoyed a close association ever since. Ancient Egyptian healers, regarded music as the "physic of the soul" and inscribed their precious chants on the medical papyri. These papyri hold the first written communications by physicians. Fifty to sixty centuries ago the Egyptian priest-physicians prescribed molds and yellow Nile mud that contained penicillin and aureomycin for infection. They also applied poultices of yellow Nile mud bound with papyri on which were written incantations and poems. The Egyptian surgeons did advanced operative procedures, including circumcision, castration, and trephining (opening the skull). These procedures are described in the papyri, and we see corroborative evidence of them in the skulls and teeth of mummies dating from that period. Imhotep, who lived about 3000 B.C., is the first physician, whose name we know.

The Chinese discovered a process for making paper at about the same time the Egyptians were writing on papyrus. The Chinese had a novel treatment for stomach and bowel dysfunction. The Chinese doctor would write some poetry or a prayer on paper and give it to the patient, who would burn it with incense and make tea of the ashes. This simple device led the Chinese to boil their drinking water. Of course charlatans got hold of the process and substituted tea leaves for the amulets.

Modern scientists believe that the boiling of tea and rice has had a profound effect on the amazing proliferation of the Chinese people throughout history. Modern public health experts advise us to boil the water in certain countries. The charred paper used in the tea worked by adsorbing the toxins from the gut. Doctors employ this principle in modern hospitals for poison ingestion cases. The gas masks issued to the "Desert Shield" troops contain charcoal. Thus the Egyptians and the Chinese showed the first connection between "healing and words."

The connection grew firmer and more complex as time passed and other cultures came into being. By the time of the Greek Classic period the musician and poet had joined the physician. The Greeks of this period had a passion for physical perfection and mental astuteness. Realizing their human imperfections they created a god, Apollo, whom they endued with all physical and mental perfection. The Greeks made him the god of healing and of music and poetry. While Apollo practiced healing *and* poetry *and* music, his two sons Aesculapius and Orpheus specialized; Aesculapius in healing and Orpheus, who invented the lyre, was the musician and poet.

Among the Greeks Hippocrates of Kos (b. 450 B.C.) stands out as the great communicator. His oath has been administered to medical students since 400 B.C. and is one of the finest codes of ethics in existence.

Later, Aristotle, the son of a physician, made many scientific observations. He was the master of all the knowlege available to him in his lifetime (c. 384-322 B.C.). He wrote treatises on *Logic, Metaphysics, Poetics,* and *Science.* He gave considerable medical advice in his treatises. All Europe followed the scientific and medical teaching of Aristotle and Galen throughout the dark ages, even though they were non-Christians. All other heathen were considered unreliable regardless of their logic.

Claudius Galen (130-200 A.D.) was a Greek physician who practiced in Rome. He wrote a large number of works on medicine, natural science and logic. Galen and Aristotle's writings were used as encyclopedias and were accepted as facts, not to be questioned. With this attitude toward medical science no progress was possible.

Saint Luke, the gifted writer of The Gospel, was a physician. He writes beautifully of historical and divine occurrences, but we know little of his medical practice. I know of no other individual physician mentioned by name in The Bible. There is much advice on hygiene, diet and cleanliness, and there are many laws governing hygienic behavior. In Leviticus Chapter 3 verse 17: "It shall be a perpetual statute for your generation throughout all your dwellings, that ye eat neither fat nor blood." Leviticus Chapter 11 describes abominations such as swine and hares and advises on how to cleanse clothing and utensils of contamination by dead animals. Leviticus Chapter 13 deals with the diagnosis and quarantine of leprosy.

After the fall of the Roman Empire, c. 500 A.D., the dark ages settled on Europe. The healing arts and the muse moved into Islam. Avicenna (980-1037) was the most celebrated Arabian physician and philosopher. A Persian philosopher and healer of the tenth and eleventh century A.D. wrote some of the world's most beautiful poetry, some of which was translated into English in 1859 by Edward Fitzgerald as *The Rubaiyat of Omar Kayyam.* Kayyam was a famous man in his time as an astronomer and mathematician but not as a poet. Indeed, few people heard of Omar Kayyam's poetry while he was alive. He believed in an earthly paradise, complete with much wine and lovely women. He showed some doubts about the wisdom of the Creator. These views reflected in Kayyam's poetry would not have been tolerated by the strict orthodox Islamic laws.

By the year 1265 Europe was beginning to wake up and Dante Alighieri was born. His "Divine Comedy," written between that date and September 14, 1321, the date of his death, has been called "the most magnificent cathedral of the middle ages." In 1295-1301 he joined the Physicians' and Apothecary's Guild.

The renaissance in literature may be said to have begun with Dante. The renaissance in the healing arts lagged far behind. It began with the discovery of the circulation of blood by William Harvey (1578-1657) and the publication of his treatise on the subject, *De Motu Cordis et Sanguinis in Animalibus* in 1628. This was an exercise in pure logic and lighted the way for all the advances in physiology and medicine since that time.

Sir Thomas Browne (1605-1682) attempted to reconcile science and religion in his *Religio Medici*. He was a great literary stylist, and a noted physician. Life fascinated him. Death revolted him. Browne states that "I am not so much afraid of death as ashamed thereof." In his *Hydriotaphia, Urn-Burial,* he shows his vast knowledge of Scriptures and history and tells of his philosophy of the soul being "snatched from the body." He ends with a quotation by the Latin poet Lucan:

> "By the swift funeral pyre or slow decay
> (No matter which) the bodies pass away."

Sir Thomas Browne believed in the immortality of the soul and the irrelevance of the body after its death.

After Harvey's discovery of the circulation of blood, the next great advance in medicine was by a gentle considerate man, Edward Jenner (1749-1823), who first ascribed the cause of angina pectoris to disease of the heart's arteries. This discovery had to be made again by Herrick in 1912 and by Samuel Levine in 1918 because of lack of communication. In the twentieth century coronary artery disease was responsible for more deaths, among Americans, than all other causes combined.

Jenner's greatest contribution to humanity was his work in immunology. He gave up a lucrative practice to pursue, without recompense, his work on smallpox vaccine. Edward Jenner is one of the pillars on which modern medicine rests. Without going into too much detail, I would say that Edward Jenner made the single most important discovery in medical history. However, he still found time to write poetry, some of it pretty fair.

Before the nineteenth century the practice of medicine was exceedingly rudimentary; however, there were several very fine writers who practiced medicine to a greater or lesser degree.

Thomas Lodge (1558-1625), a popular practitioner, is known as a fair lyric poet. Thomas Campion (1567-1620), a lawyer, physician, poet, musician, dramatist and philosopher is acclaimed as one of the nine lyric masters in English Poetry. Tobias George Smollett (1721-1771), a medical man, achieved a reputation as a novelist and poet. Oliver Goldsmith (1728-1774) tried and adorned every form of literature. He failed to earn a livelihood as a healer.

One of England's greatest poets, John Keats (1795-1821), was born in a livery stable and educated at Enfield. He was apprenticed to a surgeon for study and training in 1811 and worked there for four years. In 1815 he enrolled at Guy's Hospital where he later became a "dresser." Keats must have learned his profession well, and in 1816 he passed his examination to become an "apothecary surgeon." That year Keats came of age and abandoned the practice of medicine in favor of literature for the greater enrichment of mankind. He was to live only five more years.

John Keats's literary works have been evaluated by scholars and I can add no luster that has not already been shed on them. In February 1820 Keats coughed up blood. It was not frothy so he knew it was not pneumonia or bronchitis. It was not old black blood from retrograde nose bleed. It was bright red whole blood and Keats, the physician, knew it was arterial. This could mean only one thing, that the phthisis had eroded an artery. He had "Galloping Consumption" with only a short time to live.

The previous fall, Keats and Fanny Braune, the one great love of his life, had become engaged. Keats's brother George had run into financial difficulty, and John himself had barely enough funds to finance the winter in Italy, that he had been advised to take.

So, in the final act of Keats's drama, we have the beloved poet in a foreign land, with limited funds. He is passionately in love and fully aware that he will never see his beloved again. The muse has deserted him. His great contributions to western culture are being snipped at by Philistine reviewers. He is facing the certainty of a tediously prolonged death. John Keats had "Negative Capability," and it was now stretched to its limits.

On the Continent, Francois Rabelais (c. 1494-1553), after exhorting his reader to look beneath the surface of his frivolity for the sense in what he writes, proceeds to entertain with some of the most original stories in all literature. With his wit and ability to charm people in high places, he escaped the inquisition even though that tribunal burned one of his publishers at the stake. Beneath Rabelais' frivolity is a cry for liberty and faith in humanity.

Johann Christoph Friedrich von Schiller (1759-1805) wanted to prepare for the church but began studying law and then changed to medicine. He finished his course at Karlsschule in Stuttgart in 1780 and became a regimental surgeon. The call of literature was too much for Schiller. He wrote plays that his sovereign duke considered to be seditious. In 1792 he was made an honorary citizen of the new French Republic. His writing expresses his high ideals and his advocacy of moral and spiritual freedom. In the world's literature Schiller's *Wallenstein*, a group of plays about one of the leaders of the Thirty Years War, is without peer. All of Schiller's writing has an ethical core.

Schiller and Goethe became close friends in 1799 to the profit of each of them and German literature. In their, so called, Ballad Year (1797) Goethe and Schiller wrote some of their finest ballads, among them Schiller's *Der Taucher* ("The Diver"), *Der Handschu* ("The Glove"). The collaboration of these two great poets may have been similar to our "Poetry on Assignment."

While the American Revolution was the greatest event in the nation's history, that period, and several of the decades following it, were the darkest in the history of American Medicine. One of the great patriots and a truly great war hero, and signer of the Declaration of Independence, Dr. Benjamin Rush, conceived the idea that poison in the blood caused all human illness. He came to the conclusion that bloodletting should be the treatment for all disease. Rush had a great following because of his war record and his learned lectures and treatises. Dr. Rush cautioned his students that in bloodletting nothing could be worse than timidity. He also advised large daily doses of calomel and painful poultices and blistering with suction cups. Rush bled one of his patients 22 times in 10 days, taking a total of 176 ounces of blood. Rush died in 1813 and American Medicine thrived.

An Alabamian, J. Marion Sims, was born in 1813, the year Benjamin Rush died. Sims found that silver wire protected against infection when used as sutures to close wounds. In 1852 he won worldwide recognition when he reported on surgical operations, never done before, that he had done successfully. In 1853 he moved from Alabama to New York City and became the first doctor in the United States to practice as a specialist in diseases of women. Sims's treatise, *Clinical Notes on Uterine Surgery* (1866), was translated into several languages and was widely read in Europe, where Sims became regarded (rightly so) as America's most original and gifted surgeon.

Another Alabamian, John Allen Wyeth (1845-1922), was born in Guntersville, Alabama. He joined the Confederate cavalry and fought as a private soldier under General Joseph Wheeler and General Nathan Bedford Forrest. Union forces captured Wyeth at Chicamauga and he spent two years in a federal prison. After the war Wyeth studied medicine at the University of Louisville and returned to Guntersville to practice. His fourth patient died and Wyeth, full of guilt feelings, closed his office and went to New York City where he did graduate studies at Bellevue Hospital.

Wyeth became a famous surgeon, president of the New York Medical Society and president of the American Medical Association. He wrote a *Textbook of Surgery* that was used throughout America well into the twentieth century. A man of boundless energy, Wyeth wrote a biography of Lieutenant General Nathan Bedford Forrest that is one of the most thoroughly researched and documented works of its kind. It has recently been reprinted as *That Devil Forrest*.

John Wyeth married the daughter of J. Marion Sims. As Sims had founded the New York Lying-In Hospital, so Wyeth founded the New York Polyclinic Hospital, the first postgraduate medical institution in America. Even Wyeth's poetry is innovative. In his rhymed works he avoids the sing-song effect by separating the rhymed lines widely: A, B, C, D, A, B, C, D as in this poem:

Air Raid

Reading, at night, the shutter closed and bared
a candle by my mattress on the floor,
my Virgil open to the mellow flame,
I heard what seemed a racking change of gear—
like some truck mired outside the stable yard.
The stricken pages shook—A vast smash tore
at the room, and through the blackness came
a bestial angry grinding drone, and fear.

Wyeth also wrote poetry in the free verse mode.

Most of the healers of nineteenth century America were poorly educated and had very little training. Oliver Wendell Holmes was an exception. He was educated in law and literature and gained an early reputation as a poet. In 1833 he went to Europe and studied under the masters there. When he returned home he took his M.D. degree at Harvard and began the practice of medicine. His neighbors looked on him as a literary man and didn't take him seriously as a physician. Holmes was more interested in the scientific and educational aspects of medicine. He was an effective and lucid writer on medical and literary topics. In 1843 he read a paper before the Boston Society for Medical Improvement: *On the Contagiousness of Puerpural Fever.*

The Atlantic Monthly was founded in 1857 and Dr. Holmes gave it its name and was a regular contributor. Holmes died in 1894, one of America's great literary figures and one of the foundation stones of modern American medicine.

It would be impossible to cover the intricacies of the explosion of medical knowledge in the twentieth century. As medical learning became more complex, the quality of the literary efforts of the healers declined. The great novelist physicians —Somerset Maugham, A.J. Cronin, Frank Slaughter— after sharpening their powers of observation with a medical education, quit practicing medicine to write.

Interesting individuals appear among the poet physicians. Hans Zinsser began his education as a poet. He published a small book of poetry as an undergraduate student. After reading his poetry in book form, he felt that it was of such low quality that he decided to abandon literature and try some premedical courses. The book has been thoroughly suppressed, and it is impossible to find it.

Zinsser became so engrossed in bacteriology that he became one of the world's authorities. His textbook went through many editions. When he was asked about his occupation he would tell people that he was "a small game hunter." He continued to write poetry for such prestigious periodicals as *The Atlantic Monthly* and would sign it R.S. (Romantic Self). In 1938 Zinsser diagnosed his own malady, lymphatic leukemia. Knowing it to be fatal, he wrote his autobiography referring to himself in the third person as R.S. It is touching and interesting writing. He died in 1940. His last bit of writing was an unnamed sonnet:

> Now is death merciful. He calls me hence
> Gently, with friendly soothing of my fears
> Of ugly age and feeble impotence
> And cruel disintegration of slow years.
> Nor does he leap upon me unaware
> Like some wild beast that hungers for its prey,
> But gives me kindly warning to prepare:
> Before I go, to kiss your tears away.
>
> How sweet the summer! And the autumn shone
> Late warmth within our hearts as in the sky,

Ripening rich harvests that our love had sown.
How good that 'ere the winter comes, I die!
Then, ageless, in your heart I'll come to rest
Serene and proud, as when you loved me best.

Marianne Moore entered Bryn Mawr college in 1905. She brushed with the healing arts after a professor wrote in the margin of one of her papers, "I presume you had an idea if any one could find what it is." Crushed, she considered medicine as a career to the extent that she concentrated on biology and histology. However, she recovered and became one of America's great poets. Moore became part of a group that included Wallace Stevens, Conrad Aiken, Havelock Ellis and William Carlos Williams. Marianne Moore was the best poet in the group.

Many critics regard William Carlos Williams as the most significant poet of the twentieth century. His use of words has been compared to an anaesthetist's probing with a needle for a nerve to stimulate or sedate. He achieves poetic qualities by the short broken and staggered line. He hated all meter and especially iambic pentameter. Williams arouses no weak emotions; either you admire him greatly or you don't. Many of the finest contemporary poets swear by him.

Gertrude Stein (1874-1946) studied psychology under William James at Radcliffe. She enrolled at the Johns Hopkins Medical School where she was an enthusiastic scholar in the basic sciences, especially the anatomy courses of Dr. Franklin Mall. Stein must have done some self study under William James. She broke down emotionally when she, as a third year medical student, had to go into the obstetric wards and witness the birth process. It was during this time that she discovered that she was homosexual. In 1903 she went to France with a female friend, Alice B. Toklas. She visited the United States in 1934, then returned to Paris and remained there for the rest of her life. She was one of the most versatile of modern writers. She wrote several novels, at least one book of poetry, two biographies, and books on how to write. She also wrote an opera. Gertrude Stein is best known for her influence on artists and writers.

John McCrae is known for only one poem, "In Flanders Field," which prompted the use of the poppy as the emblem to be worn on Armistice Day (now Veterans' Day). He wrote several other poems in the same vein, but they are now virtually forgotten. McCrae was a brilliant scholar who trained in the best Canadian Universities and at the Johns Hopkins Medical School in this country. He died of pneumonia January 28, 1918 while serving as a medical officer in the Canadian Expeditionary Forces in France.

William James obtained the M.D. degree at Harvard in his late twenties and accepted a position as instructor of physiology at Harvard in 1872. From that position he moved into psychology and then philosophy. It is said that William James's psychological treatises read as interestingly as novels and his brother, Henry James's novels read like psychological studies. Neither can be overlooked in a study of the relationship existing between words and healing, if one considers psychological diseases.

Some say Sigmund Freud is "the greatest Jew since Jesus Christ." His elucidation of the subconscious, with all its complexes and the concepts of "Id," "Ego," and "Superego," is probably his greatest achievement. Even though later psychiatrists have criticized many of his theories, the impact of Sigmund Freud on the study and treatment of mental illness cannot be denied. When asked where he got his ideas he pointed to his bookshelf. It contained the works of Shakespeare, Sophocles, Goethe, and Dante. "These are my masters," he said. He might have included those pragmatic psychologists, the prostitutes of Vienna among his teachers. They taught him about id, ego, and superego.

So the oldest profession teaches the youngest offspring of the second oldest profession. We now read the poems on the papyrus poultice and the incantations in tea leaves. The great physician-writers: Hippocrates, Galen, Aristotle, Avicenna, Dante Alghieri, Rabellais, Harvey, Edward Jenner, Sir Thomas Browne, Keats, Schiller, Holmes, —Sims, Wyeth, Marianne Moore, William Carlos Williams, Sigmund Freud, may rest. There will be other healers who will listen to the dictates of the muse and other poets who will feel the surge that comes from the heart of one who has relieved suffering—

"I swear by Apollo the healer, by Aesculapius,

Hygeia, and Panacea ..."

—Hippocrates

Ron Walker

WRITING AND HEALING

Physical health may reasonably be taken as a normal state and emotional health likewise. Our current culture is not as apt at promoting emotional health as it is physical health and there has been a growing acceptance during this century that physical health is closely linked to the emotional condition; there is a close interactive process between body and mind. The body has enormous resources that maintain health and it can be argued that ill-health is an abnormality of the health promoting system (principally the immune system.) If illness or disease occurs, the body is usually able to restore health by its own immune and reparative processes. When this is not achieved, it is likely that there is damage to these processes, and there is abundant evidence now to show that emotional factors are extremely significant in the promotion and maintenance of good health. The stress resulting from the pressure and anxiety of unresolved conflict is the damaging force. Emotional ill health not only tends to impair body function, it also impairs total functioning and satisfactory self fulfillment.

Psychological trauma is a stimulus or experience that cannot be managed within the scope of the normal coping mechanisms of an individual; this results in the use of other coping or defensive mechanisms, usually by regression, and this process is less adaptive and more "costly" in terms of an individual's overall adjustment. Conflict that cannot be resolved by direct reasoning and decision is repressed to an unconscious level but continues to exert a powerful influence. Depression may be associated with this mechanism and is usually a consequence of loss—actual or threatened, real or imagined. The loss is felt as trauma, and again, regression results and in turn produces its effects on the body's functioning. Depression may produce its own direct impact on the body perhaps by the slowing down of body processes. Guilt is frequently associated with unresolved conflict, and guilt has a destructive influence on behavior and health.

More could be added to the very complex processes of mind and body, but it can be taken as a given that mental processes influence health and that stagnant regressive maladaptive psychological mechanisms play a major part in undermining health, emotional adjustment and self-actualization.

How is this condition to be overcome? There are many ways in which regression is reversed. Positive experiences of support, nurturing, care and love, all promote repair and growth. Psychotherapy is a treatment specifically designed to understand the intrapsychic problems interfering with an individual's life and by the achievement of insight promotes conflict resolution.

Can writing be beneficial in promoting health and reparation? It is a fact that writing can be a very healing process, but the reasons for this are diverse. One way that trauma can be mastered is by the repetition of a negative experience in a controlled way. Children do this in play. A trip to the hospital is re-enacted many times and often the repetition includes turning a passive experience into an active one. The child becomes the doctor. This mechanism is also associated with the awful cycle of victim becoming victimizer, especially in child sexual abuse. Writing allows an older child or an adult to achieve the same results by the repetition of the experience in the writing—whether in fiction or poetry, whether an experience is accurately and correctly described or consciously hidden by the many distortions available to the creative writer—displacement in time, place, setting and identity as well as the use of metaphor and symbol. Writing out the experience gives a feeling of mastery over something that was felt as out of control. The communication of the trauma through writing may also be associated with the release of strong feeling previously pent up, and this produces a great decrease in tension.

However it is likely that conflicts that produce significant reactions are unconscious. Traumatic events may be severely traumatic only because they cut across pre-existing unconscious conflicts and so take on enormous amounts of additional energy. This fact may make a new trauma impossible to deal with by the ordinary available resources and so produce a more intense unresolvable situation resulting in chronic regression. While the individual is convinced that the problem lies in the remembered trauma, it may actually be some previous trauma, repressed into the unconscious that makes it impossible to cope with the trauma that is blamed. It is vastly more difficult to deal with unconscious issues because of their inaccessibility. They are blocked from direct access but continue to assert their presence indirectly.

Not all conflicts produce severe adaptational problems, but they may be associated with minor health problems or minor impairments of self-fulfillment.

I believe that writing can have a function in expressing these unconscious conflicts without the conscious awareness of the writer. However by externalizing the issue, albeit in a covert manner, it is possible for the writer to obtain some degree of resolution. The child who re-enacts the hospital experience is not aware that he is gaining mastery by externalizing the inner experience and turning passive into active. So writers may believe they are "only" writing when they are in fact dealing with inner issues. I would like to give an example of this in the following poem:

GATHERING EGGS WITH GRANDPA

When you took my hand
and led me into the henhouse,
it was a ceremony to share together;
this gathering of eggs,
this robbery.

Chicken coops, stacked like bunks
along the walls, waited;
we would not speak for fear
of disturbing hens at roost.

I would tiptoe up to one,
reach out with awe
I could sense but not understand.

Even at five, I knew it was a moment
as reverent as prayer, to feel the warmth,
the pulse of the egg
as I withdrew it
and gave it to you,

before Grandma took it—
as carelessly as the plate she removed
from the shelf—before she cracked it
into the pan and served it to me
sunny-side-up.

Grandpa, I want so much
to keep you alive through me—
through the laughter of my child
and blood. I remember
those moments we gathered eggs
sense anew the mystery
and the sin.

"In Gathering Eggs With Grandpa", the writer describes an event from childhood in literal terms that appear to justify the poem's existence by itself. However there are clues within the poem that suggest more is going on than the surface meaning might suggest. The word "ceremony" in line three immediately implies that this simple event is invested in much more than a common domestic happening. "Robbery" in line five also startles a little and adds tension to the story. And "I could sense but not understand" again increases the tension and importance of the act. It is in comical relief that we find that Grandma has none of this reverence and unceremoniously cracks and cooks the egg. The last stanza opens up more meaning by connecting Grandpa with her child and then returns again to the egg gathering by referring to "the mystery and the sin." I believe this poem is dealing with unconscious oedipal fantasies—probably displaced from the Father to the Grandfather as safer. The child is working through oedipal fantasies by this activity with the Grandfather and helped by the reality restoring Grandmother. The writer, in remembering the event, is able to re-work the experience and obtain greater control and so decrease anxiety by the writing.

It would seem possible that writing serves to reduce conflict by this hidden process. Writing is influenced by unconscious drives, but the underlying communications are often hidden from the writer because of defenses and by distortions that may have been unconsciously produced. The latent meaning is even more hidden from the reader by the same mechanisms.

Psychotherapy traditionally works by making conscious what was unconscious, by providing insight, and this is the traditional way to heal emotional damage. Writing may provide a kind of subliminal insight and enable the writer to achieve some resolution of unconscious conflicts without full awareness of what is happening. Writers who can risk moving into areas where they are not necessarily aware of what is happening in the creative process may achieve healing with their writing. It is the ability to tolerate this loss of control and be "capable of being in uncertainties, mysteries, doubts, without any irritable reaching after fact and reason." This is what John Keats described as "negative capability."

Bernie S. Siegel

SHOPPING LIST FOR CHANGE:
A FIVE-PART THERAPEUTIC PROGRAM

L et me now present you with a list of things I would like to see you do every day to help you become an exceptional human being. In this way you will heal your life as well as the lives of others, and possibly cure any afflictions.

1. Keep a daily journal recording your feelings and dreams. In tests of college students and executives, those individuals who had been asked to keep journals were shown to have a more active immune system and to develop fewer colds and other illnesses during exam time and periods of work stress. Even after they stopped keeping the journals, the immune system remained more active for up to six months. Including periodic drawings may also help.

2. Join a therapy group that meets for two hours every week, where you will receive love, confrontation and discipline. It should not be a victim group. If it is a group where everyone complains every week, then don't go back. If you can't find a group specific to your needs, go to an Adult Children of Alcoholics meeting or any other group you like. The affliction doesn't have to be the same as yours; it's the attitude that is important.

3. Meditate, visualize, pray or listen to quiet music, to interrupt your day four to six times with healing intervals that allow you to refocus, destress and give your body "live" messages. These are to relax you, not to make you feel you have more work or are not doing it well. So pick what feels right for you.

4. Live one hour at a time, based on your feelings. If you are close to death, ten minutes might be the time you have to focus on. What I mean by that is not to live as if you're going to die in an hour or ten minutes, but to ask yourself at the beginning of that period of time how you feel. If you do not like how you feel, then resolve those feelings or let go of them within the time limit. This teaches you that you are in charge of your feelings. When your time is significant to you, you will make a point of not wasting it in feelings that you don't like.

5. Twice a day for fifteen minutes sit or stand naked in front of a mirror. Work with the feelings that come up—the negativity for most of us—and then learn to love what you see in the mirror just as Evy McDonald did, progressing from her image of herself as a "bowl of jello" in a wheelchair to be a part-by-part appreciation of herself, beginning with her smile, proceeding to her soft hair, and moving on to each of her body parts until she had put herself together and could honestly say that she found the whole beautiful.

Now that you've read this list you see why so many people prefer having operations. Only a truly exceptional human being will take on this work. Once you do, all these things, however, you find that you begin to live more and more in the moment, and life becomes a series of moments that you are in charge of. Then joy will enter your life and you will be in heaven without dying.

James Barfoot

JACOB COMES TO HEAR THE HEALING SONGS OF NIGHT

(from Genesis 30)

Sometimes the fallow fields become so fair
And bare such warmth that plowmen give them names
And call them "she" and delicately tear,
Reluctantly, the purple roots that rain

Damp coverings of green across the shares.
I know of one who, having walked the day,
Returned at night to listen there for rare
Exquisite songs beneath the clump and clay

Of furrowed land and found the words that wear
The world away. And where he lay full spread
Upon the earth and rising reached that care
Which held him like a sieve, he grieved and said,

"The dead we wed will come for autumn wheat
As Leah comes for mandrakes Rachel eats."

Peter Cooley

THE LAST SELF-PORTRAIT

Vincent, this is where our stars part company.
Your eyes here are taking down the thunderheads
flooding another shore, a point of vanishing
where the clouds break, the clouds break down finally.
Twice I have been there, I will not go back.
I snap shut the book of graven images
in which, time out of mind, your whitecaps wash you up.
With these words, brother, I set you straight beside myself.
Constellations swirl out of your jacket and your vest;
behind you a starry night breaks out, clarifies
dead stars swarming to life; look, golden, they explode.
Between them, Vincent, the shoreline of my own backyard
emerges, clouds lift, today is absolute and clear.
Friend, I am writing you this poem on that sky.

Sharan Flynn Tette

BLACKBIRD IN THE WALL

All morning I hunch on the sofa
and resuscitate words.
As I work, the starling which insists
on building her nest in the chimney
battles her way to light,
fluttering against the sofa-wall
like a heart.

Outside, the grace days of March
have forced cracks in winter.
Birds with tongues
have found their way out.
Hepatica buds curl close in a nest,
blue beneath their fur
like new-born rabbits.

Fighting page-blindness I fix my focus
on black words. All morning I battle
columns, struggling with shape
until I find myself lifted,
lifted by language,
while the bird behind the wall
beats her way up and out.

Jane Mayhall

LOSS OF ANEMONE

All night he tried to remember
the name of the flower, "anemone,"
it spun out in hurting paragraphs of
self-distrust, abnegated from purpose.
Lost. And he refused to go to the dictionary,
as no word to find, if you didn't know it
first. His brain like a park owned the genus,

color, transmuting papery-like petals,
white, violet, tuberous-rooted.
Fields between old Kaintuck rock fences,
moist earth. Where "daughters of the wind"
flickered on delicate stems. Precise,
and he was able to get them wrested out
of suburban yards. And back to the woods.

But night did not oblige with sleep or
knowledge, almost a weariness without
quest turned his ideas into chains. Dawn
gave signal like an emotional garbage truck,
and "wind flower" (out of syntax) broke
the thrall, and *anemone* came to mind.
Evidently by his losing, something chosen.

Theodore Worozbyt, Jr.

A BRIEF ASSAY OF COMMUNICATION

to Stephen Dunn, a reply

When our hearts depended on a word,
we had no way to say anything
immoral, even our lies were roped to an obvious truth.

Finally, somebody said right things
but too late, at the wrong time. Listen, they were only
like we are now, they knew

they had to say something. We think nothing
that isn't somehow done or spoken,
and who knows? She might forgive anyone

who can forgive himself a lifetime of lies.
Aren't the sincerely tactful
simply lovers who want to be

forgiven for the messy pronouncements
of their bodies?
This dumpy husband who grows

potatoes , his damp hand
steering toward the community
center for counseling, his church-going

wife, beer-fat and belted in
safely beside him, maybe
they have a chance so small it takes up

no more space than a caught breath
in the middle of one's dream
as the other rolls

to the wrong side of the bed.
Unintelligible, perhaps, less than a syllable
in the middle of a touchstone word like "communication."

Yes, it's an ugly word, a fifth degree
latinate abstraction black-lipped and hopeless as communism,
but only those of us who want

to make poems can believe it's words that decide
what remakes us human.
My grandfather, who couldn't spell, told me

never get between a man and a woman
who are having words.
So far that's been useful.

Nancy Lambert

these dreams are specifically concerned

these dreams are specifically concerned
as I have always been concerned
about standing naked in front of crowds
who have also come to stand naked
we always named the stuff binding bones
and our hard work the marrow
and always looked a little askance
at all the others, those of us who came
from even father than we ourselves did
and who, under the always difficult lights
emerged squalling, others more quiet
blood dripping onto the floors of sterile rooms
and through some liquid obstruction
we heard muted and uncomfortable sounds: this
was the smacking of a million tiny lips

it was here in our millions under the lights
and within the walls we built carefully
avoiding the intimations of a dark
too big for anyone's grasp
that I noticed our moving lips when numbering
in the thousands then millions all seemed to move
in unison, a chord

we fling our fingers out as if to rid ourselves
of what stays hard and small and held against
the lines of our palms laid like roads
knowing that the lines of our lives laid like roads
was never an original image

and we line the corridors to our hotel
because here at last there is no owned house
the cracks we've seen through the wallpaper
peeling away like our own skins.

Margaret Key Biggs

ABERRANTS

He told me of her aberrations
and why he had to send her away;
she had taken to walking in the night,
and carrying on conversations with the stars;
some evenings she would isolate herself

with Bach and become lost for hours;
she delighted in total nudity,
and shed her clothes for all possible moments;
she talked to herself of the insanity
of krypton gas, pollution, and acid rain,

but the final offense was her rejection
of empty words and polite nothings—
she simply refused to play the game.
I smiled feebly as he told me this,
and I wondered when they would come for me.

Vince Clemente

LENS OF A BLUEFISH EYE

If you and your friend
look through the lens,
you on one side
him on the other,
upside down.
The fish sees everything upside down,
but in time
its brain gets smart enough
to turn it around.
Brains get that smart.

Now the lens is very small, shiny
and crystal-clear.
It is also transparent,
like the wing of a
moth against the lamp
on the kitchen table—
and light can travel through it.

Where is it found—
inside the eyeball, silly.
The eyeball is there
for padding, like the cushion
on my father's favorite chair,
the child went on,
unswerving as truth—
and who dare not
believe a child!

Next time, I haul in a fierce blue
off Old Field Point,
I'll be careful not to scrape
the delicate lens,
unsettle the brain
in the business of setting
the world on its feet again.

I'll be certain to respect
the way it looks at things,
the terraqueous world

583

beyond that airy lens,
as true as the heart
pumping blood to the brain
seven and a half pounds per second,
hear the child's story again,
a lesson even Aquinas never read.

P.C. Reid

WORDS FROM THE CONCERNED

Sal sat on the porch, thinking. He'd always had a lot of spirit until recently. He could turn all the problems around if Glenda would just say something that showed she appreciated him. When she'd gotten home from work that day, she'd sniffed the air and said, "Spaghetti again, Sal?" It made him think "What's the use?"

He hadn't been to Riley's in a week; she could have mentioned that; but instead she'd started in on his poor meal planning: "I told you about the frozen chicken this morning."

"You could have pulled it out of the freezer."

"You're home all day. I can't do it all." She disappeared into the bathroom and he soon heard the water running, the second of the two showers she took every day.

Now it was dusk, and Glenda was at the little dining room table, organizing her bills of lading. They'd cut her back to three-quarter's time, but because she was the responsible type she still managed the same work load. The full aroma of the perfected simmering sauce puffed through the open window onto the screened porch where he sat on a lawn chair, a beer in hand, and stared into the yard. He was also waiting for his stepson, Chris, to get home from work. He'd put himself in Chris's path, right in line for the lecture he was certain to receive. Let them do their worst. It was true that he'd blown a couple of hours on soap operas, but he had vacuumed and he had made that great sauce.

Finally, he heard Chris's 12-speed rolling on the driveway grit, then the boy's fast steady step. Then he heard Chris's voice.

"Ah ha! Just as I thought."

Sal did not look around. "And what did you *thought*, Chris?"

"That you'd be sitting right here sucking on a beer. How many today?"

"This is the first."

"Hey, that's good."

Chris dropped his backpack beside the chair and came around behind him. The boy's arms came around his neck and hugged him from behind. Sal raised his free hand and squeezed the crossed wrists in his broad grip. "Careful, I'm in a raw mood. So how was work?"

"Pretty easy today. Orders are way down, so I had to stretch it out."

"That's not good."

"It'll pick up."

Chris left and went inside, and Sal could hear him talking with his mother in the kitchen. Then he heard the window raised higher behind him. It was Glenda. "Sal, we're going to eat in ten minutes."

"Fine. Doesn't that sauce smell great?"

Ten minutes passed, then fifteen, twenty. Chris came out, smelling of Ivory soap. "You coming in?"

Sal sighed deeply then looked up at the boy. Chris wore a freshly laundered Kelso Elevator Maintenance sweatshirt. He wore it inside out, either by style or out of consideration for Sal. Those shirts had been passed around freely once, just before hydraulic elevators came in and the Kelso contracts steadily dropped by half. Three months ago, Sal had been laid off by Kelso. He was awaiting a letter that would announce a retraining program. The letter was many weeks overdue.

"Come on, Sal. Supper."

"I'm not hungry, kid."

"Then sit with us."

He shook his head. "Not up to it."

"Spaghetti. Your specialty."

Sal snorted.

"Your all-time favorite. Kill for it, you said."

Chris started poking him, quick shots to the ribs, and Sal laughed. The kid danced away, feinting blows. Handsome kid, still full of spit after a day's work. "Okay, you win." As Sal lifted his heavy body from the chair, the aluminum and plastic squealed.

In the kitchen, Glenda was draining the pasta. "Why am I doing this?" she said.

"Your choice," he answered. "I would have done it, but you didn't seem real keen on spaghetti."

She shook her head. "Sorry. I just get tired of it."

Now he felt like a heel. Of course she was tired of it, who wouldn't be? So why couldn't he follow the plan and crack open that cook book once in a while? What trick of the mind left him blank and frightened each morning the moment he heard the front door close behind her?

At the table, he took down the spaghetti in small forkfuls. "Delicious," he said flatly.

"The best," said Glenda. "So why are you picking at it?"

"I'm just not real hungry."

"I can tell."

"I'm not pulling my weight," he said.

Glenda and Chris burst out laughing. Sal looked up. "What's so funny?"

"You," said Chris. "Sitting there hanging over your supper like it's your last meal."

"Eat, Sal," said Glenda. "You're no good to us dead."

"As if I couldn't lose a few pounds."

"With your luck, it would be your brain."

Sal nodded down at the spaghetti. "That's the truth."

The other two laughed again. Sal looked up again. "You guys are having a great time, aren't you?"

Glenda said, "It's all right, Sal. Eat!"

"I didn't pay for this. While you're yucking it up, you might remember, Glenda, how you said once that you were real glad that I was moving in, how the extra income was going to help."

"It did—for a while."

Sal winced.

Chris looked down at his plate. "That's great, Mom. Real constructive."

His mother looked at him in surprise, her eyes as round as the lenses in her glasses. "It's the truth."

"So what? You think it's so great to be always telling the truth, like it's your mission in life or something."

"It's the truth! Now don't *you* start. The money was coming in, now it's not. I can be disappointed, can't I? Is Sal the only person around here who gets to be disappointed?"

Sal stood up and walked away from the table. "I'm going out for a while."

"Good work, Mom."

"What is the big deal around here?"

"I'm just going out for a minute."

Glenda said, "So all the pouting was just an excuse to rocket off to Riley's again."

"I've got to go."

Chris jumped up. "I'll go with you!"

"So what do I do with all this spaghetti?"

Outside, Sal started up the truck, but when Chris tapped on the passenger side window, he waved him away. He tapped again, more insistently, but Sal began to back out of the driveway. Chris ran around to his side and reached across for the ignition keys, but Sal grabbed his hand first. "Okay, okay," he said. "Get in."

As they drove, the elevator tools rattled in the truck bed. "Why don't you pack those things away, Sal? They're getting rusty."

"Can we not talk? Is that all right?"

"Sure."

They drove the rest of the way to Riley's in silence, though Chris occasionally whistled old tunes in his maddeningly blithe way: "Life Is Just a Bowl of Cherries," "It's Only a Paper Moon...." Sal wondered where the hell a kid of sixteen picked up songs like those. "Could we not whistle too?"

"Sorry."

Sal stopped in the bar's parking lot and wrenched the transmission into park. He got out with a huff, but took one step into the place and stopped. At the bar, bleary, creased faces came around to encounter him. Some of the men waved, one called out that he hadn't seen him in a while. Burnt-out bores, in by ten every morning. At this hour, there were also a few knots of after-work guys, standing together and jabbering shoptalk, hammers swinging from their belts like weapons, tapes and chalk lines clipped on like badges. The Corps of the Employed. Among their number had once been two good friends of Sal's, friends he'd made at Kelso. But after the closing they'd both nearly fled from the county, they left so fast. One day the three of them were huddling, making plans about the retraining, and then the next day it seemed the two friends had packed up and left—and one of them had a big family. To no one Sal said, "I don't know why I come to this place. It depresses the hell out of me."

" 'Cause at the moment it's slightly less depressing than Mom," said Chris. "Come on, let's get a booth."

In the booth Sal said, "I could tell your Mom just how easy it would be to skip this place permanent, except that it's not much fun at the house."

"Deadly turf," said Chris. "I'll bet the workers who hang here ask you questions you're sick of answering."

Sal shrugged, wondering how to answer, or whether to answer. Sometimes the kid's awkward way of helping sounded patronizing. Sitting sideways on his side of the booth, he rolled his head towards Chris. "You know everything, don't you?"

Chris smiled queerly. "Not everything. A lot."

Sal laughed out loud. "Too much." He turned back to the bar, looking around the room. "Looks like the waitress didn't show again." He left the booth and went to the bar and called to the bartender. "Hey there, Mike!"

The bartender was down the way, at the taps. He peered up from the pint of draft he was drawing. "You been sick or something?"

"Been well! Could you bring me a couple of Buds?"

The bartender looked over at Chris. "Who're they for?"

"Both for me."

The bartender blinked slowly and nodded. When he brought the beers over, he placed them close together in front of Sal and said, "Keep them on your side of the table."

"Don't worry. We'll do them one at a time." Back at the booth, Sal took one of the bottles and placed it on the floor beneath the table. "Do the honors, Chris." Chris took the first pull, then slid the bottle across to him. He could feel the kid watching him as he took one long swig, then a second. Sal looked over at him. "So?"

Chris shrugged, then pushed his lank brown hair out of his eyes. "We should keep things in perspective. You're bringing in the unemployment."

"Measley one-forty-seven a week."

"It's yours, Sal. You paid into it for years."

Sal nodded. "That is correct. But it won't last forever, my friend. That letter from Kelso better come quick."

"It's not coming, Sal."

Sal looked at him, then nearly spoke but did not. Then he said, "I think you're right. It's not coming, is it?"

Chris took up the bottle again. "I heard some guys talking over at the company today. Kelso's on the block."

Sal sniggered. "Is that right? Figures. Jesus."

The two of them sat in silence, then Sal said, "Spill the rest. There's always something else on your mind."

The boy wagged his head, grinning a little, then abruptly slipped sideways on his bench so that the two had to turn their heads to face each other. Chris had his mother's round brown eyes. And he kept himself clean, like she did. "I think it's a good thing, really. I mean, you not getting the retraining."

"Oh, you do? That's wonderful, Chris."

"I'm serious. You could start a whole new life."

"I don't want a whole new life. I've been an elevator mechanic for nineteen years. I'm forty years old."

"You could go back to school."

"I'm forty years old."

"Technical school. People of all ages go."

"Those schools are not free. I'm making one-forty-seven a week, and the President just decided to tax that as income. We're talking one-twenty-five, take-home."

"I've got that part covered too."

Sal swung forward abruptly. He reached down and picked up the other beer and started in on it.

"Sal, we might get caught."

"Hell with it. You're making me nervous."

"Okay, but do you want to hear the plan?"

Sal said nothing.

Chris came forward himself, his expression attempting to conceal his excitement. "I think you should sue Kelso."

Sal closed his eyes, losing all taste for his beer. Lately, it always tasted like medicine, rather than the earned beverage that dissolved the burr of a day's labor.

"It's all contingency these days, Sal. Remember, you're not looking for the world. Just a good faith settlement."

"It makes me sick. It's a damned national disease."

"You think the guys at Kelso were so good to you. I hate it every time you tell me that story about the promotions you never got."

"They were hard up."

"They were driving Cadillacs, parking them right in the yard. Every brother had a Caddie, even the one who never even showed up at the office. Just get your piece of the pie, finance the plan."

Sal dropped an arm heavily on the table. "The plan, the plan! What plan?"

"The plan you, we, eventually come up with. What difference does it make?"

"I had a plan with your mother. I'm supposed to be fixing up the house, doing the housework. It's not working. Now I need another plan?"

"A better one. There's a lawyer we should talk to. He's representing a group of guys from Kelso."

"You've been doing your homework, Chris. So, while Kelso's down, we give it another kick?"

"Just enough money to finance some planning time for you. It's only fair. Hell, Sal, you never even got severance."

"It's not a union shop."

"There were benefits, and that's contractual."

Sal stopped again. "Hey, why don't you be the lawyer? Think of the money we'll save."

Chris was looking down the bar. "You want to go?"

Sal walked back to the truck so quickly that Chris had to trot to keep up.

"Sal, come on…."

"You want my answer again? It's still no." In the truck he fumed behind the wheel.

"You're driving too damned fast, Sal."

"Don't tell me what to do."

"Sal, you've got to take action. You were screwed, and you deserve some breathing space."

"Thanks."

Chris sighed. He lurched in his seat, then reached back to slap on his seat belt. "Slow down."

"Okay." He did not slow down.

"You want to know the truth? You've been living in a dream. Driving around town with your tools in back as if…"

"Do the tools bother you?" Sal hit the brakes, and the truck slid to a stop on the shoulder of the road. He leapt from his seat and walked to the back of the truck where he reached in and gripped the long, metal chest of tools and lifted it from the truck bed. There were no other cars on the road, just large silent yards on either side. Leaning way back, he swung the chest with all his strength and released it. The chest arched through the air, then hit the road in the far lane, exploding open and sending a mass of jangling tools skittering onto the far shoulder.

From the driver's side Chris called back, "That's great, Sal! I'll see you back at the house." The boy already had the truck in gear. With a shower of spray, he drove off.

At first Sal just stared after the truck. Then he waited for a while. Finally, he started walking. For the first hundred yards he thought about what he would do to Chris when he reached the house, which was a long three miles off. But as he strode around the bend and started down the narrower road, he felt the anger falling away. The road gravel scrunched beneath his workboots, chomp, chomp, chomp, and the evenly planted sycamores came up beside him and passed behind in slow progression. He could hear the rasping of his corduroys as his thighs brushed together. A mockingbird dropped into the air over the road and fluttered open, fitfully displaying its white wing feathers. It lit in a maple on the other side and, in spite of Sal's heavy feelings, began to sing joyously, solitarily. Sal's breath came faster with exertion, and then with pain, and then with sadness. He thought of Glenda, who closed her round eyes each night and slept beside him. As she slept on her side, her single raised shoulder seemed to beckon the palm of his hand, the hand that ached to touch her but held back from shame. He felt vividly, in the present moment, the deep warm change in his life that knowing her had brought. And he felt too the terror of each night when he craved to make love but feared he could not complete the act; a single awkward move, even a misunderstood word, would surely leave him soft—and how they'd loved that first year when he'd come into the home to make things easier, to be a husband to her and, to her joy, so clownishly expressed, a father to Chris. By the time he saw the long, single lane that led to his driveway, he was choking back tears.

For some reason he was thinking about himself as a boy, when he played for hours by himself in the grassless yard while his father and mother sat on the couch before the nighttime game shows. He could weep for them, and for himself, the lonely kid in the yard who couldn't make friends. Behind him at least the town receded with every step, that awful place where so many out-of-work men hung on corners, drank, preened, smoked, or visited the stupid auto parts stores to gussy up their useless trucks. He could weep for the death of his future, where he would be penniless, impotent, of no use to anyone. How good the relief of tears would feel, but the scale of that release frightened him. It would be much better, now in sight of the driveway to his home, if some wild driver would pile into the back of him before he reached his door. But he reached it physically intact.

Glenda was nowhere to be seen, thank goodness, but Chris strode directly across his path, heading for the stairs to the bedrooms. Sal had no plan of what to say, but he was surprised to find that of the two of them, Chris was the angrier. In fact, his face was livid. "What do you want?" the boy challenged. Before Sal could answer, he started up the stairs.

Words flew into Sal's mind. "I've got to figure things out for myself, Chris. I've been thinking."

Chris hurled back, "So figure. Go ahead, do it all on your own."

Sal hung back at the bottom of the stairs. "Look, kid, it's not your problem."

"Whose stupid rule is that?" Then he heard the door slam above.

So, what had he come back to, charging those three miles after his retreating truck? He should at least try to salvage the tools. He took the spare keys from the kitchen drawer and drove the truck back to the spot where he'd thrown away the tools, but someone had beat him to them. He found only one chrome wrench in the grass beside the road. The plan with Glenda was that he'd fix up the house until he found steady work. The loose hinges, the fallen sash weights ... he needed tools to fix those things. He stood for a long time, flipping the wrench over and over in his hand.

He managed to fall asleep before Glenda came to bed. With extreme gratitude he'd felt the sleep pulling him down as he looked out at the solitary street light up the road. Blessed unconsciousness. But later, he awoke and felt her lips on his neck. They moved up one side, leaving a faint moist trail.

"Glenda."

"Right. And the first time too."

Her hand was on him, a sylph touch like butterfly wings that hardened him as they fluttered. "Honey, I can't."

"Quiet, lover-boy."

He kept his eyes closed the whole time, even when her small body slipped atop his. "Time of your life coming up," she whispered, breathily.

"I can't."

"Could've fooled me."

He raised his hands, cradled one each in the hollows of her waist. Her flesh was a miracle, always had been.

"Tomorrow's Saturday," he whined. "The kid doesn't go to work."

She laughed. "Time of your life."

"Glenda, honey, I can't."

"You already are."

When he awoke the next morning he knew immediately that it was late. Cars were moving down the road, the day's wind was already active, shoving the shedding trees around. The window was open, the aroma of someone's mown grass brushing into the room. For a long time he lay, looking out at the pearl-gray sky, thinking. Finally, he rose, stood a long time beneath the shower, shaved slowly—putting off the departure from the room.

Chris was reading the paper at the kitchen table, his scraped breakfast dish before him. He kept one finger looped through the handle of a coffee mug. Glenda was at the sink, in her bathrobe, her hands at the back of her head, weaving her long brown hair into a French braid. She freed one hand long enough to wave. Chris looked up. "The bear lumbers from his lair," he said flatly.

Silently, Sal took a seat. As always, the chair whined at his weight. The air smelled of coffee and shampoo, mother and son were still damp from showers. Where did he fit in with this squeaky clean duo? With a feeble movement, he inched closer to the table.

"It's pancakes," said Glenda.

"That sounds great."

Chris moved the paper aside, regarding Sal for a moment. Then he dropped his eyes. "So, are you okay?"

Sal merely shrugged. Glenda's long narrow arm, extending from her worn robe, set a mug of coffee before him. Her hand came away, then came to rest on his head. Briefly it mussed his short, straight hair. "He's better," she said. "He had a good night."

Sal sat with his hands between his knees. He opened his mouth to speak, but the words were streaming by so quickly in his mind that he couldn't find their beginning point. He took a breath, then a plunge. "I've been thinking," he said. Neither Chris nor his mother said anything, so he took another breath and went on. "I've been thinking about what you said, Chris. But…" But what? Where were the words? He could make anything with a drill or a saw, but making words…. "But I need a little more time to think it through." Yes. But why more time? "I guess it's sure now that I need to find another job, a different kind maybe. But I'm not sure which one yet. Once I figure that out, then I'll know if I need training or not."

Chris nodded. "Makes sense."

At the stove he heard Glenda say "Good!" He waited. "Fall's coming," she said. "You're still going to tighten up the windows and the rest, aren't you?"

"The windows. Insulate the doors, everything."

"Didn't you used to work in the yard with your dad?" asked Chris.

"I used to … hang out in the yard," said Sal, reddening.

"I mean the trees."

Sal reached back, stretching, though he didn't need to. "You mean the fruit trees."

"Something about that. Anyway, why not fix up the yard? I hate the yard. There's hardly a blade of grass out there, and the big trees are all broken."

"I could definitely do some work in the yard. I mean, it needs it."

"The whole damned place is falling apart," said Glenda. "I know that."

It wasn't easy. As he paced the house, pad in hand, the whiteness between the scrawled lines of his list seemed to blind him. He kept sighing to himself, as if he hadn't enough breath. Where was the purpose, the plan that would drive this decision forward? The doors, following weeks of dry weather, shut snugly in their jambs. How many weeks until the dampness that would reveal their swelling points? What to do first, what second … what to *do*. When he was on a payroll, they told him what to do, laid the whole day out before him. After lunch, Glenda peered quickly at his list and said, "Prioritize." The office manager. He almost but did not quite ask her to sit down with him and the list. By the early afternoon, he had at least managed a rough list of tasks and a separate list of the tools he would need, but who would lend them to him? At two, he watched a baseball game and fell asleep in his chair. When he awoke, his heart began pounding at the thought of the long hours until dinner. He should get up and cook. What should he cook?

At four, Chris came in from a pickup basketball game, the front of his shirt patched with sweat. Sal had succeeded in boiling a pile of elbow noodles and stirring in tuna and mushroom soup. Through the window he saw Chris watching him while spinning his basketball on the tip of one finger. "Hey, Salvador. Let's take a tour of the grounds."

They walked side by side around the nearly perfect square of yard, Chris asking questions, Sal answering—shortly, at first, then more and more fully. "Fall's the best time for seeding," said Sal. "That's sure. Rent a tiller, dig everything up to six inches, then lime it and manure it and till again. Then you roll it, spread the seed, and lay down straw. The straw holds it and keeps most of it away from the birds."

"What kind of grass?"

Sal considered, walking evenly. "There's bluegrass, but it drinks a lot and has to be cut all the time. The fescues are nice, but they're temperamental sprouters and the seeds real expensive. They usually cut it with bluegrass, or even rye. There's zoysia—the kind you plant in plugs. It takes over everything, though. It'll get into the ground cover near the fence."

"What about the trees? The neighbors want that dead limb off the elm."

They stopped before what was actually a maple, the largest of a line of big trees that formed a ragged west boundary to the yard. High up, one thick bare limb arched into the neighbor's yard. "That's one dead branch, all right." He stepped closer, resting one hand on the trunk bark of the maple. From the base he could just see the uneven line of small holes in the dead limb where the bark had peeled away. "Borers are already at it," he said. "Unless they're the problem."

Chris nodded. "So, what about the lawsuit idea? What do you think now?"

Sal kept his eyes on the tree's bark. "About the same, Chris. It's not my style. I mean, I had a lot of good years there ..."

From the porch, Glenda called Chris to the phone. After the boy had left, Sal stayed to stare longer at the dead branch. Across the back of the hand that rested on the bark, a single large black ant was stumbling through the coarse hair. Peering closer, Sal spotted a shiny stream of ants moving in the valleys of the bark, some moving beneath his palm and reappearing on the other side, traveling up and down. He followed the stream down to the ground and discovered several small holes in the exposed nubs of the roots. Then he could see fine sawdust deposited in small conical piles here and there under the rough grass blades, and then similar piles of fine soil. He tore away tufts of grass from around the base of the tree, discovering silt and sawdust wherever he looked.

Later, back in the kitchen, he took out the baked casserole and sprinkled a layer of crushed potato chips atop it. Then he put it back in to bake a while longer. At dinner, he told them about the carpenter ants that were slowly eating the big maple, but Chris seemed distracted, and though Glenda listened he began to suspect she was faking her interest. Perhaps they didn't want to hear about ants; maybe they wanted to hear something different from him. And what might that be? He left his dinner half eaten, then sat through two sit-coms before all the excited commercials began to make him feel even more inadequate. He ended up trying to beat Glenda to sleep. But as he lay in the darkness, the invading ants kept crawling through his mind. When she came in later, he was on his side and staring. He pretended not to watch her, but he was distracted by her undressing. She had turned on the lamp beside the bed, and now walked about, dreamily discarding layers of her clothing. In brief high-cut panties, she stood before the mirror and slowly unravelled the long French braid until her hair came free and rippled across her shoulder blades. She moved him, everything about her—her gracefully aging breasts, curving down to round centers with the nipples pointing up; the extra little puckers of flesh; the fact that she kept her glasses on even when she was virtually naked.

He took a breath. "The kid's mad that I won't sue Kelso."

She moved about, putting things away, folding clothes. "He'll get over it," she said.

"Did he tell you about the tools?"

"Uh huh."

"They were gone when I went back."

She shrugged. "That might be good."

He closed his eyes. Within him, pain was everywhere. Then he felt her beside him, then felt himself neatly tipped onto his back. She straddled him, settling herself upon him and arching her back in a long luxuriant stretch. "Oh, it's all so difficult, isn't it?" She laughed, privately, then looked down at him. "Men. Men and their stuff."

"What stuff?"

"Do I know?" She took his two hands and brought them up to her breasts. "I'm cold. I do appreciate your warm hands."

"Warm hands, cold heart."

She smiled, off somewhere in her thoughts. Under his hands, her breasts settled into the shapes of his palms. "That time in the parts store," she said. "He told me about that."

He looked up at her, puzzled. His breathing was shakey, but he kept his hands obediently upon her. "What time?"

"That time when the guy behind the counter told Chris to go back home and figure out what he wanted, and then he started to walk away?"

Sal nodded. "Oh, yeah. He kept saying brace for bracket, or something. Chris, I mean."

Glenda took off her glasses and tossed them onto the rug. "And you reached across the counter and grabbed the guy before he could walk off. You said 'This kid's a good friend of mine. You're not going anywhere until you understand what he wants'." She smiled down at him. "Did you really do that?"

Sal reddened. "Something like that. I'm not sure how it went exactly."

Glenda kept smiling, looking dreamy, then leaned down upon him. She ran her tongue from his collarbone to his earlobe. Into his ear she whispered, "I wish I'd been there."

They started to kiss, but he couldn't get hard. Whole parts of him felt dead. "What is it?" she said, rolling away. She rolled a good foot away, he noticed.

"Sorry."

The lamp was still on. She squinted at him, her face a shadow with the lamp behind.

"This list business," he said. "It seems so … puny."

"Puny is making my house nice? I mean, our house?"

He had said the wrong thing. It hadn't even been what he'd meant to say. He tried again. "I want to make an important contribution, that's what I'm saying."

She shook her head. "So, make a less important one in the meantime. What's the big deal?"

"The money, the …"

"The men stuff again." She rolled onto her side, her back to him.

This time he reached up and cupped her shoulder, though it did not seem at all to be beckoning to him. "It's not easy," he said. "There's a lot of pain all the time."

She said, "I know, I know. I know all about pain. Tell me, Sal. Do you think you might be liking it a little?"

He awoke later. Outside the window a full moon had risen above the trees. It must have been its brightness that had awakened him. Fully awake now, he watched it rise. Surely the ants were busy in the moonlight. He stared out, remembering that as a child he'd often had deep, disturbing dreams under a full moon. He tried to remember those dreams, but grew quickly tired again, and then fell asleep, and then dreamed. He dreamed that he was back in his childhood home, out in the yard late at night. He was sitting up in a tree and staring across the yard at his parents, both silhouettes facing an unseen television in the warm light of the house. He awoke immediately after the dream; it was still night, but the moon had travelled on.

The dream unsettled him, because he remembered that he had, very often, climbed the big tree in his childhood yard and, just as in the dream, had stayed up there, sitting on a limb. He got up to think about that, about how often he had sat out there on that limb. As he paced the quiet hallway outside the bedrooms, then stole about in the rooms downstairs, he remembered why he had stayed in that tree. He had been waiting to be missed. He had waited for one of his parents to look around, then rise, and then come out into the yard and call for him. But they never did. Usually, he eventually gave up and came in, where he would be greeted off-handedly, or not at all. But once, he had waited a long time. Finally, his parents had risen, walked about for awhile, then turned off the lights and gone to bed, leaving him alone in the yard outside the darkened house. Now, in the dark living room of his present home, he ran his hands along his own thick sides, testing. He felt so strange, like a child in a huge body.

He was up and out before Glenda and Chris the next morning. He read the paper over breakfast at Woolworth's, waiting for Vinnie's Nursery to open. Later, he dogged Vinnie Petriano all around the nursery—from the counter, past the stacked sacks of topsoil, and even into the hothouse. "It's a goner," said Vinnie. "You never really get rid of carpenter ants."

"I hear you can make life miserable for them, make them pack up and move out."

"Sure! Got a month or two?"

"So happens I do. Doesn't anything work?"

Vinnie stopped at a shelf and looked over the bottles and paper cannisters. "There's some systemic stuff. I guess it eventually makes the wood taste bad or something."

"I was thinking about a metal spike. Drive it into the trunk and just keep whacking it. You know, vibrations."

"Really? I never tried that. Could work. My guess is you do it at different times. If you get into a pattern, they just adjust. They're amazing. I have a lot of respect for ants." The phone rang and Vinnie answered it. At the same time he took down a shrink-wrapped package with a plastic spigot and several little green rods. Sal read the back of the package while Vinnie yammered on to someone about roses.

When Vinnie hung up, Sal followed him back to the front counter. "So maybe this systemic stuff, and my spike idea?"

"Why not? And I'd keep the ground covered with Diazon, so everytime they come up for air they get singed."

Sal nodded, flicking the edge of the shrink-wrapped package. "And what about soaking the holes in the ground."

Vinnie shrugged. "You say you got the time. Let me know if it works. Maybe we'll be famous someday!"

Sal borrowed tools from his next door neighbors, the couple who wanted the limb removed. With a hacksaw, he cut off the curved end of an old lug wrench, then drove the end of it into the maple's trunk until the tip stuck in the hardwood. For ten minutes, he pounded the end of the rod, the sullen thwacks echoing through the surrounding yards. Then, as dusk came on, he pointed the garden hose, the nozzle focused for highest intensity, at one ground hole after another. The water ripped into the topsoil, but no matter how long he held the hose in place the water never backed up. There was a whole metropolis of ants down there, a nearly limitless network of tunnels. He imagined the successive gallons rapidly percolating down into the thousands of intricate chambers. He imagined the alarmed ants, scrambling, drowning, hurtling in thousands through other still dry chambers. When his patience gave out, he moved the hose to another hole. It was nearly dark when he attached the plastic spigot to the hose and plunged the systemic dripper into the soil. When he'd set it properly, he sprinkled Diazon liberally around the base of the trunk. At last, he patted the tree and said, aloud, "Good night, old girl."

The connection he'd lost with Chris was hard to find again. Their words went out towards each other in the same space, but like loose strings that fluttered in the breeze they failed to knot. One night, they found themselves out on the porch, alone, and Sal mentioned that school must be starting soon.

"In a week," said Chris.

"That soon! I didn't realize." Fall was coming; a good time to plant grass.

Chris nodded, walking about with an empty juice bottle in his hands. Finally, he sat down across from Sal and leaned forward with his elbows on his knees. He put a finger in the mouth of the bottle, and rolled it about on its base on the patio cement. "I wasn't sure I was going back. I don't have to, you know."

"Sure. It's a free country."

"No, I mean I can stay on and still bring in money." He looked up at Sal.

Sal looked back at him for a moment, then took a breath. "I get it. You mean, money for the family."

Chris said nothing. Sal nodded, nodded again. "Any chance you might never go back?"

"No. I'd go back after you've landed work. It's just a matter of time."

Sal pulled at one earlobe, the one that Glenda had said he was making longer. "I'll talk it over with your Mom."

"If you say so. Isn't it my decision, though?"

Sal looked out into the yard for a moment, then slowly turned his gaze on Chris. "Ninety percent. But I'll talk it over with your Mom. We owe it to her."

Sal stood at the base of the maple and raised the short-handled sledgehammer. Under the rising half-moon, he whacked the spike's end. He kept at it until he broke a fine sweat on his brow and had to slip off his flannel shirt.

"What a racket!"

He looked around and saw Glenda standing on the patio, watching him with her arms crossed. He waved and she waved back, then went inside. He whacked a while longer. Under his hand, the ants picked about—in a manner that he hoped seemed irritated. Up above, the dead limb reached for the moon. On an impulse, he dropped the sledgehammer and walked to the shed for the axe and a single section of ladder.

With the ladder propped against the trunk, he began to mount, then continued though he felt sillier and more awkward at every rung. The limb was higher than he'd thought. With some difficulty, he got his feet right in the deepest fork of the maple and leaned back against one of the whole limbs. At this angle, he could raise the axe and bring it down low on the dead limb. Maybe if he could open up the wounded part, he could get at the ants more directly. He could almost imagine the tree's relief at the removal of the dead weight, the hastening of its healing.

But before he landed the first blow, he looked back at the house through the dim twilight, wondering if either Chris or his mother was watching. He could see them both passing back and forth before the kitchen window, probably getting a late supper on the table.

Sal raised the axe and began to chop. The blows landed uncertainly at first, then began to cut a deeper V in the dead limb. It was still very solid, but at the center the wood came away in chunks, and the steady whacks echoed in the quiet dusk. Half way through he paused to wipe his brow with his t-shirt sleeve. He could see that he'd penetrated to the rotten marrow of the branch. It was powdery, pulpy in parts. With another look to the house, he set to work for the final chopping. He didn't stop, though his arms ached, until the last fibers began to crack under the weight of the drooping limb. Finally, with a loud, prolonged rasp the long limb dropped, twisted loose from its own falling weight, then fell wholly to the earth, where it bounced and twisted and broke into even smaller sections.

Gasping, Sal leaned back against the supporting limb and fought for breath. He could see neither Glenda nor Chris in the house. All around, the yards were filling with quiet. Not a leaf stirred, as if the trees were watching. The air was full of waiting. Sal, panting in the maple, felt the silence slipping into him. He could swear that it nourished him. With the axe still gripped in his hand, he felt powerful, and with that powerfulness he swore to heal, heal all around him with axe or word or tool or touch, heal all or die trying. He would saw the branch wound flat and dress it with creosote. He would....

"Hey, Paul Bunyan! Are you hungry or what?"

The sound of Glenda's voice startled him. He looked down to discover her standing at the base of the tree and looking up at him. How long had she been down there?

"You here?"

"I came to watch the show!"

Go down there to her, he told himself. He could just see her smile, and the half moon flashing off her glasses. *Take her in your sweaty arms and tell her she's the best thing that ever happened to you. Go now, now!*

Dale Edmonds

TIPPY, HITLER, MY FATHER,
AND THE FLIGHT OF THE RED KITE

I was out in my back yard with Bobby Keith, trying to get his kit airborne, when I heard my grandmother calling "Buddy, Oh, Buddy," from the back porch.

I hated to be called "Buddy"—my grandmother's pet name for me—especially in front of a friend, and I hated to be interrupted when I was playing. We'd been fooling around with the kite, which was brand new and bright red, for more than an hour, but we couldn't get it to fly properly. First, we didn't have enough tail. Then, we had too much. Then, the bridle broke. Then, the wind quit on us. Finally, though, we were all set. Only my grandmother was about to spoil everything. She probably wanted me to come in and pick up my room or something dumb like that.

"Buddy, Oh, Buddy," she called, more urgently.

I was holding the kite by the stick crossing. Bobby, about ten feet away, was holding the string, which was wrapped around a ruler.

"Off we go, into the wild blue yonder," Bobby yelled.

"Roger. Willco," I yelled back. "Over and out."

We started running at the same time, Bobby a little faster than me. When the string became taut, I tossed the kite into the air, and up it went.

When I saw the kite clear the telephone wires in the alley, I turned and trotted a few steps toward the back porch. "What is it, Granny?" I yelled.

She said something I couldn't understand. She didn't have a very loud voice, and Bobby was jabbering away as he played out the string.

"What?" I cupped my hand behind my ear and moved a few steps nearer.

"Tippy's dead," I heard her say.

"No!" I screamed and started running toward her.

Tippy was my dog, a mixed German Shepherd and collie. A couple of months earlier, my parents had given him to the K-9 Corps after he'd bitten a chunk out of the leg of the paper boy (that chunk joining a long string of others bitten out of various portions of the anatomies of yard men and door-to-door salesmen). Every night since my father had driven off with Tippy, I had made a nest for him under my bed covers and talked to him and petted him until I fell asleep. Some nights he was fighting the Germans, some nights the Japs. Whatever theater of war he was in, though, he was a great hero and was awarded every medal I could think of.

Every day since Tippy had left I badgered my father for information about his whereabouts. My father always said, "They'll let us know, Son." Finally, after a month of my badgering, my father said, "You know, Son, Tippy's just like a soldier. They can't tell us anything about him, because it might give away troop movements. We'll just have to be patient." I knew that "Loose Lips Sink Ships," so my father's words silenced me. But, every morning when I woke up the first thing I thought was that *this* would be the day that I would hear about Tippy.

The last thing in the world I dreamed that I would hear, though, was that he was dead.

Some words must have tumbled out of me as I dashed up the back porch steps, but whatever they were my grandmother ignored them.

"I heard it on the radio," she said, in an excited voice. "They broke into 'Widder Brown' with a news bulletin."

At eleven I should have realized that, however heroic Tippy had been, his death wouldn't merit a radio news bulletin. But all I could think of was that my dog was dead.

"They gotta send us his body," I blurted out. I had decided long ago that when Tippy did finally die, twenty or thirty years in the future, I'd bury him under the chinaberry tree in our back yard.

This remark got my grandmother's attention. "Of course they won't send us his body," she said, peering at me. "They'll bury him in Germany."

I had a sudden vision of Tippy leading an assault upon the remnants of the German Army that were making a last-ditch stand around Berlin. Then it hit me anew that my dog was dead.

"They gotta send him *here*," I sobbed. "I wanta bury him under the chinaberry tree."

My grandmother took me by the shoulders and shook me. "Buddy," she said. "What *are* you raving about?"

"They've gotta send Tippy *home*. He's my dog, I love him—"

She shook me again, harder. "Buddy, listen to me. What did you think I said?"

"You said Tippy was dead."

"I said *Hitler* was dead," she said firmly. "Adolph Hitler, the German dictator. He's the one that's dead, not Tippy. I heard it on the radio. They broke into 'Widder Brown' with a news bulletin."

Tippy was alive! He was still with the K-9 Corps somewhere, fighting the Germans or the Japs. When the war was over, he'd come home and be my dog again.

I pulled out of my grandmother's grasp and ran down the porch steps toward Bobby, who was flying the kite at the far end of the back yard.

"Hitler's dead!" I yelled, running up to him. "Hitler's dead!"

Bobby threw up his hands: "Yay!"

The ruler with the kite string wrapped around it flew out of his hand, hit the ground, bounced along it for a few yards, then struck the fence, where it jammed between two palings. I ran after it, but just as I reached it, the last of the string unwound and flew just out of reach of my clutching fingers.

Bobby and I stood there watching as the kite soared upward, a red diamond against the white of the clouds and the blue of the sky.

Forty years later my father lay dying in a nursing home in Columbus, Ohio. He was very weak, but he still could talk. Rather, he still could listen to me talk. He liked for me to tell him stories about our life in Fort Worth, when we were still a family.

He particularly liked to hear stories about World War II, when he was working the swing shift at the bomber plant, and we were the happiest we ever were. He got a paycheck every week, as opposed to the fitful and uncertain returns from his usual work as a real estate salesman. Also, his work schedule meant that he had to stay out of honky-tonks five nights a week. He tried to take up the slack on Saturday night, true, but even then he was so exhausted that he was nothing like the ferocious drunk he had been before the war and would become again after the war.

So, I sat in the chair by my father's bed in the nursing home in Columbus and told him again the story about Tippy and Hitler and the red kite. He always got a kick out that one. When I finished the story, my father smiled faintly and whispered, "Red ... white ... and blue ..."

"That's right, Dad, just like the flag."

He was trying to say something else, so I waited. Finally he got it out: "We won, Son."

"The war? We sure as heck did. Only Tippy never came home."

My father shook his head and mouthed "No."

We never heard a word from the K-9 Corps about Tippy. My father said that in all the confusion at the end of the war they must have lost his records. I grieved terribly for awhile, but then my parents bought me another dog, a cocker spaniel named Tuffy, who was my dog until I went away to college. During my junior year in high school our family dissolved, amid much misery and bitterness. My parents divorced. My mother and I stayed in Fort Worth, while my father drifted around the country for several years before finally settling in Columbus.

He had sunk as low as you can get at that point, maybe a hair above Skid Row, but not much more than that. Then he had a massive heart attack. A doctor told him that he could either stop drinking or die. He stopped drinking. Fear of death accomplished what family, friends, AA, and the law couldn't accomplish, in spite of decades of effort.

After he dried out, my father got in touch with me. It was the first time I'd heard from him in five or six years. I was extremely wary at first. Too many times in the past he had convinced me that he'd "straightened out" and begged money from me, only to backslide egregiously. But, this time he didn't ask for money. After much soul-searching, I decided to give him one more chance. I flew up to see him in Columbus and discovered that he had, indeed, at age sixty-four, finally "straightened out." About time, you might say, and you'd be right.

In any case, my father lived the last eighteen years of his life in sobriety and decency, and we managed to establish a cordial, if not warm, relationship. Neither of us ever spoke of the alcoholic horror of the past. If we talked about the past at all, it was in terms of mellow reminiscence. We somehow managed to extract nuggets of light from the dark slag of the past.

"I'll bet Tippy made a great soldier," I said, reluctant to let go of the particular nugget I'd extracted. "Don't you think he did, Dad?"

My father looked at me and seemed about to speak, but at that moment a nurse came in to give him a shot. As I watched her expert manipulation of his frail body, suddenly I had one of those intuitive flashes in which latent suspicions mesh with luminous clarity. It hit me with such force that I had to get up from my chair and go out in the corridor for a drink of water.

When I got back to the room, the nurse was just leaving. My father had closed his eyes, waiting for the shot to work. It wouldn't take long. I walked over to the bed and bent over him.

"Dad," I said, "can you hear me?"

He opened his eyes and looked into mine.

"Dad, you didn't give Tippy to the K-9 Corps, did you?"

He gazed steadily into my eyes. In a moment he mouthed "No."

"You took him to the dog pound."

He nodded once, then opened his mouth, struggling to speak. I bent over, my ear close to his mouth.

"We had to, Son," he whispered. "He got too mean ... your mother and I ... we wanted to ... spare your feelings ..."

His mouth closed, and then his eyes, and he was asleep.

A nurse called me at my motel room early the next morning. My father had died peacefully in the night.

He had made arrangements for cremation several years before. All I had to do was go to the funeral home that morning and sign some documents. Before I did this, though, I was left alone for a few minutes in the chapel with my father's body.

I stood looking down at him in the coffin. I wished I had said this to him the night before, but this would have to do: "It's okay, Dad," I said. "About Tippy."

Then I went out to the office, signed the documents, and told them to go ahead with the cremation.

Late that afternoon I sat in an airplane window seat with the discreet brown box which held my father's ashes in my lap. As the plane banked above Columbus and turned for the flight South, I looked out the window to my right.

From horizon to horizon, the sky was filled with bright red kites, thousands of them, flying bravely in place, amid the billowing clouds.

I looked down at the box in my lap. "And it's okay, Dad," I murmured. "About everything else."

"Pardon?" said the man in the seat on my left.

"Sorry," I said, "just talking to myself."

With one hand I reached into the pocket on the seat back in front of me and pulled out a copy of the airline magazine. My other hand rested, palm down, on the box in my lap, in what could be considered an attitude of benediction.

CHAPTER VIII

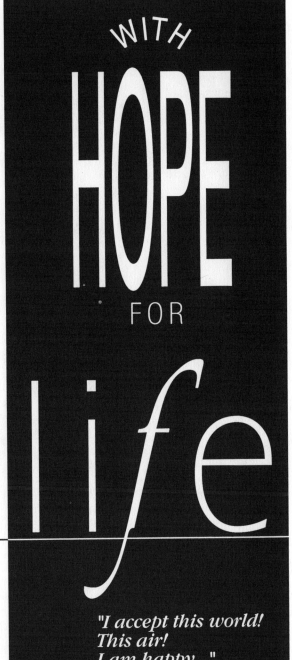

WITH

HOPE

FOR

life

"I accept this world!
This air!
I am happy..."

Liubov Sirota - "Fate"

Adol'f Kharash
Science Director, Professor of Moscow State University

A VOICE FROM DEAD PRIPIAT'

I first met Liubov' Sirota late in January 1988 in Kiev, in an area of the city called Troeshchino where, in November of 1986, a group of people settled after evacuating Pripiat', the satellite city of the Chernobyl nuclear plant. They warmly greeted our Moscow University group of students and professors in the Zemliaki club, where the children from the deserted city were taking classes in dance and drawing and the adults were meeting to recall what had been and plan what would come.

The residents of Pripiat' very much appreciated any kind of attention. It was no joke that for almost two months after the catastrophe not a single word of the event—not in the central press or tv or radio—was said about the fate of the city which was in an hour forever deserted by over 50,000 inhabitants. But even if a few knew of its existence (since it was a "special purpose" city and was classified "secret"), nobody knew that this was the nearest city to the Chernobyl nuclear plant, only three kilometers away. I myself learned about the existence of this city only in June, 1986, when I went to the site. The inhabitants of Pripiat' had not been aware of the explosion. The majority of them had suspected nothing, took no precautions, and were exposed to the fallout from the Chernobyl catastrophe for thirty-six hours.

The City of Ghosts, was what the city was called in the poems of another of our acquaintances from Troeshchino, a friend of Liubov' Sirota, Vladimir Shovkoshitny. He had formerly worked in the Chernobyl nuclear plant and was one of the first to volunteer with the cleanup of the aftermath of the catastrophe.

Liubov' Sirota and her little son lived in the neighborhood of Pripiat' closest to the nuclear plant. The night of the April 25th was very warm and clear. Liubov' couldn't sleep. She went outside to get some fresh, fragrant April air. She was one of the first—one of the few—people in Pripiat' to see above the Chernobyl plant the evil flash of light, the star Wormwood (in Russian, *Chernobyl*), which two thousand years ago was prophesied in the Book of Revelation, and which that night incinerated—abruptly—people's hopes and plans. If she had only known then that she should have closed her eyes and run, not looking back, away from this dawn glow, from this air rich with spring blossoms.

"Nobody knew anything."

This is how I see Liubov' even today, though I have often met with her after that remarkable evening in Troeshchino she was the embodiment of defenselessness and of limitless baffled anger.

"Nobody knew anything."

She was the first one to try to explain to us, the uninitiated, who came from well-protected, undisturbed Moscow, what had actually happened in Pripiat' that night and in the following thirty-six hours of anxious waiting. Now, three years after we met

607

in Troeshchino, I can see the Pripiat' of that time in the light of my endless pondering and in the pain of Liubov' Sirota's voice:

> Has day died?
> Or is this the end of the world?
> Morbid dew on pallid leaves.
> By now it's unimportant
> whose the fault,
> what the reason,
> the sky is boiling only with crows ...
> And now—no sounds, no smells.
> And no more peace in this world.
> Here, we loved ...
> Now, eternal separation
> reigns on the burnt out Earth ...

"At the Crossing"

On the copy she gave me Liubov' Sirota entitled her collection of poems, "A Voice from Dead Pripiat': The voice of the burnt-out Earth." This is the name she might give her burden. The destruction of Pripiat' is the destruction of the promised land; it is a metaphor of universal destruction, a prophecy and sign of the Apocalypse. For the latter inevitable and universal catastrophe there will be in reality no one who can be called guilty. Any merely human cause is utterly petty, trifling, not worth mentioning. But for earthly tragedies earthly beings must pay the price. The earthly flesh of human beings is heavy, an inexorable burden without which the spirit, while it exists in this world, cannot survive. The perishable flesh prevents the spirit from freeing itself from earthly cares and from soaring into cosmic space. It drags it down to the deserted hearth, forces it to grieve without consolation for the fate of relatives and neighbors, to look into the eyes of children in which an unchildish despair is fixed. Again and again, we torture ourselves with the living pictures of that fine warm summery April day, when the people—unsuspecting—opened the windows of their apartments, strolled about in the streets, took the sun on the river beaches, celebrated weddings, picnicked in the nearby forests, eating ice cream which was sold in the street, the children frolicking, thrusting their bare arms up to the elbows into the foaming streams of radioactive water which was streaming profusely through the city streets. And again and again one is horrified by the hideous traces left on the face of our native planet.

Again and again one seeks in torments the guilty and laments for the victims. This is why Liubov' Sirota's apocalyptic insights are not for an instant abstract or passion-less, even prophesying as they do the end of the world. These insights are deeply personal and quite mortal. They are penetrated by physical pain and inscribed with the grief for the casualties and concern for the lives and fates of mortal, living people and also by angry accusations against other people—also very much alive and mortal—who did not rush to help, did not warn of the danger, did not prevent the fatal outcome.

In one of the films of Rolan Sergienko, who created a cycle of films on the Chernobyl catastrophe, fact is uniquely combined with artistic expressiveness. Liubov' Sirota participated in making one of the films, *Threshold*. One scene, shot in Pripiat' April 26, 1986 by a young local cameraman named Nazarenko, shows a sunlit street filled with people in the midst of their festive Saturday holiday, women strolling carelessly, wearing light, loose dresses, infants in their strollers, bareheaded men relieved of their workday burdens. Suddenly two strange and gloomy figures appear. They look like characters from a science fiction film about an invasion from another planet: two militiamen with shiny protective clothing fully covering their bodies, wearing gloves, hoods, and tightly-sealed military respirators. A passerby who meets them stands still as if petrified, looking at this fantastic vision, not trusting his own eyes, as if he had seen them in a dream. Or perhaps this is what our terrifying reality is—a dream.

"Nobody knew anything," repeats Liubov' Sirota, but this does not apply to everybody—not to those who in one way or another knew about the April tragedy. The citizens of Pripiat', who in one way or another knew about the April tragedy. The citizens of Pripiat', who should have been informed in the first place so that they could immediately take care of their own safety, didn't know anything about it. But those who made decisions knew everything about the catastrophe—or almost everything. The posthumously published notes of academician Legasov prove that by four o'clock a.m. of April 26, 1986, in the Kremlin, a thousand kilometers from carefree and defenseless Pripiat', they already had sufficient information about all elements of that night's catastrophe at the Chernobyl nuclear plant. Those authorities took care to have the militiamen dressed in special protective clothing; the unsuspecting citizens were given only counseling. The official declaration by the important bureaucrats from the Ministry of Health declared that the evacuation was carried out in time and that none of the city's inhabitants had suffered any harm. Their fears and concerns were declared unnecessary, groundless, labelled with the sinister psychiatric term "radiophobia."

The event in Chernobyl inspired special documentary films such as Rolan Sergienko's movies and also the writings of the poets from Pripiat'. The works in this genre are difficult to understand even without a consideration of their factual basis. The poem "Radiophobia," which stands out in the poetic work of Liubov' Sirota, belongs to this genre.

"Don't promote this terrible word 'radiophobia!' "

This was the first request made to us that evening in Troeshchino by the citizens of Pripiat'. For those who were at the epicenter of the Chernobyl cataclysm, this word is a grievous insult. It treats the normal impulse to self-protection, natural to everything living: moral suffering, anguish and concern about the fate of children, relatives and friends, and one's own physical suffering and sickness as a result of delirium, of pathological perversion. This term "radiophobia" deprives people who became the victims of Chernobyl of hope for a better future because it dismisses as unfounded all their claims to care for their physical health including adequate medical care, food, decent living conditions, and just material compensation. It causes an irreparable moral harm, inflicting a sense of abandonment and social deprivation that is inevitable in people who have gone through such a catastrophe.

Does this term console anyone? Yes, of course. First, it calms public opinion, suggesting that there is only a handful of victims of Chernobyl. And what are tens or hundreds of thousands of people, or even several million, in such a large country, or measured against all of humanity? A handful of super-sensitive individuals who gave in to panic. But most importantly, the term excuses the authorities from worrying. It relieves them of responsibility for the destructive effects of the Chernobyl catastrophe on human organisms and helps them to "conserve" huge material resources.

> They did not register us
> and our deaths were not linked to the accident.
> No processions laid wreaths,
> no brass bands melted with grief.
> They wrote it off as
> lingering stress,
> cunning genetic disorders ...
> But we—we are the payment for rapid progress,
> mere victims of someone else's sated afternoons.

These lines are addressed to the Ministry of Health which protects State interests, as are the following lines:

> What has become of the world
> if the most humane of professions
> has also turned bureaucratic?
>   "Radiophobia"

Representatives of the most humane of the professions—medicine—have demonstrated in the Chernobyl catastrophe the most amazing bureaucratic cynicism into which a human soul can be frozen, a cynicism that transforms a human being into a faceless dead statistic, a piece of information without feelings, without a face.

In one of Sergienko's films, at the international conference in Kiev, the representative of the Ministry of Health confidently spoke in a ringing youthful voice about the consequences of Chernobyl for the population of Byelorussia [now Belorus]. The number of cancers resulting from the radionucleides will increase, he said, but by no more than 75,000. And what is 75,000 in such a huge republic? Other representatives of this agency went even further, calculating the post-Chernobyl average incidence of oncological illnesses for the whole European region of the USSR, as well as for the population of whole country. The resulting numbers immediately seem comforting.

In a newspaper interview with academician Leonid Il'in, who is chair of the National Commission on Radiation Defense and who was leading the campaign of consolation, one finds a most curious metaphor. Speaking of one of the "tongues" of radiation spread by the cloud of energy, this prominent scholar remarked that this tongue licked only once at the city of Pripiat';. What an image, and how harmless it sounds: to lick. Isn't it a beautiful image? Such a nice little tongue, especially if one takes into consideration that this tender touch was applied to a city of 58,000 people.

How many felt the result of this touch? Simple mortals like Liubov' Sirota, her son, her friends and neighbors. One, two, three thousand? In the face of the all-powerful law of large numbers one can of course ignore such a tiny quantity. No, the medical bureaucrats are not timid. They who sit in the armchairs of the ministry are not radiophobes. They laugh at the fears of the man on the street. They are not afraid of radiation, especially when this radiation licks other, far-off cities and villages.

But someone is surely supposed to be afraid for this world. Someone is supposed to value human life. And who will grieve for the losses? Let us all together fear radiation. Long live radiophobia!

> *Radiophobia,*
> may you be omnipresent!
> Not waiting until additional jolts,
> new tragedies,
> have transformed more thousands
> who survived the inferno
> into seers—
> Radiation phobia might cure
> the world
> of carelessness, satiety, greed,
> bureaucratism and lack of spirituality,
> so that through someone's good will,
> we don't mutate into non-humankind.

The poet's pen uses this term, taken from the lexicon of psychiatry with its meaning reversed, to designate not a pathological disturbance of the reason, but a humanistic mission that only a few can carry out, a transformation like that which takes place in Andrei Tarkovskii's two last films: *Nostalgia* and *The Sacrifice*.

The "radiophobic tradition" in humanistic art consists of people who in the eyes of a sober, rational human being show all the signs of madness, who commit strange acts that other madmen have put them up to, and who save the world from nuclear catastrophe. So who are these madmen? And who is the sober, pacific, calm citizen who moves not a finger to help himself and his friends. Who is normal and who is mad?

That meeting in Troeshchino went on late into the long winter night. "Look, he's fallen asleep," suddenly said Liubov' Sirota, looking at her son who napped in a corner. "He's tired. *Before the war* he sat in front of the TV until long after midnight." [These words have a special meaning: 'before the catastrophe' as they are used by those who happened to be in the area contaminated by radioactive rain of cesium, plutonium, and strontium. People call that period in history which began for them on the night of April 25th, 1986 and which stretches into the present, "the war."]

"My apartment is not in order," Liubov' Sirota excused herself when I unexpectedly visited her one week later in her small two-room apartment in Kiev in the Kharkov district. She added bitterly, "I'm still young, a little over thirty, but have no energy to clean the floors properly, no energy." This is also the voice of Liubov' Sirota, the voice of motherly worries and cares, the voice of physical exhaustion which came unwanted.

A very heavy burden became the fate of children and adults who were also burned by the invisible fire of Chernobyl.

> This how we live.
> The body is heavier and heavier,
> the spirit is subtler and narrower.
> It can enter the deserted house;
> it circles like a bird above Pripiat' in the night ...
> and you often wish that it would leave the inept body
> and not days but years flow away
> and numberless are the losses.
> But one has to live,
> and for the sake of the children,
> accumulate anger,
> to efface the old age in children's eyes
> with the hope for a cure.

These lines are not printed in the copy of the collection Liubov' gave me. She wrote these lines by hand on the last page as a personal gift from the poet. *But one has to live*. Others should read this reminder from a person who is burdened with suffering, this reminder I appreciate especially from the poet from Pripiat'. This talisman was a friend's gift and it helps to overcome all troubles in times of despair and hopelessness acts as soon as you remember it and touch it. We all have to carry burdens in our own way, even if these are not as heavy as the burden of Liubov' and her fellow-citizens. And the sin of grumbling about life, precisely this is the sacred burden:"

> the heavier
> the dearer!

"Burden"

A soul weighed down with suffering: this is the image which poetic intuition meets again and again, an intuition reached through the Chernobyl experience, an image inevitably born of suffering. The similarity of experience explains the fact that this image appears in the poetry of another poet of deserted Pripiat', Liubov' Kovalevskaia.

> And though it is not easier to leave
> the body weighs half as much
> and the soul weighs more.
>
> (From the collection
> *Defense and Defenselessness: Kiev, 1989*, p. 64.)

"The sacred burden of the soul, how to carry it when the body weakens and your arms fall? The soul of a human being is a hundred times heavier than the body. It is so heavy that one person cannot carry it: and therefore we humans, while we are alive, should try to make each other's souls immortal. You should try to immortalize my soul and I, yours, and someone else a third person's, and so on into infinity."

This is the law of eternity. It was discovered by one of the heroes of the remarkable Georgian writer, Nodar Dumbadze, who spent many months in the hospital after a heart attack. The same image, born of suffering, but this time with the complete instruction for action: entrust the weight of your soul to another person and he will help you to carry it.

In her poems Lyuba entrusts her soul to other people. She believes that people will carry on this burden and help her, as she herself is ready to help everyone on earth. The source of her faith is a crystal-clear spring of love, friendship, comradeship, mutual understanding, which penetrates her lyrics from the beginning to the end. The lyrical hero of her poems is never lonely. Near him, and together, eye to eye, or shoulder to shoulder, in one impulse, embracing, touching compassionately, in sad recollection, in happy premonition, always someone else is present.

At times this someone is the beloved, a person to whom one speaks, or a relative, a friend, a neighbor, co-worker—sometimes all who feel and experience together with the poet the tragedy: victims of the Chernobyl tragedy, all who were enlightened by terrible tragedy, all people, humanity. We are with you, dear reader; while people live on earth, hope is alive, the hope for a better future. This is what the poet's hand wrote on the copy of *Burden* that I have. The voice of dead Pripiat' with hope for a better future. From dead Pripiat' with hope for life. From dead Pripiat' the voice of living suffering, of a living soul, of living hope. This hope is the underlying current of the creative impulse that inspires the poetry of Liubov' Sirota, the sacred meaning of her lyrics. I am enormously happy that this voice will sound for thousands of Americans whose friendly help will no doubt ease the uneasy burden a poet. Perhaps this is also a small foreshadowing of the message about the better future for which Liubov' Sirota hopes.

Translated by Arkady Rovner
with Paul Brians and Birgitta Ingemanson

Liubov Sirota

TO PRIPYAT

1.

We can neither expiate nor rectify
the mistakes and misery of that April.
The bowed shoulders of a conscience awakened
must bear the burden of torment for life.
It's impossible, believe me,
to overpower
or overhaul
our pain for the lost home.
Pain will endure in the beating hearts
stamped by the memory of fear.
There,
surrounded by prickly bitterness,
our puzzled town asks:
since it loves us
and forgives everything,
why was it abandoned forever?

2.

At night, of course, our town
though emptied forever, comes to life.
There, our dreams wander like clouds,
illuminate windows with moonlight,

live by unwavering memories,
remember the touch of hands.
How bitter for them to know
there will be no one for their shade
to protect from the scorching heat!
At night their branches quietly rock
our inflamed dreams.
Stars thrust down
onto the pavement,
to stand guard until morning ...
But the hour will pass ...
Abandoned by dreams,
the orphaned houses
whose windows

have gone insane
will freeze and bid us farewell! ...

3.

We've stood over our ashes;
now what do we take on our long journey?
The secret fear that wherever we go
we are superfluous?
The sense of loss
that revealed the essence
of a strange and sudden kinlessness,
showed that our calamity is not
shared by those who might, one day,
themselves face annihilation?
... We are doomed to be left behind by the flock
in the harshest of winters ...
You, fly away!
But when you fly off
don't forget us, grounded in the field!
And no matter to what joyful faraway lands
your happy wings bear you,
may our charred wings
protect you from carelessness.

Translated from the Russian by Leonid Levin and Elisavietta Ritchie

Liubov Sirota

To Vasily Deomidovich Dubodel, who passed away in August 1988,
and to all past and future victims of Chernobyl.

They did not register us
and our deaths
were not linked to the accident.
No processions laid wreaths,
no brass bands melted with grief.
They wrote us off as
                lingering stress,
cunning genetic disorders ...
But we—we are the payment for rapid progress,
mere victim (of someone else's sated afternoons.
It wouldn't have been so annoying for us to die
had we known
our death would help
to avoid more "fatal mistakes"
and halt replication of "reckless deeds"!
But thousands of "competent" functionaires
count our "souls" in percentages,
their own honesty, souls, long gone—
so we suffocate with despair.
They wrote us off.
They keep trying to write off
our ailing truths
with their sanctimonious lies.
But nothing will silence us!
Even after death,
from our graves
we will appeal to your Conscience
not to transform the Earth
                into a sarcophagus!

***

Peace unto your remains,
unknown fellow-villager!
We'll all end up there sooner or later.
Like everyone, you wanted to live.
As it turned out,
you could not survive ...

Your torment is done.
Our turn will come:

prepare us a roomier place over there.
Oh, if only our "mass departure"
could be a burning lump of truth
in duplicity's throat! ...

May God not let anyone else
know our anguish!
May we be extinction's limit.
For this, you died.
Peace unto your remains,
my fellow-villager
from abandoned hamlets.

Translated from the Russian by Leonid Levin and Elisavietta Ritchie

Liubov Sirota

BURDEN

How amazing
in my thirtieth year
not to live
but instead
stumble along—
all bygone years
both happy and deadly,
heavy, wet, like logs,
crowd in the soul
as if in a tomb!

The soul does not sing
but rather becomes satanic;
ails
rather than aches …
So it is harder to breathe.

I am not to fly!
Though the shallow edge
of heaven is over my porch.
Already the roads have tired me,
hobbled me so—
I can no longer soar!

Faces reflect in the heavens,
faces of those
to whom I have said farewell.
Not one can be forgotten!
No oblivion!

The soul, it seems—
is a difficult memory.
Nothing can be erased,
nothing subtracted,
nothing canceled,
nothing corrected! …

… Even so,—the burden is sacred,
the heavier
the dearer!

Translated from the Russian by Leonid Levin and Elisavietta Ritchie

Liubov Sirota

RADIOPHOBIA

Is this only—a fear of radiation?
Perhaps rather—a fear of wars?
Perhaps—the dread of betrayal,
cowardice, stupidity, lawlessness?
The time has come to sort out
what is—radiophobia.
It is—
when those who've gone through the Chernobyl drama
refuse to submit
to the truth meted out by government ministers
("Here, you swallow exactly this much today!")
We will not be resigned
to falsified ciphers,
base thoughts,
however you brand us!
We don't wish—and don't you suggest it!—
to view the world through bureaucratic glasses!
We're too suspicious!
And, understand, we remember
each victim just like a brother! ...
Now we look out at a fragile Earth
through the panes of abandoned buildings.
These glasses no longer deceive us!—
These glasses show us more clearly—
believe me—
the shrinking rivers,
poisoned forests,
children born not to survive ...
Mighty uncles, what have you dished out
beyond bravado on television?
How marvelously the children have absorbed
radiation, once believed so hazardous! ...
(It's adults who suffer radiophobia—
for kids is it still adaption?)
What has become of the world
if the most humane of professions
has also turned bureaucratic?
Radiophobia

may you be omnipresent!
Not waiting until additional jolts,
new tragedies,
have transformed more thousands
who survived the inferno
into seers—
Radiophobia might cure
the world
of carelessness, satiety, greed,
bureaucratism and lack of spirituality,
so that we don't, through someone's good will
mutate into non-humankind.

Translated from the Russian by Leonid Levin and Elisavietta Ritchie

Liubov Sirota

AT THE CROSSING

A century of universal decay.
In cyclotrons nuclei are split;
souls are split,
sounds are split
insanely.

While behind a quiet fence
on a bench in someone's garden
Doom weighs
a century of separation
on the scales.

And her eyes are ancient,
and her palms are taut with nerves,
and her words clutch
in her throat ...

Nearby and cynical, death
brandishes a hasty spade.
Here, whispers are worse than curses,
offer no consolation.

Yet out on the festive streets
the mixed chorus
of pedestrians and cars
never stops.

The stoplight
winks with greed,
gobbles the fates of those it meets
in the underground passageways
of eternity.

How long
the bureaucrats
babbled on
like crows
about universal good ...
Yet somehow
that universal good
irreversibly

seeps away.
Have we slipped up?

In the suburbs, choke-cherries
came out with white flowers
like gamma, fluorescence.
What is this—a plot by mysterious powers?
Are these intrigues?
We have slipped up!

Choke-cherries are minor.
They are not vegetables ...
Here, tomatoes ripened too early:
someone just ate one—the ambulance
had to be called in a rush.
We have slipped up.

We came to the sea—
the eternal source of healing ...
And—we were stunned.
The sea is an enormous waste dump.
What happened?
Have we slipped up?

How masterfully
the blind promoters
of gigantic plans
manipulated us so far!
Now the bitter payment
for what we so easily
overlooked yesterday.

Has day died?
Or is this the end of the world?
Morbid dew on pallid leaves.
By now it's unimportant
whose the fault,
what the reason,
the sky is boiling only with crows ...
And now—no sounds, no smells.
And no more peace in this world.
Here, we loved ...
Now, eternal separation
reigns on the burnt out Earth ...

Liubov Sirota

These dreams are dreamed
ever more often.
Ever more often I am sad for no reason,
when flocks of crows
circle over the city
in skies, smoky, alarmed ...

Translated from the Russian by Leonid Levin and Elisavietta Ritchie

Liubov Sirota

FATE
(Triptych)

1.

I am working—
as if with my final strength,
as if from my final days
I look at eternity.
The moment of farewell
has made my head spin ...
I adore you—
random passersby!
To me—you are no one,
but you give me the plot,
the smile,
the glance laced with bitterness ...
Your astonished looks follow me, surprised
I love you for no reason.
Yet maybe
I can see more clearly
from the silence,
bareness of abandoned hamlets—
nothing more absurd than feuds,
nothing more splendid than confession,
how petty are success and luck,
how lowly the yearning for riches.
Like last year's snow, you can't buy
at any price the sense
                          of brotherhood.
What happiness—
to come home,
to repay debts to friends and kin,
without thinking
your last duty is
to bow over your smoldering home!

2.

I accept
this world!

I embrace
this air!
I am happy
it is not simple
for me
to become
your happiness ...

3.

I am working—
as if with my final strength,
as if from my final days
I look at eternity.
But only with you
is the hour of daybreak kind.
And only with you
is every evening splendid.
Indeed can it be
I have only a handful of days
left to live—
to be burnt up in one short month?
Now,
when I can love so much,
when my world is so majestic and bright!
Life went up in smoke from somebody's campfire
(this world has inquisitors to spare!).
Everything burned,
burned up.
　　　Even the ashes
were not always left behind ...
But the stubborn soul still lives
yet again resurrected from ashes!
I live with abandon!
I live, breathing you!
And for you, I am ready to go
into the inferno again!
But with merciful hands you extinguish
the fatal fire under me.
My beloved,
may God protect you!
May the flame of the redeemed soul shield you!

Translated from the Russian by Leonid Levin and Elisavietta Ritchie

Liubov Sirota

Your glance will trip on my shadow
and the shadow
will thrust itself
into the leafy shade.
The pale sun will shine over us,
a lantern
scorched by the burning question ...
Caught by the gravity of the light,
breathing is choked, lips are pressed,
and there is no answer,
no answer
to this light in the violent night.
But freed from gravity our shadows
shook the jasmine bush,
they will drift apart,
breathe night haze at our backs.
And the yellow leaf will fall exhausted,
it will take unbearably long to inhale.
As if the wisdom of autumn
were to catch us by surprise ...

Translated from the Russian by Leonid Levin and Elisavietta Ritchie

LIFE ON THE LINE BIOGRAPHICAL SKETCHES

Dannie Abse (London, England) is a physician who is in charge of the chest clinic in the Central London Medical Establishment. A fellow of the Royal Society of Literature, Abse is the author of 15 books of poetry, 11 plays, three novels, five radio plays, recordings, and numerous articles on medicine.

Anya Achtenberg (New York, NY) has published in *American Poetry Review, Southern Poetry Review, The Madison Review, etc.* Her first book, *I Know What The Small Girl Knew*, was published in 1983 by Holy Cow! Press. She has taught creative writing and literature with children as well as adults and is currently working with young adults who have dropped out of high school.

B.B. Adams (Newburgh, NY) is an associate professor of English at Pace University in New York City and Director of Business Communications for the Lubin Graduate School of Business at Pace. Her book on Laura Riding, *The Enemy Self*, was published by UMI Research Press, Ann Arbor, Michigan in January, 1990. She has also published essays on Riding, Joseph Conrad, and various literary subjects. Her poetry has appeared in *The Nation, Wooster Review, Modern Poetry Studies,* etc. Her short stories have appeared in *Madison Review, Other Voices, Fiction 83*, etc. She writes poetry reviews for *Chiron Review* and *Lake Effect.*

Linda Allardt (Pittsford, NY) is an associate editor of State Street Press. She teaches creative writing at Eastman School of Music.

Maggie Anderson (Kent, Ohio) is the author of four books of poems, most recently *A Space Filled With Moving*, published by the University of Pittsburgh in 1992. Anderson is a 1990 recipient of a poetry fellowship from the National Endowment for the Arts. She teaches at Kent State University in Ohio where she helped to organize a Gathering of Poets in 1990 to commemorate the 20th anniversary of the 1970 shootings there.

Frank Anthony (Windsor, VT) is President of the New England Writers/Vermont Poets Association, editor of *The Anthology of New England Writers*, and Special Consultant for *Dream International Quarterly.* He has recently published in *Anemone, Negative Capability,* and *Northern New England Review.* His "Legendry" interviews have appeared in *Northwest Review, American String Teacher*, and *Dramatics Magazine.*

Marion Arenas (Wyckoff, NJ) was born and reared in New York City but has lived in Japan, Peru, Colombia, and Egypt. She has been an editor of the New York City literary journal, *Box 749* and has taught poetry writing in a continuing education setting in Ridgewood, New Jersey. She works as a volunteer, counseling persons with AIDS at the Gay Men's Health Crisis in New York City and lives in northern New Jersey with her husband. She has published in *Stone Country, The New York Times, Poets On*, etc.

Gary Aspenberg (New York, NY) has a first collection of poems, *Bus Poems* appearing from Broken Moon Press of Seattle in the spring of 1993.

Jeannine Atkins (Whatley, MA) won a recent PEN Syndicated Fiction Award. Her stories have appeared in *The North American Review, Boston Review, Fiction Network, Descant*, etc.

Mary Alice Ayers (Miami, FL) teaches English in South Dade. Recent work has appeared in the *Paris Review, the Literary Review,* etc.

Betsy Barber Bancroft (Birmingham, AL) is the author of four books of poetry. The most recent, *Belonging, A Retrospective Journal of the South* was published by NSU Press of Louisiana. She was the first Poet in the School in Alabama, serving during the 1972-73 school year. She was awarded the Award of Merit by the Alabama State Historical Commission for "Preservation of Alabama's Heritage Through Poetry." She has appeared on radio and television in many southern towns and cities and served for a year as Poetry Editor of the *Village Press.*

Mary Jo Bang (Chicago, IL) spent three years living in London where she completed a B.A. in Photography at the Polytechnic of Central London. Her degree work, which combined color still-life photographs with autobiographical poems, was awarded a "Distinction." She has published in *Earth's Daughter's, Poets On, Echoes,* and *Kalliope.* She has recently edited a collection of contemporary women's poetry for The Oscars Press in London.

James Barfoot (Montgomery, AL) is an associate professor at Auburn University at Montgomery where he teaches poetry writing and religious studies. His poems have appeared in the *Anglican Theological Review, The Christian Century, Christianity and Literature, Religion and Intellectual Life,* etc.

Meg Baxter (Fairhope, Al) is a retired teacher, poet and short story writer.

Phyllis Beauvais (Roxbury, CT) is a poet and psychotherapist. Together with her husband, Dr. Richard Beauvais, she is the founder of Wellspring, an innovative psychiatric treatment center for emotionally disturbed adolescents and adults located in Bethlehem, Ct. She has published in *Poetry, The New Yorker, Prairie Schooner,* and many other journals and anthologies.

Libby Bernardin (Columbia, SC) was the 1986-87 recipient of the South Carolina Arts Commission Literary Fellowship. She has edited two volumes of writing by South Carolina teachers, the most recent,*Out of Unknown Hands.* A poem was included in *Negative Capability's* 1991 poetry awards issue, and three poems were included in a recent issue of *Charleston Magazine.* A former newspaper reporter and business editor, she teaches at the University of South Carolina.

Richard G. Beyer (Florence, AL) is an award-winning photographer as well as a poet. The former president of the Alabama Writers' Conclave and the Alabama State Poetry Society, he is the managing editor of *Negative Capability* and the author of a book of poems entitled *The Homely Muse* (The Pinpoint Press, Florence, AL)

Margaret Key Biggs (Port St. Joseph, FL) has taught school for over three decades. She writes fiction and non-fiction, but her first love is poetry. She has published five books: *Swampfire, Sister To The Sun, Magnolias and Such, Petals From The Womanflower* and *The Plumage of the Sun.*

Robert Bixby (Greensboro, NC) is the editor of *Parting Gifts* (March Street Press, 1987) and has published in the *Greensboro Review, Nightsun, Oxalis,* etc.

Cathy Blackburn (Little Rock, AR) has had poetry published in *The Texas Review, Negative Capability, The New Laurel Review,* etc. She was chosen by Marge Piercy to participate in an advanced poetry workshop at the Omega Institute. She teaches English at Pulaski Academy.

Karen Blomain (Allentown, Pa) teaches Creative Writing in the Professional Writing Program at Kutztown University and is a poetry consultant for the Geraldine R. Dodge Foundation and a member of the Literature Panel of the Pennsylvania Council on the Arts. Her publications include two chapbooks, *Black Diamond* (Great Elm Press, 1987), and *The Slap* (Nightshades Press, 1990). She co-authored a textbook, *Writing the Rainbow* (Kendall Hunt, 1988), and edited an anthology, *Coalseams* (University of Scranton Press, 1992). A new collection of poems, *Borrowed Light,* (1992) is published by Nightshade Press. Her awards include one from the Academy of American Poets, two Fellowships to Blue Mountain Center, a residency at the Djerassi Foundation, two Individual Artists Fellowships from the Pennsylvania Council on the Arts, two Pen Syndicated Fiction Project Awards (1989 & 1990) etc.

E.P. Bollier (New Orleans, LA) is a professor of English at Tulane University in New Orleans.

Gloria Brame (Atlanta, GA) has published poetry and prose in numerous literary magazines. Her first book (non-fiction) was published by Villard in 1992.

John Brand (Greenley, CO) teaches literature at the University of Northern Colorado and has served parishes in west Texas and northeastern Colorado.

Paul Brians (Pullman, WA) is a professor of
English at Washington State University. He has published numerous articles on nuclear war in fiction and a book entitled *Nuclear Holocausts: Atomic War in Fiction 1895-1984* (Kent State University Press). He also edits the newsletter of the International Society for the Study of Nuclear Texts and Contexts.

Kim Brigford (Southport, CT) has published in *The Georgia Review, The Quarterly, North Dakota Quarterly, New Orleans Review, The Laurel Review,* etc. She won the National Society of Arts and Letters National Career Awards Competition in Poetry, and from 1986-1988, she held a Jacob K. Javits Fellowship in English awarded by the U.S. Department of Education. She won a recent Tennessee Williams Scholar in Poetry at the Sewanee Writers' Conference. She teaches at Fairfield University in Connecticut.

Claudia Smith Brinson (Columbia, SC) has published in *Kalliope, Iowa Woman,* and *Crescent Review.* She was a recipient of the National Pen Women's biennial literary scholarship. She is a senior writer for *The State* newspaper in Columbia, SC.

Ruth Brinton (Seattle, WA) has worked in public relations, theater administration and corporate (for profit) accounting. She won the 1989 Louisa Kern Literary Award. She is an editorial assistant for the *Seattle Review* and teaches writing at North Seattle Community College. Her work has appeared in *Seattle Review, Poetry Seattle, Washington English Journal,* etc. Her reviews appear regularly in *The Literary Center Quarterly.*

Michael Dennis Browne (Benedict, MN) has a fourth collection of poetry, *You Won't Remember This,* forthcoming from Carnegie Mellon University Press in the winter of 1992. Other publications include *Smoke From The Fires* and *The Sun Fetcher* (Carnegie-Mellon, 1985, 1978), *Tri-Quarterly,* and *The Virginia Quarterly Review.*

Joseph Bruchac, III (Greenfield Center, NY) is a storyteller and writer of Abenaki, English and Slovak ancestry. His poems and stories have appeared in more than 400 magazines and anthologies, and he is the author of two published novels, 14 collections of poetry and two non-fiction books. The winner of an NEA Creative Writing Fellowship, a CCLM Editors Fellowship, a Rockefeller Foundation Humanities Fellowship, two New York State CAPS Poetry Fellowships, a PEN Syndicated Fiction Award and the Cherokee Nation Prose Award, his work has been translated into German, Danish, French, Italian, Dutch, Polish, Swedish, Czechoslovakian, Macedonia, Russian, and Frisian. He is also the editor of a dozen different anthologies of poetry and fiction and the author of *Survival This Way: Interviews with American Indian Poets.* Bruchac is the Director of the Greenfield Literary Center in Greenfield Center, NY.

John J. Brugaletta (Fullerton, CA) is the editor of *South Coast Poetry Journal* and a professor of English at California State University, Fullerton. He is the author of *The Tongue Angles* published by Negative Capability Press in 1990 and *Tilling The Land* (1992) has just been released by The Mellen Poetry Press..

Cullene Bryant (Edmonton, Alto, Canada) is a member of the Canadian Author's Association. She has been published in the *Alberta Poetry Anthology, Other Voices, Prairie Dreams,* etc.

Michael J. Bugeja (Athens, Ohio) writes a monthly poetry feature for *Writer's Digest.* He is the author of *The Visionary* (Taxus Press), *Before I Go* (Amelia Press) and *What We Do For Music* (Amelia Press).

Janet Burroway (Tallahassee, FL) is the author of plays, poetry, children's books, and seven novels including *The Buzzards, Raw Silk, Opening Nights,* and the forthcoming *Cutting Stone.* Her text, *Writing Fiction,* is used in more than 300 colleges and universities in the U.S. She is the McKenzie professor of Literature and Writing at the Florida State University in Tallahassee. "Homesick" was originally a part of the author's autobiography in The Gale Contemporary Authors series.

Gerald Cable, (Vashon, WA) died in January, 1988 of cancer. He had poems published in *Ironwood, Shenandoah, Abraxas, Plainsong, Cimarron Review, Nebraska Review, Prairie Schooner, Southern Poetry Review, Connecticut Review, Cream City Review, South Coast Review, Another Chicago Magazine, Pennsylvania Review, Unmuzzled Ox,* and *In the Dreaming,* an anthology of Alaskan writers. He earned a Masters of Fine Arts at the University of Alaska in 1982. He finished a book length manuscript of poems shortly before he died.

Marilyn Elain Carmen (Aisha Eshe) (Philadelphia, PA) has been widely published in the United States and Canada. In the U.S., her poetry has appeared in such journals as *Heresies, Black American Literature, Forum, Iris, Sing Heavenly Muse,* and *Shooting Star Review.* Short fiction has appeared in *Hurricane Alice, Home Planet News* and *Little Magazine: Cuaderno.* Her non-fiction narrative entitled, "Recovery as an Art" will be included in Crossing Press's *Our Many Pathways.* Carmen is the recipient of the 1990 Pennsylvania State Council of the Arts Grant, based on an excerpt of *Blood at the Root* recently published by Esoterica Press. She is currently working on the sequel to *Blood at the Root* entitled *A Long Way From Home.*

Sal Cetrano (Ridgewood, NY) is a teacher in Brooklyn, NY. His work has appeared in *Kansas Quarterly, Outposts Poetry Quarterly, Wind,* and *Reseda Review.*

Michael Chitwood (Chapel Hill, NC) is a science writer and editor for the Research Triangle Institute. He is a recipient of a recent writing fellowship from the North Carolina Arts Council.

Vince Clemente (Setauket, NY) is a poet-editor whose books include *Snow Owl Above Stony Brook Harbor, Broadbill of Conscience Bay, Songs from Puccini, From This Book of Praise,* and *Paumanok Rising.* His work has appeared in *The New York Times Newsday,* and in many literary journals and anthologies. Founding editor of *Long Pond Review* and West Hills Review: A Walt Whitman Journal, he is a professor of English at Suffolk Community College as well as a trustee of the Walt Whitman Birthplace.

Leo Connellan (Norwich, CT) has published 12 books of poetry and has won many awards including a grant from the National Endowment for the Arts and the Shelly Memorial Award from the Poetry Society of America. His poems have been recorded by the Library of Congress. He is poet-in-residence at Eastern Connecticut State University.

Colleen Connors (Northwood Narrows, NH) teaches writing at the University of New Hampshire. Recent poetry has appeared in *Bitterroot.*

Tina Marie Conway (Boulder, CO) is a recent recipient of a Creative Writing Fellowship in Literature from the Colorado Council on the Arts and Humanities. Her work has appeared in *Black Ice, The Florida Review, Slipstream, Permafrost* and the anthologies: *The Luxury of Tears* and *North of Wakulla.*

Peter Cooley (New Orleans, LA) has lived in the Crescent City for the past 16 years and is a professor of English at Tulane University. He has published five books of poetry: *The Company of Strangers, The Room Where Summer Ends, Night Seasons, The Van Gogh Notebook,* and *The Astonished Hours.* His work also appears in *The Morrow Anthology of Younger American Poets.*

Jack Coulehan (Setauket, NY) is a physician, epidemiologist, and medical ethicist who has recently moved from the University of Pittsburgh School of Medicine to join the faculty of the State University of New York at Stony Brook. His published medical writing ranges from epidemiological studies of illness among American Indians to essays on doctor-patient communication and symbolic healing. He co-authored a widely-used textbook on medical interviewing for health-professionals. In 1988-89, he participated as a fellow in an NEH-funded Institute for Humanities in Medicine at Hiram College in Ohio. He is the author of *The Knitted Glove* published by Nightshade Press in 1991 and has been published widely in many journals, including *Kansas Quarterly, Prairie Schooner, Negative Capability, South Coast Poetry Journal,* and *The Journal of the American Medical Association.* He was awarded a Pennsylvania Council for the Arts creative writing grant in 1989.

Tom Crawford (Cloverdale, OR) has been published in *If It Weren't for Trees* (Lynx House Press 1986) and *I Want to Say Listen* (Ironwood Press, 1980).

Brian Cronwall (Saint Paul, MN) is a writer, teacher, and political organizer.

Barbara Crooker (Fogelsville, PA) has published over 440 poems in such magazines as *America, The Christian Science Monitor, Yankee,* and *Country Journal.* Her work has appeared in 32 anthologies and five chapbooks. She has won two Pennsylvania Council on the Arts Fellowships in Literature; the NEA and *Passages North* Emerging Writers competition and was a Fellow at the Virginia Center for the Creative Arts in 1990.

Danielle D'Aunay (Mobile, AL)

David R. Dahl (Santa Barbara, Ca) Is a Vietnam veteran. He earned a California Arts Fellowship in 1989 and has published in *Abraxis, Exquisite Corpse, Poetry Motel,* etc.

Ruth Daigon (Mill Valley, CA) is editor of *Poets On.* She is the author of *A Portable Past* and *On My Side of the Bed* and has been published in *Realities Library,* 1986 and *Omnation,* 1978.

Bernadette Darnell (Amesbury, MA) teaches writing at Northern Essex Community College in Haverhill, MA, and writes for the local paper.

Lynne H. deCourcy (Oxford, Ohio) is the author of *The Good Child* (Still Waters Press, 1990) and *The Time Change* (1991) from Ampersand Press. She has received fellowships from the Ohio Arts Council and the National Endowment for the Arts.

Mary R. DeMaine (Minneapolis, MN) holds a Ph.D. from the University of Minnesota in Ancient Art and Archeology with a specialty in Ancient Glassmaking. She has recently completed a novel and edited a small press poetry publication.

Carl Djerassi (Stanford, CA) is a member of board of directors of Cetus Corp., Vitaphore, Inc., and Monoclonal Antibodies, Inc. Founder and president of resident artists' colony, Djerassi Foundation, Woodside, CA. Among numerous awards and honors he received the National Medal of Science, 1973, for synthesis of first oral contraceptive, Award in the Chemistry of Contemporary Technological Problems, 1983; Roussel Prize, 1988, Gustavus John Esselen Award for Chemistry in the Public Interest, 1989' award from National Academy of Sciences, 1990, for industrial application of science. His writings include *The Futurist, and Other Stories,* MacDonald Futura, 1988; *Cantor's Dilemma* (novel), Doubleday, 1989; *The Pill, Pygmy Chimps, and Degas's Horse: An Autobiography,* MacMillan, 1991.

Rita Dove (Charlottesville, VA) is a professor English at the University of Virginia. She is also the Commissioner, Schomburg Center for the Preservation of Black Culture, New York Public Library. She won a Pulitzer Prize in poetry in 1987 for *Thomas and Beulah.* Publications include *Fifth Sunday* (short stories), Callaloo Fiction Series, 1985; *Grace Notes* (Norton, 1989), *Thomas and Beulah* (Carnegie-Mellon, 1986), and *Ploughshares.* She serves as advisory editor for the *Gettysburg Review* and *Tri-Quarterly.*

Leon Driskell (Louisville, KY) is a professor of English and Creative Writing at the University of Louisville and an advisory editor for *Negative Capability.*

Richard Eberhart (Hanover, NH) served as honorary president of the Poetry Society of America. Educated at Dartmouth, Cambridge, and Harvard, he has been Poet-in-Residence at Dartmouth since 1956. His books include *The Quarry, Shifts of Being, Fields of Grace, Chocorua, Florida Poems, The Long Reach* and *Maine Poems..*

Dale Edmonds (New Orleans, LA) is a professor of English at Tulane University. He has published in *Negative Capability, South Coast Poetry Journal,* etc.

Sue Saniel Elkind (Pittsburgh, PA) has published in *Kansas Quarterly, Negative Capability, Centennial Review,*etc. Her published books include: *No Longer Afraid,* (Lintel); *Waiting for Order,* (Naked Man Press); *Dinosaurs and Grandparents,* (MAF Press); *Another Language,* and

Bare as the Trees, (Papier-Mache Press.) She received the Esther Scheffler 1987 poetry award for the best poem in *Centennial Review* and founded the Squirrel Hill Poetry Workshop in 1977.

Sandra Engel (Utica, NY) received her M.A. in English from the University of New Hampshire and her Ph.D. from University of Iowa.

Angie Estes (San Luis Obispo, CA) is a professor of English at California Polytec State University. She is the author of *Boarding Pass* published by Solo Press in 1990.

Frank Finale (Pine Beach, NJ) is the editor of *Without Halos*. He has published in the *Anthology of Magazine Verse, New York Quarterly, The Brooklyn Review, Blue Unicorn*, and numerous other journals.

M.F.K. Fisher (Glen Ellen, CA) has published *The Art of Eating: Five Gastronomical Works*, Vintage, 1976; *A Cordiall Water: A Garland of Odd and Old Receipts to Assauge the Ills of Man or Beast*, Little, Brown, 1961; *The Story of Wine in California*, University of California Press, 1962; *Maps of another Town: A Memoir of Provence*, Little, Brown, 1964; (author of introduction) Robert Louis Stevenson, *Napa Wine*, J.E. Beard, 1965; *The Cooking of Provincial France*, Time-Life, 1968; *With Bold Knife and Fork*, Putnam, 1969; *Among Friends*, Knopf, 1971.

Alice B. Fogel (Washington, NH) teaches writing at the University of New Hampshire and Keene State College. She has recently published in *Ironwood, Amaranth*, and *Puckerbrush*.

Jeanne Foster (Berkeley, CA) teaches at St. Mary's College in Moraga, California. She has published one book of poems, *A Blessing of Safe Travel, Quarterly Review of Literature* (Princeton, 1980), and a chapbook, *Great Horned Owl*, (White Pine Press, 1980. Her poems have appeared in *American Poetry Review, Hudson Review, The Nation, Paris Review*, and others. Two long poems appeared in *Ploughshares*, (Winter 1991) edited by Gerald Stern. She has a doctorate in the field of Literature and Religion and is an ordained minister.

Kenneth Frost (New York, NY) is a poet and former teacher.

Nan Fry (Bethesda, MD) teaches in the Academic Studies Department at the Corcoran School of Art in Washington, D.C. A book of her poems, *Relearning the Dark*, was published by Washington Writers Publishing House. In 1988, Sibyl-Child Press published *Say What I am Called*, a chapbook of riddle-poems which she translated from the Anglo-Saxon and for which she received a Maryland State Arts Council grant. Individual poems have appeared in publications such as *Antietam Review, Kalliope, The Little Magazine, Negative Capability*, and the anthology *Pocket Poems* (Macmillan, 1985)

Anne George (Birmingham, AL) is the author of several books of poetry and the publisher of Druid Press (Birmingham, Alabama).

Daniela Gioseffi (Andover, NJ) won a NYSCA of NEA award/grant for poems contained in her collection, *"Eggs in the Lake,"* (Boa Editions). She has published a novel, *The Great American Belly*, from Doubleday and stories and poems in major press books as well as in leading magazines such as *The Paris Review, Choice, Antaeus* and *The Nation*. A collection of award winning prose and poetry, *Women on War; Global Voices for Survival*, edited by Ms. Gioseffi was published by Touchstone, Simon & Schuster, 1988. Her translations of the Latin American poet, Carilda Oliver Labra, with a foreword by Gregory Rabassa, is another recent publication. She is a member of PEN, The National Book Critics Circle, The Poetry Society of America, and a Board Member of The Writers and Publishers Alliance where she helps to nominate the *Olive Branch Awards*. Her poetry and prose appears in texts for the teaching of writing from Harper & Row, Houghton Mifflin, and D.C. Heath.

Andrew Glaze (Miami, FL) has the following publications to his credit: *Reality Street* (St. Andrews Press, 1990), *Earth That Sings* (Ford Brown, 1985), and *Reality Street*, recently published by St. Andrews Press in 1992. His poetry has also appeared in the *New York Quarterly, Poetry. The Atlantic, Negative Capability, New Yorker*, etc.

Judy Goldman (Charlotte, NC) has recent poems in *Southern Review, Crazyhorse, Gettysburg Review, Shenandoah, Prairie Schooner* and *Yankee*. Her first collection of poetry, *Holding Back Winter,* won a NC Poetry Council Award and is in its third printing.

Susana Gomes (Scarborough, Ontario, Canada) is currently working on a novel entitled *Recluse.*

W.C. Gosnell (Northampton, MA) has published in *Black River Review* and *Sounding East.*

Roger Granet (Morristown, NJ) is a Clinical Associate professor of Psychiatry at Cornell University Medical College and in private practice. A book of poetry, *The World's A Small Town* is new from Negative Capability Press.

Pamela Gross (Seattle, WA) has published in *Poetry, Antioch Review, Georgia Review, Commonweal,* and *Raccoon.* Her first collection was published by Ion Books, Memphis, Tennessee in 1990.

Isabella Halsted (Amherst, MA) teaches basic writing and leads creative writing groups in Western Massachusetts, where she also edits the newsletter of the Peace Development Fund. Her poems and short fiction have appeared in *Croton Review* and *Peregrine.* She has been a resident fellow at Ragdale Foundation and the Virginia Center for the Creative Arts, where a growing collection of stores about Africa first began to take root.

Ralph Hammond (Arab, AL) is Alabama Poet Laureate: 1991-1995. He is a former mayor, past President of the Alabama State Poetry Society and the Alabama Writer's Conclave and was recently awarded an honorary D. Litt. from Livingston University. He is currently the 1st V.P. of the National Federation of State Poetry Society. He has published 16 books.

Joseph Harris (Aiken, SC) served for a number of years as the headmaster of an Episcopal school. He has published widely in such journals as *The Georgia Review, Saturday Evening Post, American Poetry Anthology, The Yearbook of American Poetry,* etc.

Penny Harter (Sante Fe, NM) teaches English and Creative Writing at Santa Fe Preparatory School.

Nancy Peter Hastings (Las Cruces, NM) is the editor of *Whole Notes* and has had poems published in *Poetry, Cafe Solo, Plainsongs, The Connecticut River Review, Earthwise,* and in several anthologies.

Ellen Herbert (Falls Church, VA) teaches English composition at George Mason University. Her short fiction has been published in *Sanskrit, Thema, Pennsylvania English, The Iris,* and *The Carolina Literary Companion.* Her novel-in-progress won first place in the 1989 Florida State Writing Competition.

Wendy S. Hesford (Oberlin, OH) is a Visiting Lecturer in the Expository Writing Department at Oberlin College. Her poetry has been published in *Abraxus, Dreamworks,* and *Poet Lore* among others. She has also published articles on the dynamics of feminist teaching.

Jeffrey Hilliard (Cincinnati, OH) is an Associate Editor of *Cincinnati Poetry Review* and an assistant professor of English at The College of Mount St. Joseph. His book of poems, *The Shadow Family,* was published by Cincinnati Poetry Review Press in October, 1989.

Judith Hirshmiller (St. Francis, WI) is the author of *Bowler Poems* and *The Poetry of a Nurse* which addresses matters related to her nursing profession.

Roald Hoffman (Ithaca, NY) is the John A. Newman professor of Physical Science at Cornell University where he is engaged in teaching and research in theoretical chemistry. He won the 1981 Nobel Prize in Chemistry and is the author of two books of poetry.

David Hood (Mebane, NC) teaches honors English at Eastern Alamance High School and is completing a doctorate at the University of North Carolina at Chapel Hill. His poetry has appeared in *International Poetry Review* and *The Sun* of Chapel Hill.

Nall Hollis (Arab, AL) the cover artist, was born in Alabama but divides his time between Arab, Alabama and his villa "The Cocoon" (built by the late French artist Jean Dubuffet) in Vence, France. A University of Alabama graduate, Nall is an artist with total dedication to the call of art forms. Few artists in history have achieved Nall's success by the age of 40. Equally gifted in oil and watercolor and design, Nall has been called "the greatest drawer in the world today." To find an equal, one must return to the drawings of Rembrandt and the 16th century German master drawer, Albrecht Durer. Since 20, Nall has exhibited more than a hundred one-man shows in leading museums and art galleries and corporate offices in such cities as Paris, Brussels, Washington, Huntsville, Nice, New Orleans, Birmingham, Beruit, Miami, Cannes, Avignon—the number is endless. Reviews and critiques of his shows have received the highest acclaim. Art collectors, worldwide, as well as museums, are purchasing and adding Nall art work to their collections. Already, at 40, Nall is Alabama's most honored artist. An illustrated volume of his work, *Nall—1971-1986,* was recently published in Torino, Italy.

Ingrid Hughes (New York, NY) has published poems in *The Massachusetts Review* and *Mudfish.* She recently completed a novel about coming of age during the Vietnam War, and the effect of the war on her generation.

Connie Hutchison (Kirkland, WA) graduated from Pacific Lutheran University and taught science and math. She has studied poetry with Nixeon Civille Handy and completed the Certificate in Writing Program with Nelson Bentley at the University of Washington. She is Associate Editor of *Brussels Sprout,* a haiku and art journal.

David Ignatow (East Hampton, NY) has won a number of awards for his poetry—the Bollingen Prize in 1977, and earlier, two Guggenheim fellowships, the Wallace Stevens fellowship from Yale University, the Rockefeller Foundation fellowship, the Shelley Memorial and the National Institute of Arts and Letters awards. He is president emeritus of the Poetry Society of America and has taught at several universities and is the author of thirteen books of poetry and two other prose books.

Birgitta Ingemanson (Pullman, WA) is an associate professor of Foreign Languages and Literatures and Director of Russian Area Studies at Washington State University. She has done extensive research on Alexandra Kollontay and is currently studying the cultural history of Vladivostok.

Susan Jacobson (Pittsburgh, PA) is a Certified Nursing Assistant on an orthopedic unit. She served four years as Poet in the Classroom for the Pittsburgh Public and area schools and three years as Poet in Residence for the Western Pennsylvania School for the Deaf.

Judson Jerome (Yellow Springs, OH) wrote a poetry column for *Writers Digest* for many years and edited their annual *Poet's Market.* He is a former English professor and the author of numerous books of poetry.

Alice A. Jones practiced Internal Medicine for a number of years before doing a second residency in Psychiatry, which she now practices in the San Francisco Bay Area. She has completed a book manuscript entitled *The Knot.* Poems have appeared in *Poetry, ZYZZYVA, The New England Review, Chelsea,* and *The Gettysburg Review.*

Rodney Jones (Carbondale, IL) holds a fellowship from the National Endowment for the Arts and teaches at the University of Southern Illinois at Carbondale.

Sandi Kadlubowski (Pittsburgh, PA) is an artist and a potter.

Marilyn Kallet (Knoxville, TN) is Director of Creative Writing at the University of Tennessee, Knoxville. Her essays on May Sarton, Cathy Song and Joy Harjo have appeared in *Before Columbus Review, Belles Lettres,* and *American Book Review.*

Susan A. Katz (Monsey, NY) worked as a Book Review Editor for Menke Katz and *Bitterroot* for the past six years. Her most recent publications include *An Eye for Resemblances,* (a poetry/painting responsive collaboration) (University Editions, 1991) and *Teaching Creatively By Working The Word* co-edited with Judith A. Thomas and published by Prentice Hall in 1992

Adol'f Kharash is the Science Director and a professor at Moscow State University.

Herb Kitson (Titusville, PA) is an Associate professor of English at the University of Pittsburgh at Titusville. He has been a participant at the Bread Loaf Writers Conference and has received two poetry-related NEH grants—one at New York University and one at the University of Arizona. Kitson has two chapbooks with M.A.F. press—*Slow Watch For Children/Fast Watch For Adults* and *On the Way To Where; Satori Poems*—and has had poems in *Bitterroot, Black River Review, Lucky Star, Negative Capability, The New York Quarterly, Poetry North Review, Ransom, Real, Riverrun, Studies in Contemporary Satire, Sunrust,* and *Thirteen.*

Mary Sue Koeppel (Jacksonville, FL) is the editor of *Kalliope,* a journal of women's art. She recently won the 1992 Esme Bradberry Contemporary Poets' Award. Her work has been published in *Poets for a Livable Planet* and *Clockwatch Review.* Prentice Hall published her first book, *Writing.*

Norbert Krapf (Roslyn Hts, NY) a native of southern Indiana and a professor of English at Long Island University. His poetry collections include *Lines Drawn from Durer* and *A Dream of Plum Blossoms.* He is the editor/translator of *Shadows on the Sundial: Selected Early Poems of Rainer Maria Rilke* and *Beneath the Cherry Sapling: Legends from Franconia.*

Carolyn Kremers (Fairbanks, AK) is the author of *Place of the Pretend People,* a collection of poems and essays which received a Special Citation from the PEN/Jerard Fund Award for emerging women writers of nonfiction, New York, NY, 1991. She teaches writing and literature at the University of Alaska Fairbanks.

Melissa Kwasny (San Francisco, CA) is the author of the novel, *Modern Daughters and the Outlaw West,* (Spinsters Book Company). She teaches in the California Poets in the Schools program. Her poems have been published in many regional periodicals and anthologies, most recently in Breitenbush Press's *Season of Dead Water: Poems About the Alaskan Oil Spill.*

Nadine Lambert (Hattiesburg, MS) is in graduate school at the University of Southern Mississippi.

Nancy Lambert (Van Nuys, CA) has had poems and essays appear in *L.A. Weekly, Chiron Review, Practicing Angels: An Anthology of San Francisco Bay Area Poetry,* and elsewhere. In 1990, she received the Kay Deeter Award for poetry from *Fine Madness.*

Henry Langhorne (Pensacola, FL) is a physician.

M.S. Leavitt (Westbrook, MN) has published in numerous publications, including *Potato Eyes, Orphic Lute, Bone & Flesh* and *Deviance.*

Cynthia Lelos (East Freetown, MA) worked as a clinical psychologist in Boston for many years after graduating from Harvard University. She won two awards from entering the Mass. Poetry Society's national poetry contest of which one was for "Sweet Parsley."

Arlene G. Levine (Forest Hills, NY) lives and teaches in the New York City area. Her writing has appeared in *The New York Times* and various magazines including *Z Miscellaneous* and *Frogpond.* She was the recipient of a New York Times Company Foundation Scholarship.

Lyn Lifshin (Niskayuna, NY) has recently had a film made about her that bears the title of a recent book, *Not Made of Glass,* published by Beacon Press in 1978, *Tangled Vines* is being reprinted by Harcourt Brace Jovanovich. Two additional books are: *The Doctor Poems* by Applezaba and *Naked Charm* by Illuminati.

Joseph Lisowski (St. Thomas, USVI) is the author of *Tremors: A Dialectic in Poetry* (Univ. of Virgin Islands.) He translated the poems of Wang Wei in *The Brushwood Gate* published by Black Buzzard Press in 1984. He is a professor of English at the University of Virgin Islands and has published recently in the *Kansas Quarterly* and *Negative Capability.*

Maryrica Lottman (Charlottesville, VA) has published in *Quarry Magazine, Lake Effect, The Farmer's Market, Aim Magazine,* and elsewhere. In 1983, she was awarded the Henry Hoyns Fellowship in fiction at the University of Virginia.

Sandra Love (Yellow Springs, OH) is Director of the Antioch Writers Workshop. She won the Ohio Arts Council individual artist fellowship, participated in the artists-in-education program sponsored by the same council, won the Elizabeth Enright award for a short story at Indiana

University, taught in the Antioch Writers' Workshop, and is the author of four children's novels for the 8-12 and 12 and up category of young readers.

Glenna Luschei (Atascadero, CA) who's first book, *Carta al Norte,* was published by Papel Sobrante, Medellín, Columbia in 1967. Twenty-two years later she found herself teaching students from Medellín as poet-in-residence at California Men's Colony, San Luis Obispo. During the intervening years she has also been active in the small press community. Her journal, *Café Solo,* is now celebrating its twenty-fifth year. She has served as Chair of COSMEP and also has acted as literature panelist of the NEA At present she is an avocado rancher. She is the author of a dozen books, chapbooks, and special editions.

Susan Luzzaro (Chula Vista, CA) teaches at Southwestern Community College. She has been published in the *American Poetry Review, Centennial Review, Malahat Review* and other magazines. In 1989, she was awarded First Place in Poetry by the Los Angeles Arts Council.

Paul Martin (Allentown, PA) has published in numerous journals, including *Kansas Quarterly, Passages North, Nimrod, Green Mountains Review*; also in several anthologies, including *Carrying the Darkness: Poetry of the Vietnam War* and *Passages North Anthology*. Recently published a chapbook, *Green Tomatoes*, by Heatherstone Press, Amherst, MA. He teaches at Lehigh County Community College, Schnecksville, PA.

Jane Mayhall (New York, NY) has been published in *Southern Rev, Pivot, New Yorker, Manhattan Poetry Rev, Confrontation* and *The American Scholar.*

Rebecca McClanahan (Charlotte, NC) is the author of *Mother Tongue* and *Mrs. Houdini* (University Presses of Florida), is the recipient of a 1989 North Carolina Writers Fellowship. is She is Poet-in-Residence for Charlotte-Mecklenburg Schools and has given readings at the Poetry Society of America and at Lincoln Center as part of the Writers' Nights series. She has also edited several collections of children's writings, including *I Dream So Wildly: An Anthology of Children's Poetry* (Briarpatch Press). State University.

Wilma Elizabeth McDaniel (Hanford, CA) was born to a family of Oklahoma sharecroppers, part Cherokee, in 1918. She spent a lifetime as a farm worker and at the age of eight, began writing poems. After nearly a half a century of writing in near-solitude, she began to show her poems, and in 1973, her first book was published. Since then, she has published fiction and poetry in many magazines and collections (including *Sister Vayda's Song*, published by Hanging Loose).

Daniel McDonald (Mobile, AL) is a poet & professor of English at The University of South Alabama in Mobile.

Peter Meinke (St. Petersburg, FL) is a professor of Literature at Florida Presbyterian College. His poems have appeared in *Motive, Antioch Review, Ladies' Home Journal, The Christian Century, Red Clay Reader* and other magazines.

Anne Meisenzahl (Brooklyn, NY) is an art teacher and curriculum writer.

Robert Mezey (Claremont, CA) has taught briefly at several universities. His publications include *Evening Wind*, 1987; *Selected Translations*, 1982; *The Lovemaker, White Blossoms, Favors, The Mercy of Sorrow* and *A Book of Dying.*

Elizabeth Michaels (New Orleans, La) is a graduate student working on her Ph.D. in English.

Judi Kiefer Miles (Farmingdale, NJ) teaches writing at Brookdale Community College, Lincroft, NJ, coordinates an annual writers' conference and literary series, and facilitates a weekly writing group. She created Summer Poets at the Shore and Writers Read featuring local poets; poetry broadcast on local cable TV. She has published in *Writer's Digest, Earth's Daughters, Widener Review, Reach of Song V, Cape Rock, Without Halos, US#1, Worksheets, Journal of New Jersey Poets, Orphic Lute*, etc.

Carol Miller (Oyster Bay, NY) has published in the *Wisconsin Review, Commonweal, Confrontation, The Cape Rock*, etc. She has published five collections of her poetry on a circa 1900 Chandler & Price foot-treadle press, doing the type-setting and binding by hand.

Wendy Mitchell (San Rafael, CA) was born in London, works as a technical writer. Publications include, *Negative Capability, Stone Country, Bitterroot,* and *Pudding.*

Berwyn Moore (Erie, PA) has poetry and reviews published in *Shenandoah, New Virginia Review, Poetry Miscellany, Mid-American Review, Kansas Quarterly,* etc. Her manuscript, *Proving the Earth's Movement with Shadow,* was a finalist in the Wesleyan New Poets Series and the Anhinga Poetry Prize in 1989. She teaches at Gannon University in Erie, PA.

Janice Townley Moore (Young Harris, GA) teaches in the English Department at Young Harris College. Recent poetry has been published in *The Bedford Introduction to Literature, Artemis, Blue Pitcher,* and *A Carolina Literary Companion.* She is poetry editor of *Georgia Journal.*

Richard Moore (Belmont, MA) has published five books of poetry, beginning with *A Question of Survival* (University of Georgia Press, 1971) and including *The Education of a Mouse* (Countryman Press, 1983). His poems and reviews appear in countless magazines including *Atlantic Monthly, Parnassus, The New Criterion, American Poetry Review* and *Sewanee Review.* A pilot and intelligence officer in the Air Force from 1950 to 53, Moore received a Fulbright Scholarship to study modern German poetry, and has taught at Boston University and Brandeis University. His recent novel, *The Investigator* was published by Story Line Press.

John T. Morris (Cullman, AL) received his M.D. degree from John Hopkins School of Medicine. He has been published in *The John Hopkins Magazine, Alalitcom,* and other small press journals. His most recent book is, *Miniature Miracle,* published by Honeysuckle Imprints.

Christopher Moylan (Long Island City, NY) teaches poetry and writing at New York Institute of Technology. A graduate of Harvard and Boston University, his poems have appeared in *Tempo Presente* and *Trame* (Italy), as well as *Rhino* and *Teaching English in the Two Year College.*

Alice Connelly Nagle (El Cerrito, CA) has published in the *Berkeley Poetry Review, Boston Literary Review, Five Fingers Review, Santa Clara Review, Visions International, Zone 3* and other magazines. A chapbook, *Jou ey of the Rooms,* was published as a 1990 *Poetry Atlanta Signature Series* winner.

Guillermo de Borja Narvacan IV "Gumby" (Houston, TX) is a senior at Spring Hill College in Mobile, Al. He is studying advertising and fine art and hopes to be a graphic artist.

Rochelle Natt (Great Neck, NY) has worked as a professional singer, a teacher, an artist, and a tarot reader.

Joan New (Gainesville, FL) is a lecturer in the creative writing program at the University of Florida. Her chapbook, *Knocking Down Pears,* has been published by the Nightshade Press. Other recent poems have appeared in *Earth's Daughters, Zone 3* and *Warren Wilson Review.* Her latest book, *The River Bend,* has been published by North Carolina Wesleyan College Press in 1992.

Kathleen Newroe (Santa Fe, NM) works as librarian for the Nizhoni School for Global Consciousness. Her most recent publication is "High Desert Garden," a poem in the anthology *Heart of the Flower.*

Robert Noreault (Massena, NY) has published in *Negative Capability* and *The Wallace Stevens Journal.*

Mary Beth O'Connor (Ithaca, NY) is a poet and fiction writer. She's an assistant to the Feminist Women's Writing Workshops, Inc. and is working on her M.F.A. degree. She's been published in *Common Lives/Lesbian Lives, New Directions for Women, Nimrod,* and *Sunrust.*

Joyce Odam (Sacramento, CA) is the author of *Lemon Center For Hot Buttered Roll* (Hibiscus Press, 1975). She has published in *Blue Unicorn, Impulse* and other small press magazines.

Mary Oliver (Provincetown, MA) is the author *House of Light* (Beacon, 1990), and *Dream Work* (Atlantic Monthly Pr, 1986), etc. Her poetry has appeared in numerous publications including *Poetry* and *Amicus.*

William Packard (New York City, NY) is editor of *New York Quarterly* and author of *The Art of Screenwriting, The Poet's Craft, The Art of the Playwright, Saturday Night at San Marcos,* and *Evangelism in America.*

Mario René Padilla (Santa Monica, Ca) won a 1991-92 Fulbright award for writing and dissertation research at the *Universidad Complutense* in Madrid. His poetry and translations have appeared in *Visions International, Negative Capability, The Amaranth Review, Chiron Review, Echoes Quarterly, etc.* He is an award winning composer, having received an ASCAP award for writing the music and scenario for the ballet *Harbinger of Evolution* which received its world premiere in 1980 by the Los Angeles Ballet Co.

Carolyn Page (Troy, Maine) is a poet-potter-reviewer and co-edit's *Potato Eyes* magazine.

Linda Parsons (Knoxville, TN) has been published in *The Georgia Review* and *The Iowa Review.* She won the 1990 AWP (Associated Writing Programs) Intro Award in Poetry. Her musical *Lambaréné, t*he story of Albert Schweitzer, was given a staged reading at Paper Mill Playhouse in New Jersey in June 1991.

Deborah Partington (Northhampton, MA) has published in the *Lullwater Review* out of Emory University and *Spectrum,* the University of Massachusetts' literary publication. She is a member of Amherst Writers and Artists. Prior to writing she was a professional calligrapher and now earns a living by editing and teaching technical writing.

Kathleen Patrick (St. Louis Park, Minnesota) is a poet and fiction writer. She is the recipient of a 1991 Loft-McKnight Fellowship in Poetry.

Lisa Peck (Chicopee, MA) is a student at Holyoke Community College.

Walter Peterson (Pittsburgh, PA) teaches (among other places) at the Young Writers Summer Institute at the University of Pittsburgh. He is part of the Pittsburgh Poetry Exchange. His first chapbook *Rebuilding the Porch* (Nightshade Press) was published in 1990.

Pfeiffer-Towner (Iowa City, IA) is a painter who has had exhibits in Chicago, New York, and Iowa, where she now lives. Her drawings have been published in *Fiddlehead, Caliban, Rhino, Literary Review, Format,* etc.

Marge Piercy (Wellfleet, MA) is the author of several books of poetry including *Breaking Camp, Hard Loving, To Be of Use, The Moon is Always Female, Available Light* as well as several novels including *Going Down Fast, Small Changes, Woman on the Edge of Time, The High Cost of Living* and others. The University of Michigan Press published a volume of her essays, reviews and interviews entitled *Parti-Colored Blocks for a Quilt,* as part of their Poets on Poetry Series. A book of critical essays on her work was recently published by Negative Capability Press.

Susan Policoff (Berkeley, CA) has fiction published in *West Branch, Moving Out, The Alaska Quarterly Review, Sequoia,* and other magazines. Three of her stories won a prize from *Permafrost,* She was runner-up for the *1988 Iowa Short Fiction Award.*

Laura Pollard (San Francisco, Ca) has recently published in *The Birmingham Poetry Review, Rhino,* and *The Rockford Review.* She was a fellow at Dorland Mountain Arts Colony.

Pamela Portwood (Tucson, Arizona) is a freelance writer and editor, specializing in art criticism and public-access television. Her poems have appeared in *Without Halos, Mildred, Haight Ashbury Literary Journal, Survivor* and *Thirteen.* She is the co-editor of *Rebirth of Power: Overcoming the Effects of Sexual Abuse through the Experiences of Others,* an anthology of poetry and prose published by Mother Courage Press.

Clark Powell (Mobile, AL) is a high school teacher and a columnist for the *Mobile Press-Register.*

Marjorie Power (Olympia, WA) is a native of Connecticut. She is the author of *Living With It,* Wampeter Press, 1983. Her numerous publications include *Poet & Critic, Artful Dodge, Plainsong,* and *Crosscurrents: A Quarterly.*

Anna Rabinowitz (New York, NY) has published in *The Best American Poetry 1989, Sulfur, Caliban, The Cream City Review, Southwest Review, Sonora Review, Denver Quarterly* and *Mudfish*. Her first manuscript, *Lifelines*, was a finalist in 1990 for the AWP Award and for the CSU Poetry Prize.

Robert M. Randolph (Wimberley, TX) has a Ph. D. in English and a M.A. in Theology. He recently taught in Finland on a Fulbright.

Alison Reed (Nashville, TN) is editor of *Cumberland Poetry Review* and a leader of a poetry group in Nashville. She is a sculptor, painter and pianist. She has been published in numerous publications in the United States as well as Canada, the United Kingdom and Australia. She has two books, *The First Movement* and *Bid Me Welcome*.

P.C. Reid (Boston, MA) has won several awards including the *Colorado Quarterly's* national fiction contest, and *The Literary Review's* Charles Angoff Award (poetry). He was awarded a grant to support a novel manuscript from the Mary Winston Rinehart Foundation, was one of nine finalists from a field of 3,000 entries for the Charles Nelson Algren Award for Fiction (Chicago Tribune), and a semifinalist for the Anhinga Press Poetry Prize. Other stories and poems have appeared in *The Webster Review, Pequod, Voices International,* and *Outposts,* a British quarterly.

Joanne M. Riley (Higgins) (Aberdeen, WA) has published two books of poetry: *Pacing The Moon* (Chantry Press) and *Earth Tones* (Seattle University Press). Her work appears regularly in small press journals. She is Youth Services Librarian for the Timberland Regional Library in southwestern Washington State.

Elisavietta Ritchie (Toronto, Canada) is the author of *Flying Time: Stories & Half Stories* (Signal Books), and seven collections of poetry including *Tightening The Circle Over Eel Country*, winner of the Great Lakes Colleges Association's "New Writer's Prize for Best First Book of Poetry 1975-76", and *Raking The Snow* (Washington Writers Publishing House 1982 winner; etc.) Four stories were PEN Syndicated Fiction Project winners. She conceived and edited *The Dolphin's Arc: Poems on Endangered Creatures of the Sea*. She has read at the Library of Congress, and elsewhere. Under the United States Information Agency auspices, she has read throughout the Far East and the Balkans.

Elspeth Cameron Ritchie (Washington, DC) is currently the unit director of an inpatient psychiatry ward at Walter Reed Army Medical Center.

Kathryn Roach (Salt Lake City, UT) has had three ten-minute plays produced by TheatreWorks West as part of Utah Shorts, and stories accepted for publication by *Voices, Spectrum,* and *13th Moon*.

Katrina Roberts (Keene, NH) is a graduate of the Iowa Writers' Workshop.

Margaret Robison (Shelburne Falls, MA) taught as a "Poet In The Schools" and has also taught writing to women in prison. She is working on a book about her recent stroke and her ongoing recovery.

Charles B. Rodning (Mobile, AL) is associate professor of surgery and anatomy in the College of Medicine, University of South Alabama. He is a member of the Haiku Society of America, the Sumi-e Society of America, the Alabama State Poetry Society, and the Academy of American Poets. He is the author of several books of poetry and has published in both literary and medical journals throughout the United States.

Evelyn Roehl (Seattle, WA) is the author of *Whole Food Facts* (Healing Arts Press, Rochester, Vermont) and former managing editor of the *North Country Anvil* magazine. Her writings have also appeared in *Iowa Woman, Tidewater, What We Will, Zeitgeist, Faminews, The Scoop, The Winoman,* and *PCC Sound Consumer*. She founded and edited *YUM! Your Usable Magazine* for three years and is currently owner-operator of Flying Fingers Typing & Graphics in Seattle, Washington.

Rosaly DeMaios Roffman has been published in *Living Inland* (Bennington, 1989), *Wings of the Rainbow* (Eapsu, 1984) and *Laurel Rev, Aegean*. She is a professor of English at Indiana University of Pittsburgh.

Marianne Rogoff (Bolinas, Ca) has won the Wilner Award and a Marin Arts Council grant. Recent stories have appeared in *My Father's Daughter: Stories By Women (Crossing Press, 1990), Santa Clara Review,* and the anthology *Out of Season*. She has taught creative writing at San Francisco State University and the California College of Arts and Crafts.

Conrad Rosenberg (New York, NY) is a an associate professor of clinical medicine at New York University.

Liz Rosenberg (Binghamton, NY) has published stories in *The Atlantic Monthly, Prairie Schooner, Seattle Review* and elsewhere. She has published a book of poems, *The Fire Music* (U. Pittsburgh Press) as well as three children's books with Harper/Collins. She teaches English and Creative Writing at SUNY Binghamton.

Geri Rosenwieg (Chappaqua, NY) was born and grew up in Ireland, worked as an R.N. in London and came to America in 1960. Her first book is *West of Ireland & Other Poems,* Linwood Publishers, Stone Mountain, Georgia. Her poems have appeared in *Verse, West Hills Review, Greensboro Review, Images, Gryphon, Riverrun, Poet Lore, The Small Pond, Blue Unicorn, Xanadu, Dog River Review, Poetic Justice, Croton Review, Christian Science Monitor, Taurus, Creative Loafing, Aura/Lit Arts, Poet & Critic,* and *Inlet*. She also won the Maclachan Award: West Hills Review, 1988.

Stephanie Sallaska (Edmond, OK) teaches in the creative writing program at the University of Central Oklahoma in Edmond. Her work has appeared (or will) in *Anything That Moves, Up Against the Wall, Mother, Z Miscellaneous, New Plains Review, Poems for the New Decade* and *Four Poets of Oklahoma*.

James Sallis (Ft. Worth, TX) has a new novel, *The Long-Legged Fly,* published by Carroll & Graf. he has recently finished *Difficult Lives,* a study of paperback novelists and is completing a translation of Raymond Queneau's novel *Saint Glinglin* for its first English-language publication. Recent work appears in *Pequod, APR, Chariton Review, Ellery Queens's Mystery Magazine, The Georgia Review, Washington Post Book World, High Plains Literary Review*.

Liza Schafer (Brooklyn, NY) works as a writer and editor for Scholastic Inc.

Pat Schneider (Amhurst, MA) is director of Amherst Writers & Artists, and AWA Press. Her plays, poems, and fiction have been widely published in such journals as *The Minnesota Review, Sewanne Review,* etc. She has a recent libretti recorded and performed in Carnegie Hall by the Atlanta Symphony Orchestra.

Amy Jo Schoonover (Mechanicsburg, OH) was named Ohio Poet of the Year in 1988 for her (fourth) book, *New & Used Poems*. She has recently published in *The Lyric* and in *Hiram Poetry Review* and *Voices International*. She is contest chairman for the National Federation of State Poetry Societies.

Joan Vannorsdall Schroeder (Roanoke, VA) has published in the op-ed pages of the New York *Times*, the Washington *Post*, the Baltimore *Sun*, etc. She has won several prizes and has been published in *Yankee, Virginia Country,* and *Potato Eyes*.

Mark Scott (Highland Park, NJ) recently completed his doctorate at Rudgers. He was a finalist in the *National Poetry Review* and *Western Humanities Review* competitions as well as winning a Academy of American Poets' Prize.

Jan Epton Seale (McAllen, TX) has published in *The Chicago Tribune, Newsday,* and *The San Francisco Chronicle* through PEN Syndicated Fiction Projects and in *Concho River Review, New Mexico Humanities Review, Yale Review, Texas Monthly* and *New America*. She is the author of two books of poetry, *Bonds* and *Sharing the House,* (RiverSedge Press) and is one of four poets featured in *Texas Poets in Concert: A Quartet* published by the U. of North Texas Press.

Joanne Seltzer (Schenectady, NY) is the author of three chapbooks: *Adirondack Lake Poems* (The Loft Press, 1985), *Suburban Landscape* (M.A.F. Press, 1988) and *Inside Invisible Walls* (Bard Press, 1989). Her poems have been widely published in literary magazines and anthologies where she has published short fiction, essays, reviews and translations of French poetry.

Karl Shapiro (Davis, CA) has taught at the Johns Hopkins University, the University of Nebraska, and until his recent retirement, at the University of California, Davis. He is a past editor of *Poetry* and *Prairie Schooner* and is the author of numerous books of poetry including: *Person, Place, and Thing, To Abolish Children, White-Haired Lover, The Poetry Wreck, Adult Bookstore,* Pulitzer Orize winning, *V-Letter, The Bourgeois Poet, Collected Poems: 1940-1978, New and Selected Poems 1940-1986* and *The Old Horsefly released from Northern Lights in 1992. His two volumes of autobiography are The Younger Son* and *Reports of My Death. His critical studies include In Defense of Ignorance* and *The Poetry Wreck*, and he has written a novel entitled *Edsel*. Shapiro was awarded the Bollingen Prize in 1992.

Vivian Shipley (North Haven, CT) directs the creative program at Southern Connecticut State University and runs an active reading series for writers. Her most recent book of poems, *Poems Out of Harlan County* was published by Ithaca House.

Bernie Siegel (New Haven, CT) holds membership in two scholastic honor societies. Phi Beta Kappa and Alpha Omega Alpha. He is a pediatric and general surgeon in New Haven. In 1978, he started Exceptional Cancer Patients, a specific form of individual and group therapy utilizing patients; dreams, drawings, and images. ECaP is based on "carefrontation," a loving, safe, therapeutic confrontation, which facilitates personal change and healing. He is the author of *Love, Medicine & Miracles* and *Love, Peace, & Healing*.

Jim Simmerman (Flagstaff, AZ) is the recipient of writing fellowships from the Arizona Commission on the Arts, the Bread Loaf Writers' Conference, the Fine Arts Work Center, The National Endowment for the Arts, and the Port Townsend Writers' Workshop. He directs and teaches in the creative writing program at Northern Arizona University.

Liubov Sirota (Troeshchino, USSR) is a poet.

Judith Skillman (Bellevue, WA) is the author of *Worship of the Visible Spectrum* (Breitenbush Press, 1988). She received a 1990 grant from the Washington State Arts Commission and has published in *Poetry, North West Review, Iowa Review, Poetry Northwest*, etc.

Nathan Slack (Philadelphia, PA)

Gerry Sloan (Fayetteville, AR) is on the music faculty of the University of Arkansas. His work has appeared in *Kansas Quarterly, North Dakota Quarterly, The Nebraska Review,* and *Negative Capability* as well as Alan Pater's *Anthology of Magazine Verse & Yearbook of American Poetry*.

Vivian Smallwood (Chickasaw, AL) is the recipient of numerous poetry awards including the Grand Prize of the National Federation of State Poetry Societies Competition, the Wilory Farm Poetry Contest, and the World of Poetry first place award.

Sybil Smith (Norwich, VT) has published in *New England Review/Bread Loaf Quarterly, Epoch, The Poetry Review, Southern Poetry Review, New Virginia Review, Cumberland Poetry Review, Worcester Review, 13th Moon, Negative Capability, Salthouse, Panoply, Peregrine,* etc. She works as a psychiatric nurse.

James Snydal (Bainbridge, WA) has been published in *Mill Hunk Herald, Talapus, Bogg, Poetry Wales, High Plains Lit Rev, Exhibition,* and ONTHEBUS, etc.

Laurel Speer (Tucson, AZ) has several books which include *The Sitting Duck, Lovers and Others,* and *A Bit of Wit* (poetry) and stories collected in *The Hundred Percent Black Steinway Grand, The Self-Mutilation of an Aged Apple Woman,* as well as plays. She writes a regular poetry feature for *Small Press Review*.

B.A. St. Andrews (Syracuse, NY) has published in *The New Yorker, Paris Review, The Christian Science Monitor, Commonweal, Carolina Quarterly* . He works in the College of Health Related Professions, State University of New York Health Science Center, Syracuse, NY.

William Stafford (Lake Oswego, OR) worked for the Church of the Brethren and for Church World Service, and taught in Kansas, Iowa, California, Indiana and Oregon, where he served for many years as professor of English at Lewis and Clark College in Portland. He retired from teaching in 1980 and devotes much of his time to giving workshops and reading from his poetry throughout the U.S. He has received a National Book Award for poetry, a Guggenheim Fellowship and the Shelley Memorial Award. He served as Consultant in Poetry to the Library of Congress in 1970-71.

David Starkey (Florence, SC) teaches English at Francis Marion College. His recent poetry appears in *The Beloit Poetry Journal, Cimarron Review, The Gamut, Kansas Quarterly, Puerto Del Sol, Writers' Forum*, etc.

Marian Steele (Pacific Palisades, CA) is a cell and molecular biologist at the professorial rank in a major university. She has a substantial publication record and has received a Guggenheim Fellowship as well as other awards and distinctions.

Lamont B. Steptoe (Camden, NJ) is the author of four books of poetry, *Crimson River, American Morning/Mourning, Small Steps and Toes* with Bob Small and *Mad Minute*, a collection of Vietnam war poetry. Steptoe is the founder of *Whirlwind Press* and is a photographer. He has read at the Geraldine R. Dodge Festival, the Library of Congress, the National Library of Nicaragua, at universities throughout the United States. Steptoe's poetry has appeared in *Chiron Review, the Mickle Street Review, the Painted Bride Quarterly, Big Hammer, Bulpeen, Branch Redd Review, Konch, 1/2 Dozen of the Other, Brother to Brother, Asphodel, Paper Air, Long Shot Review, Blue guitar and Shooting Star Review*. Two recent books entitled, the *Hotness of Blood* and *Uncle's South China Sea-Blue Nightmare*. Currently, he is the poetry consultant for the Spoken Arts Series at the Painted Bride Art Center in Philadelphia.

Gerald Stern (Iowa City, IA) has published *Selected Poems, Lovesick* (H&R, 1990, 86), *Paradise Poems* (Random House, 1984), etc.

Edward William Stever (Ridge, NY) is the author of *Transparency* (Writers Ink Press, 1990). He has published in *Pearl, Wide Open Mag*, and *Slipstream*.

David Stringer (Ypsilanti, MI) has published in *Blue Unicorn, Passages North, Green River Review, Full Circle*, etc. He has won a Hopwood Award for poetry from the University of Michigan and is a high school teacher.

Dorothy Sutton (Richmond, KY) is on the graduate faculty (creative writing and Modern British and American literature) at Eastern Kentucky University. She conducts poetry workshops at the annual Creative Writing Conference and is on the Editorial Board of *Scripsit* literary magazine. She has won grants, awards, and fellowships from the Atlantic Center for the Arts, Kentucky Foundation for Women, Kentucky and Ohio Arts Councils, Appalachian Writing Association, and Virginia Center for the Creative Arts. She was the Robert Frost Scholar in Poetry at Bread Loaf Writers' Conference in 1988.

Sharon Flynn Tette (Stanley, NY) has published in *Yankee, Cumberland Poetry Review, Painted Bride Quarterly, Lake Effect, The Syracuse Herald-Journal-American* and *Echoes*, etc.

Madeline Tiger is a Master Poet/Trainer, AIE Program, NJ State Council on the Arts. Her recent books include: *My Father's Harmonica* (Nightshade Press) and *Mary of Migdal* (Still Waters Press). She has published in *Gopherwood Review, Oxford Magazine, Paterson Literary Review, Shenandoah, Visions, West Wind Review, Onionhead, The Bridge* and in the following anthologies: *Blue Stones & Salt Hay* (Rutgers University Press), *Cradle and All* (Faber & Faber) *The Unmade Bed of Married Love* (Harper/Collins).

Tom Timmons (Greenfield, MA) is working on a novel-length prose poem fairy tale currently titled "Death Jamming and the Juice."

Barbara Unger (Woodside, CA) is a professor of English at the Rockland Community College. She is the author of *Basement: Poems 1959-63* (Isthmus Press, 1975), *The Man Who Burned Money* (The Bellevue Press, 1980). *Inside the Wind (Linwood Publishers, 1986), Dying For Uncle Ray* (Kendall/ Hunt 1990) and *Learning to Foxtrot* (Bellvue, 1989).

John Updike (Beverly Farms, MA) was a member of the staff of *The New Yorker* from 1955 to 1957, to which he contributed poems, short stories, essays, and book reviews. He is the author of over thirteen novels of which his fiction has won the Pulitzer Prize, the National Book Award, the American Book Award, and the National Book Critics Circle Award.

Pamela Uschuk (Gig Harbor, WA) was the winner of the 1989 *Ascent* Poetry Prize from the University of Illinois, as well as a prizewinner in the 1989 Chester H. Jones Competition and the University of South Alabama's 1989 White Rabbit Poetry Contest. Her poems have appeared in numerous journals and anthologies, including *Poetry, Pequod, Commonweal, Tendril, Calyx, Another Chicago Magazine*, and *48 Younger American Poets*. Her non-fiction has appeared in *The Bloomsbury Review, High Plains Literary Review*, and *Cutbank*. She was Writer in Residence spring semester 1990 at Pacific Lutheran University in Tacoma, Washington and has resumed teaching poetry through Marist College at Green Haven Maximum Security Prison for men.

Peter Viereck (S. Hadley, MA) is the author of *Hospital Window* the opening poem of his forthcoming new book, *Last Poems: Tide and Continuities*. His latest poetry book is *Archer in the Marrow*, W. Norton, NY, 1987. His earlier poetry book, *Terror and Decorum*, Greenwood Press, Westport, CT, was awarded a Pulitzer Prize. His prose books include *The Unadjusted Man* and *Conservatism from John Adams to Churchill*, both published by Greenwood Press. Author of half a dozen poetry books and half a dozen history books, Viereck is a professor of history at Mt. Holyoke College. His verse drama, *Opcomp* will be forthcoming from Negative Capability Press.

Diane Wakoski (East Landing, MI) has published over sixteen collections of poems. Among her most recent collections of poetry are *The Collected Greed, Parts 1-13* (1984), *The Rings of Saturn* (1986), *Emerald Ice: Selected Poems 1962-1986* (Black Sparrow Pr 1990, 1988) and Medea the Sorceress (Black Sparrow Press, 1991). The University of Michigan published her criticism of *Toward a New Poetry* (1980). She is Writer in Residence at Michigan State University.

Ron Walker (Mobile, AL) is a psychiatrist and psychoanalyst and associate editor of *Negative Capability*.

Sue Walker (Mobile, AL) is the editor and publisher of *Negative Capability* and a professor of English at the University of South Alabama. She is the author of *Travelling My Shadow* and *Shorings*, published by South Coast Press, Ca.

Eugene Walter (Mobile, AL) helped found *The Paris Review and worked as an assistant editor of Botteghe Oscure. His work includes Jennie the Watercress Girl; The Likes of Which; Love You Good, See You Later; The Byzantine Riddle* (fiction) and *Monkey Poems, Shapes of the River; Singerie-Songerie, The Pack Rat* (poetry). He has won a Lippincott Fiction Prize, a Sewanee Rockefeller Fellowship for poetry, and an O. Henry citation.

Pamela Wampler (Zionsville, IN) has published in *Black Warrior Review, Crazyhorse, Prairie Schooner*, and several other literary journals. She works as a writer and editor.

Marine Robert Warden (Riverside, CA) began writing poetry seriously in 1975 at age 48. His other published works include: *Beyond the Straits, 1980; Love and the Bomb Don't Mix, 1982; Lullabies from Cochiti, 1983*. He works as a physician in Riverside.

Ron Weber (Alexandria, VA)

Gerald Weissmann (New York, NY) has published essays in three books *The Woods Hole Cantata, They All Laughed At Christopher Columbus*, and *The Doctor With Two Heads*.

Sharon White (Leeds, MA) work has appeared in *Paragraph, The North American Review, The Bloomsbury Review, Wingbone, Poetry from Colorado*, and other magazines. She has received grants from the National Endowment for the Arts and the Colorado Council on the Arts.

Peter Wild (Tucson, AZ) teaches at the University of Arizona and is currently doing research on Art for Art's Sake critic John C. Van Dyke.

Kennette H. Wilkes (Huntsville, AL) has published in *Nimrod, Negative Capability, Phoenix, Green Fuse, etc. She has won numerous poetry awards including a Hackney Award for poetry in 1991 and has taught English in America and abroad.*

Barbara Williams (Toronto, Ontario) is a British-born Canadian poet. She recently served as guest curator for the exhibition, *Anne Langton, Gentlewoman Artist.*

Bayla Winters (Burbank, CA) is the author of *Sacred & Propane* (Croton Rev Pr, 1989). She has published in *Cream City Rev, Potato Eyes, Flesh & Bone, Phoenix*, etc.

Harold Witt (Orinda, CA) is the author of *Beasts in Clothes* (Macmillan), *Now, Swim* (The Ashland Poetry Press), *Winesburg by the Sea* (Thorp Springs), and *The Snow Prince*, published by Blue Unicorn, of which he is co-editor. His poems have appeared in hundred of periodicals and in more than fifty anthologies, including *Strong Measures* (Harper & Row) and *Desert Wood*: an Anthology of Nevada Poets.

Blanche Woodbury (Anyplace, USA) is the pseudonym for a woman still surviving the trauma of incest. "My Brother" was published by Harper and Row in *I Never Told Anyone: Stories and Poems by Survivors of Child Sexual Abuse.*

Allen Woodman (Flagstaff, AZ) grew up in Alabama and Florida. He teaches creative writing at Northern Arizona University. He has published over thirty stories in magazines, and his work has been cited in *Best American Short Stories* and The Pushcart Prize series. His first collection of short-story stories, *The Shoebox of Desire*, received good reviews in *The New York Times Book Review, The Short Story Review*, and elsewhere. He is also the author of several children's books with award-winning poet David Kirby.

Theodore Worozbyt, Jr. (Clarkston, GA) is a regular contributor to *Poetry* and has recently published in *Prairie Schooner, Poet & Critic, Northwest Review, South   Poetry Review*, etc.

Lila Zeiger (Great Neck NY) has been published widely, in many magazines and anthologies, since her first appearance in *The Paris Review. (Kayak, New Republic, Georgia Review, Southern Poetry Review, Yankee, Tangled vines, Light Year*, etc.) Her collection, *The Way To Castle Garden*, appeared from State Street Press in 1982. New York State CAPS Grant, in 1983, several Mac-Dowell fellowships, PSA annual awards and others. She received a 1990 Witter Bynner Foundation Grant of $5000 for a writing workshop called "Here and Now" which she leads in an AIDS Day Treatment Program in New York City.

AUTHOR INDEX

645

ABOUT THE EDITORS:

Sue Walker received her M.Ed., M.A. and Ph.D. degrees from Tulane University in New Orleans, Louisiana. She is currently a professor of English at the University of South Alabama in Mobile, Alabama where she teaches courses in advanced poetry writing, contemporary poetry, modern drama, the modern novel and professional writing. She received an Individual Writer's Fellowship from the Alabama Council on the Arts and a Newcomb Fellowship from Tulane University. She is the founding editor of the international literary journal, *Negative Capability* and publisher of Negative Capability Press. She is co-editor of *Ways of Knowing: Critical Essays on the Work of Marge Piercy*. Her poetry books include *Traveling My Shadow* and *Shorings* published in the fall of 1992 by South Coast Press, Fullerton, California.

Rosaly Roffman studied in New York City, Hawaii and Japan and presently teaches mythology, creative writing, and Oriental Literature in Translation at Indiana University of Pennsylvania where she is an associate professor. She has been the recipient of a Cummington School of the Arts Award, a National Endowment Grant, an Edward Albee Writing fellowship and University Awards to study "archetypes and symbol-making" at The Jung Institute. Her poems have appeared in magazines, journals, and chapbooks. She was the editor of the first poetry publication in Honolulu, Hawaii, *Threepenny Papers*. In 1990, she was awarded the Distinguished Faculty Award in the Arts for Poetry.